FREEZING FERTILITY

T0314053

BIOPOLITICS

MEDICINE, TECHNOSCIENCE, AND HEALTH IN THE TWENTY-FIRST CENTURY SERIES

General Editors: Monica J. Casper and Lisa Jean Moore

Missing Bodies: The Politics of Visibility
Monica J. Casper and Lisa Jean Moore

Against Health: How Health Became the New Morality
Edited by Jonathan M. Metzl and Anna Kirkland

Is Breast Best? Taking on the Breastfeeding Experts and the New High Stakes of Motherhood
Joan B. Wolf

Biopolitics: An Advanced Introduction
Thomas Lemke

The Material Gene: Gender, Race, and Heredity after the Human Genome Project
Kelly E. Happe

Cloning Wild Life: Zoos, Captivity, and the Future of Endangered Animals
Carrie Friese

Eating Drugs: Psychopharmaceutical Pluralism in India
Stefan Ecks

Phantom Limb: Amputation, Embodiment, and Prosthetic Technology
Cassandra S. Crawford

Heart-Sick: The Politics of Risk, Inequality, and Heart Disease
Janet K. Shim

Plucked: A History of Hair Removal
Rebecca M. Herzig

Contesting Intersex: The Dubious Diagnosis
Georgiann Davis

Men at Risk: Masculinity, Heterosexuality, and HIV Prevention
Shari L. Dworkin

To Fix or to Heal: Patient Care, Public Health, and the Limits of Biomedicine
Edited by Joseph E. Davis and Ana Marta González

Mattering: Feminism, Science, and Materialism
Edited by Victoria Pitts-Taylor

Are Racists Crazy? How Prejudice, Racism, and Antisemitism Became Markers of Insanity
Sander L. Gilman and James M. Thomas

Contraceptive Risk: The FDA, Depo-Provera, and the Politics of Experimental Medicine
William Green

Personalized Medicine: Empowered Patients in the 21st Century
Barbara Prainsack

Biocitizenship: On Bodies, Belonging, and the Politics of Life
Edited by Kelly E. Happe, Jenell Johnson, and Marina Levina

Toxic Shock: A Social History
Sharra L. Vostral

Managing Diabetes: The Cultural Politics of Disease
Jeffrey A. Bennett

Feeling Medicine: How the Pelvic Exam Shapes Medical Training
Kelly Underman

Freezing Fertility: Oocyte Cryopreservation and the Gender Politics of Aging
Lucy van de Wiel

Freezing Fertility

Oocyte Cryopreservation and the
Gender Politics of Aging

Lucy van de Wiel

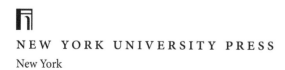

NEW YORK UNIVERSITY PRESS
New York

NEW YORK UNIVERSITY PRESS
New York
www.nyupress.org

References to Internet websites (URLs) were accurate at the time of writing. Neither the author nor New York University Press is responsible for URLs that may have expired or changed since the manuscript was prepared.

An earlier version of part of chapter 2 was previously published in Lucy van de Wiel. 2015. "Frozen in Anticipation: Eggs for Later." *Women's Studies International* 53 (November–December): 119–28. https://doi.org/10.1016/j.wsif.2014.10.019. Reprinted with permission.

Library of Congress Cataloging-in-Publication Data
Names: Van de Wiel, Lucy, author.
Title: Freezing fertility : oocyte cryopreservation and the gender politics of aging / Lucy Van de Wiel.
Description: New York : New York University Press, [2020] |
Series: Biopolitics: medicine, technoscience, and health in the twenty-first century series | Includes bibliographical references and index.
Identifiers: LCCN 2020015028 (print) | LCCN 2020015029 (ebook) |
ISBN 9781479877584 (cloth ; alk. paper) | ISBN 9781479817900 (paperback ; alk. paper) |
ISBN 9781479803620 (ebook) | ISBN 9781479868148 (ebook)
Subjects: LCSH: Ovum—Cryopreservation. | Human reproductive technology. | Cryopreservation of organs, tissues, etc—Political aspects. | Human reproduction—Age factors. | Feminism.
Classification: LCC QP261 .W54 2020 (print) | LCC QP261 (ebook) | DDC 612.6/2—dc23
LC record available at https://lccn.loc.gov/2020015028
LC ebook record available at https://lccn.loc.gov/2020015029

New York University Press books are printed on acid-free paper, and their binding materials are chosen for strength and durability. We strive to use environmentally responsible suppliers and materials to the greatest extent possible in publishing our books.

Manufactured in the United States of America

10 9 8 7 6 5 4 3 2 1

Also available as an ebook

For Caroline Smart and Lesley Gamble

CONTENTS

Introduction   1

1. Making Fertility Precarious: Egg Freezing and the
Politicization of Reproductive Aging   27

2. Freezing in Anticipation: Fertility Planning with
Eggs for Later   60

3. Frozen Eggs and the Financialization of Fertility:
Distributing Reproductive Aging in the
Reproductive-Industrial Complex   88

4. Aging Embryos and Viable Rhythms: The Visualization
and Commercialization of Time-Lapse Embryo Selection   119

5. Postfertile Conceptions: Egg Freezing and the Reinvention
of Older Motherhood   143

6. Oocyte Futures: The Global Flow of Frozen Eggs   180

Conclusion   217

Acknowledgments   237

Glossary   241

Notes   243

Bibliography   279

Index   321

About the Author   335

Introduction

When I imagine my eggs, I think of them as grey and shiny, like slippery helium balloons clustering in the thousands within organs lit up and awake. I think of eggs enfleshed in follicular cavities, folding again and again into a sponge of cells and yellow bodies, pulsing patiently with only an occasional burst: membrane breaking at the touch of engorged fimbrae, fallopian fingers brushing the ovarian skin. After stories and statistics, after computer animations and camera registrations of organs shining against surgical light, my eggs become palpable within two pulsing opals, shielded by hipbones, roused with embodied symbolism. Hypnagogic, I dream them into being—a fiction of the body.

Celebrated as empowerment and criticized as exploitation of women, egg freezing is a contested new reproductive technology that has brought the human egg into the public eye with renewed prominence. The technology, and the eggs and bodies it pertains to, have been widely featured in popular culture and public debates about whether or not women should (be allowed to) freeze their eggs and, if so, at what ages. Eggs have become some of the most culturally determined cells in the human body, represented in declining fertility statistics and referenced in tropes of the "biological clock" and "ticking ovaries." Egg freezing has made headlines throughout the mediascape—from the *Guardian* to *Cosmopolitan*—particularly when egg freezing cocktail parties and Apple's and Facebook's offer of egg freezing as an employee benefit provoked international media hypes. More broadly, frozen eggs have become a familiar sight in popular culture. A giant egg floated above the dancing nurses and gynecologists of Amsterdam's first egg bank at the Amsterdam Gay Pride, and millions watched Kim freeze her eggs in the popular reality show *Keeping up with the Kardashians*. As more women began freezing their eggs, they encountered them through medical imaging techniques like ultrasound or photomicrography and made new types of reproductive choices about the extracted cells in informed-consent contracts. In each of these ways, and many more, eggs are brought into discourse in ways that affect not only the women who freeze them but also the wider public.

The egg has a rich symbolic history, in which it has figured as a sign for life, death, and regeneration in many civilizations around the world. Long before human eggs were described within the tradition of European biology, creation myths across the globe identified the "cosmic" egg as the origin of the world, or humankind—from the ancient Greek cosmogonies in which the world springs from an egg, to Finnish epics that sing of an egg that broke in two and created the earth and the sky, to the numerous legends in Oceania that ascribe the birth of the first human to birds' eggs.[1] This cosmogenic significance of the figure of the egg was also referenced in the first medico-scientific postulation that all animals are conceived from eggs, described in William Harvey's *On the Generation of Animals* (1651). His work opens with a frontispiece that depicts Zeus holding an egg with the famous dictum *"Ex Ovo Omnia"* (everything from the egg).[2] Almost two centuries later, this notion was confirmed—at least where mammals were concerned—when, in 1826, Karl Ernst Von Baer killed a dog, cut open her ovaries, and became the first human to observe a mammalian egg, thereby lodging the egg more solidly in the anatomical model of the female body. In turn, the theoretical possibility of dislodging eggs from human bodies emerged with the development of tissue culturing at the *fin de siècle*.[3] The notion that cells could live outside of the body raised popular interest in the speculative idea of human *in vitro* reproduction. Stories about "babies in bottles" proliferated, most famously in biofuturist Aldous Huxley's dystopian *Brave New World* (1932), which opens with a technologized origin story featuring "racks upon racks of test-tubes" in which "detached and ripened eggs were kept," from which new citizens would be created.[4]

Whereas tissue culturing had externalized human cells, the birth of Louise Brown (1978), the first baby conceived through *in vitro* fertilization (IVF), solidified the notion that the egg could also be successfully fertilized outside of the woman's body. After that first controversial birth, a further eight million have followed, and IVF has become routine practice.[5] The popularity of IVF has brought the egg into vision—first to gynecologists, many of whom, until the extraction of eggs became familiar clinical practice in the early 1980s, had never seen a living human female gamete.[6] Later, the visual of an egg being fertilized *in vitro*, whether by a flock of sperm or by a hand-held needle inserting a single sperm in the ICSI procedure, became ubiquitous as a stock image of IVF, and reproductive technologies more broadly, in popular media.[7] Much as genes became a "prominent iconic vocabulary in turn-of-the-millennium public culture *because there is a rapidly expanding range of things that can be done to them*," eggs have become the subject of public awareness as their particular existence in time and space has become alterable in new ways with IVF and, more recently, with egg freezing.[8]

As the 20th century witnessed the advent of the extracorporeal egg's fertilization, its cryopreservation has been hailed as the harbinger of a 21st-century "reproductive revolution" on a par with the introduction of the contraceptive pill.[9] Egg freezing, or oocyte cryopreservation (OC), is effectively an IVF procedure with a prolonged period of cryostorage after the eggs' extraction from the body, but before their fertilization. While the eggs are in the freezer, stored at −196°C in liquid nitrogen tanks, they are thought to be unaffected by the passage of time. Those eggs that survive the freeze-thaw process may be used for fertilization when a pregnancy is desired. Initially used primarily as a technique to aid women with a cancer diagnosis who were confronted with imminent fertility loss, egg freezing may also be used to circumvent the effects of age-related infertility—and it is this application that is the focus of this study.

Freezing Fertility critically examines the technology of egg freezing, and its construction in public discourses, in relation to a notion that is relatively undertheorized in the study of culture: aging. As a reproductive technology that is employed for so-called fertility preservation rather than immediate childbearing, egg freezing both prompts the articulation of existing age normativities and reconfigures the temporal logic of reproductive aging. I investigate the implications of egg freezing for contemporary thinking on bodily temporality by analyzing a selection of cultural objects—varying from sparkly online platforms to heart-breaking court cases and intimate autobiographical accounts—that are emblematic of each stage of the procedure. Accordingly, *Freezing Fertility* follows the journey of the egg: starting from the initial anticipation of reproductive aging in relation to *in vivo* eggs and moving on to the accumulation of *in vitro* eggs after extraction, the selection of fertilized eggs with time-lapse embryo imaging, the novel forms of older motherhood following the implantation of fertilized frozen eggs, and, finally, the global impact of egg freezing as a condition of possibility for the transnational flows of eggs that can emerge once cryopreservation renders the egg newly mobile.

Although public discourses typically frame egg freezing as an individual reproductive choice for women who may want to have children later in life, in this book I explore how the emergence of egg freezing also reveals widespread cultural negotiations about the new norms that govern reproductive aging and the timing of childbearing when eggs become freezable. On the one hand, we are witnessing a discursive and infrastructural shift that rationalizes egg freezing by rendering fertility increasingly precarious and making women responsible for proactively managing its potential decline at specific moments in the life cycle. Multi-million-dollar investments in organizations that target young women to preserve "peak fertility," the mainstreaming of egg freezing as a health benefit covered by Fortune 500 companies, and the rise of "Fertility MOT" tests offered by fertility clinics all evidence this development. On the other hand, the introduction of egg freezing has also elicited the reaffirmation of existing age-related normativities—whether in national regulations prohibiting fertility treatment after 45 or in popular discourses denouncing childbearing beyond "normal reproductive years"—in the face of their potential transgression with frozen eggs.[10]

Freezing Fertility engages the dynamic between these two developments by analyzing the changing contemporary constructions of the relation between fertility and aging—a relation that has become both more alterable and more politically charged with the emergence of the freezable egg. Oocyte cryopreservation presents a situation in which bodies age while frozen eggs, and the reproductive potential they embody, are understood to be unaffected by the passage of time. This study explores what is at stake—culturally, politically, commercially—in the encounter between lived and frozen time by following the egg as it exists inside and outside the body, in freezers or in photographs, in glass or as glass, in time or out of time. In *Freezing Fertility*, egg freezing functions as a prism onto a broader gender politics of aging, which both transforms and solidifies as OC practices reconfigure the ways in which reproductive cells and bodies are understood to live in time.

In order to situate the popularization of egg freezing, this introduction first considers its historical emergence and subsequently outlines the conceptual framework for rethinking notions of fertility and aging in relation to the frozen egg. This lays the foundation for *Freezing Fertility*'s consideration of how the clinical possibility of OC, and the concomitant emergence of frozen eggs, provide the occasion for contemporary reimaginations of reproduction and regeneration that have been associated with eggs for millennia.

The Emergence of the Frozen Egg

Described as the "holy grail of fertility medicine," egg freezing technologies have been a long time in the making.[11] Sperm and embryos have been routinely frozen for decades, but the cryopreservation of eggs has proved challenging. In the 1950s, the first woman birthed a child after being inseminated with previously frozen sperm. Three decades later, an Australian girl named Zoe was the first to be born after a frozen embryo transfer.[12] Although egg freezing only gained popularity after the turn of the millennium, the first babies—they were twins—created from frozen eggs were born as early as 1986, only a couple of years after Zoe, and also in Australia.[13] Notwithstanding this early achievement, egg freezing continued to be difficult, primarily because the egg—the biggest cell in the human body at 0.1 millimeters—has a relatively large liquid volume, which is sensitive to freezing damage from ice crystal formation. So while embryo and sperm freezing soon became routine clinical practice, the early successes of OC were not easily reproduced, and further clinical attempts to use frozen eggs for human reproduction were largely suspended as if "cast under a voluntary moratorium."[14]

Meanwhile, IVF became increasingly popular in the 1980s and 1990s, particularly as a treatment for age-related infertility. Although IVF was originally designed as a method to avoid tubal infertility by circumventing the fallopian tubes and instead allowing fertilization to occur *in vitro*—indeed, Lesley Brown, who carried the first IVF baby, had been unable to conceive for nine years because her fallopian tubes were blocked—assisted reproductive technologies were increasingly used to treat age-related infertility.[15] Lisa Harris describes how this focus reflects the fact that IVF was becoming a particularly market-driven sector—both in the United Kingdom, where Thatcher's rule coincided with the rise of private, for-profit IVF clinics alongside public NHS facilities, and in the United States, where healthcare was more privatized across the board.[16] The US IVF sector was also particularly affected by anti-abortion ideologies that curtailed federal funding for embryo research. As a result, US fertility research became more reliant on clinical IVF cycles, often paid for by patients themselves. Consequently, Harris argues, both IVF practice and research became organized around market rationales, reflecting the demands of patients who could afford to undergo ART (assisted reproductive technology) treatment. This group mostly consisted of relatively older women, who were "often professionals, disproportionately white, . . . delayed childbearing and had the best odds of affording IVF care."[17] Although low-income women with limited education, who were disproportionately women of color, had almost twice the infertility rates—often tubal infertility—compared to their affluent, highly educated white counterparts, IVF has primarily focused on the age-related infertility of the women who can afford treatment.[18]

Spurred on by the potential demand for female fertility preservation in the context of growing IVF markets geared towards treating age-related infertility, legal restrictions on embryo research, and demographic trends of later childbearing, new approaches to freezing eggs were developed from the 1990s onwards.[19] At first, efforts focused on freezing eggs very slowly to limit cryodamage, but eventually vitrification emerged as the most promising approach. Vitrification entails freezing the eggs so rapidly that the liquid in the cells does not form ice crystals, but transforms into a glass-like state. These vitrified eggs, then, do not so much exist *in vitro* (in glass), but rather are *vitreum* (as glass) within the liquid nitrogen tanks. In fact, the vitrified egg is no longer held by the glass referenced in IVF (*in vitro* fertilization), but is rather stored on a thin film strip. It was the postmillennial development of this alternative container, the Japanese Cryotop system, that proved pivotal in raising the eggs' post-thaw survival rates up to 90%.[20] These high survival rates, and their reproducibility in clinics across the world, have transformed egg freezing into a technology that is used not only for women with malignant diseases but increasingly also for the purpose at the center of this study: anticipating age-related infertility.

It is important to note that nonhuman animals are also implicated in the development of human egg freezing, whether as model species for research or through the use of animal products in cell culturing—

notably fetal bovine serum (FBS). This serum is commonly sourced through an unanaesthetized puncture between the ribs directly into the beating hearts of late-term fetuses taken from slaughtered cows who are pregnant (an estimated 8% of cows).[21] Over 800,000 liters of serum are produced from more than 2 million fetuses annually, and it is widely used in cell and tissue culturing, including some OC studies, as a growth medium.[22] Kuwayama's abovementioned Cryotop study, for example, reported on the freezing of eggs from cows and humans and used FBS for developing the former. Although FBS is not typically used in clinical egg freezing practices, publications announcing some of the first human babies born through vitrification describe the use of this serum.[23] In these "always asymmetrical" cross-species relations of oocyte cryopreservation, the frozen egg thus emerges from a broader interspecies organization of "living and dying, and nurturing and killing" and the "hierarchy of deaths" that underlie them.[24]

Following its improving success rates, egg freezing has become a widely popular technology. Although OC cycles only make up a small percentage (1.5% in the United Kingdom) of all IVF cycles, the number of women freezing their eggs has increased every year, and awareness of the technology is widespread among the general population, particularly as it is frequently featured in popular media.[25] An increasing number of clinics across the world have introduced egg freezing, especially after the American Society for Reproductive Medicine (ASRM) lifted the "experimental" label of the procedure and the European Society for Human Reproduction and Embryology (ESHRE) considered it ethically acceptable in 2012. This study focuses primarily on the popularization of egg freezing in the Euroamerican context and draws on case studies from the United States, the United Kingdom, and the Netherlands.

Many of the novel clinical, financial, and infrastructural developments in egg freezing that are central to this study emerged first in the relatively unregulated fertility industry of the United States—whether it is fertility companies selling egg freezing insurance or cryobanks shipping frozen eggs internationally. The highly regulated national contexts of the United Kingdom, with its unique legal framework regulated by the Human Fertilisation and Embryology Authority (HFEA), and the Netherlands, where Parliament barred women's access to egg freezing for several years, give insight into the constraints and controversies surrounding egg freezing. In the United Kingdom, egg-storing regulations were first drawn up in 1990, and the ban on using frozen eggs for fertilization was lifted at the turn of the millennium. Soon after, in 2002, Emily Perry, the UK's first frozen egg baby, was born. In the Netherlands, elective egg freezing was not formally permitted until almost a decade later, in 2011. This was the result of a two-year political debate, which started in 2009 when the Amsterdam Medical Centre (AMC) proposed to offer OC to healthy women for age-related fertility preservation.

US IVF is characterized by a permissive regulatory regime and a largely for-profit fertility sector.[26] IVF costs are significantly higher than in other countries, and assisted reproduction has become a "luxury" market, in which many people are excluded from treatment because of its cost. Those who do access IVF and egg freezing are, unsurprisingly, disproportionately wealthy, well educated, and white; perhaps more surprisingly, this trend persists even in states where treatment costs are covered by insurance.[27] The US fertility sector has attracted substantial private equity and venture capital investments; particularly egg freezing start-ups have received significant capital investments and are reshaping the fertility industry through mergers and acquisitions of traditional IVF clinics, the organization of care through online platforms, and employer insurance packages for ART treatment.[28]

In the Netherlands, almost all IVF clinics are situated in public hospitals and egg freezing, accordingly, primarily takes place in a nonprofit context. Dutch national health insurance covers three cycles of IVF for women under 43, but egg freezing is only covered for "medical" reasons; women who wish to circumvent age-related infertility have to pay out of pocket. The Dutch egg freezing ban and both minimum and maximum age limits for OC are in keeping with the relatively restrictive regulation of ARTs in the Netherlands. For example, in Amsterdam, egg freezing is only allowed after 30 years, reflecting the Dutch tendency not to "over-medicalize" bodily problems (e.g., one third of deliveries take place at home, which is unique in the Western world).[29]

The United Kingdom combines both private and public reproductive healthcare systems. IVF emerged in the wake of the postwar establishment of the National Health Service (NHS) for universal healthcare. A spirit of altruistic voluntarism characterized both the large number of egg donors and the (often unpaid) medical professionals who contributed to the underfunded development of IVF for nearly a decade before Louise Brown's birth in 1978.[30] Subsequently, under Thatcher's neoliberal rule, IVF became "a bellwether of health privatization," and the 1980s saw the rapid rise of lucrative private IVF clinics and semiprivate fertility treatment offered alongside NHS facilities.[31] Today, particularly the private fertility centers promote and specialize in egg freezing for age-related infertility; NHS-only services make up only 22% of all clinics in the United Kingdom.[32]

Yet the analysis does not confine itself to these particular national contexts. The cultural objects under scrutiny in this study may circulate transnationally, exemplify a broader discursive logic, or operate in the complex geographies of on/offline dynamics and data distribution. Film and news media are broadcast internationally. Online platforms may be accessed globally. The standardization of techno-clinical systems linked to egg freezing—whether automated vitrification or algorithmic embryo selection—facilitates their use in various local contexts. Practices like cross-border frozen egg donation are defined by their transnational nature and cause not only gametes but regulations, norms, and clinical practices to travel across the globe. So while I situate these cultural objects in specific sociocultural and geopolitical contexts, their locus is often more networked, distributed, and dynamic than the frame of the nation-state permits.

OC Critiques and Controversies

As is the case for most new reproductive technologies, egg freezing has been widely criticized, but also hailed as a means of improving women's reproductive self-determination. And indeed, egg freezing may be of great benefit to people at different life stages by offering a means to (potentially) retain the reproductive capacity of one's eggs in spite of the passage of time, allowing further possibilities for undergoing IVF with one's own eggs later in life and establishing biogenetic relationships with the potential future children born as a result. Women who have chosen to freeze their eggs indicate that the primary motivations for undergoing the procedure are the absence of a partner with whom a family can be formed,[33] avoidance of future self-blame and concern about the biological clock,[34] and irreconcilable social, professional, and biological time pressures.[35]

Yet, notwithstanding egg freezing's potential benefits, the choice to freeze one's eggs also requires gauging the reproductive potential of the frozen eggs against the procedure's health and financial risks, all of which are mediated through discourses that may themselves be contested and informed by third-party interests.[36] Another downside is that the possibility of egg freezing may also entail assuming responsibility for *not* doing so, thereby reframing certain experiences, such as age-related infertility, as the outcome thereof. The financial and cultural capital, time investment, health status, and favorable regulatory and medical context required for undergoing the procedure moreover mean that such choices are not equally accessible, and may therefore contribute to further stratification of reproduction in general, and the timing of childbearing in particular.

In line with this concern, most studies suggest that women who freeze their eggs in anticipation of age-related infertility are relatively well-to-do. Because egg freezing is expensive and not covered by national insurance plans when used for this type of "fertility preservation," it is unaffordable for most people. Beyond affordability, Cahn and Carbone point out that the demand for OC by childless women in their late thirties also reflects existing class- and race-specific trends in relationship formation and average age at first birth, resulting in a situation in which white, middle-class, highly educated women are overrepresented in the group for whom egg freezing becomes relevant in the first place.[37]

Following from this, egg freezing aligns with the critique of IVF developed by Dorothy Roberts, who describes it as a further extension of high-tech reproductive interventions that are geared towards encouraging the reproduction of the most privileged in society. Meanwhile, nonreproductive technologies and policies have been used to discourage less affluent and less privileged women from having children.[38] Charis Thompson has coined the term "selective pronatalism" for this practice of differentially restricting access to reproductive or nonreproductive technologies in keeping with settler-colonial, racial, religious, or class hierarchies.[39] Indeed, Bhatia and Campo-Engelstein highlight that ESHRE's recommendation that egg freezing should be allowed because "there are demographic reasons for welcoming the birth of any extra child born to women who are socially, economically, and physically able to give it a good start in life" reflects a selectively pronatalist attitude towards egg freezing as a technology that can encourage particular groups of people to have children.[40] In the private sector, fertility insurance offered for workers in high-status Fortune 500 companies likewise aligns with this selectively pronatalist frame.

Yet this pronatalist framing is complicated by the fact that, although privileged women are more likely to undergo OC, egg freezing is not a reproductive technology in the strict sense of the word. Given that currently only approximately 5% of women return to use their eggs and only 20% of those women end up having a baby conceived from the eggs, OC is hardly driving up birth rates among the privileged.[41] While OC's marketing to, and uptake among, middle-class women aligns with ideologies that selectively promote elite reproduction, egg freezing has equally been criticized as having the effect of further postponing motherhood and encouraging women in high-status jobs to focus on their careers rather than become mothers. In other words, the reproductive and non-reproductive qualities of egg freezing complicate the pronatalism and antinatalism implicit in the uptake and promotion of this technology.

Some feminist and bioethics scholars have advocated the availability of egg freezing because it benefits women in making reproductive choices and improves gender parity in timing childbearing,[42] with others suggesting that egg freezing can improve reproductive autonomy by offering a way for women to "choose when to become a mother."[43] Yet academic studies of OC have more commonly raised concerns about egg freezing as an individual choice that may detract attention from the sociocultural factors that contribute to a situation in which childbearing becomes problematic and egg freezing appears as a solution, including the (temporal) organization of education, labor, relationship patterns, and their intersection with race, class, and sexuality.[44] The framing of egg freezing as an individual choice suggests an expansion of women's reproductive rights, when in fact, Lisa Ikemoto argues, its "empowerment" serves to "fuel demand" within a logic of free market individualism, while ignoring the structural factors that help determine the safety and autonomy of women's reproductive choices, including poverty, racism, and heterosexism.[45] In other words, critics have asserted that egg freezing is an "expensive and physiologically risky procedure that offers an individualist solution to social reasons for delayed childbearing" and have instead called for the need to address the structural inequalities underlying these social issues through such measures as parental leave, child care, wage equality, and comprehensive health insurance.[46]

These critical positions respond to two different developments in the gender politics of reproductive aging, which problematize women's reproductive decision making in contrasting ways. On the one hand, critics like Goold and Savulescu speak out in favor of OC in response to negative news reports admonishing "career women" for "delaying" having children by freezing their eggs, moral outrage about technologically assisted older motherhood—but not older fatherhood—and calls to ban egg freezing for "social" reasons.[47] They criticize the widespread affirmation of normative reproductive age limits that the introduction of egg freezing provoked in media, regulatory, and medical discourses, which have limited women's access to the procedure or the resultant frozen eggs. On the other hand, critics who advocate social change rather than biotechnological fixes like OC typically object to the neoliberal responsibilization of women implicit in the idea that one can "extend fertility" and "stop the biological clock." The suggested alterability of reproductive aging evades structural change and instead provides an individualized coping mechanism for social structures that do not offer supportive conditions for women to have children, or financially encourage them to reproduce later in life.[48]

So while egg freezing's introduction may intensify the naturalization of reproductive aging norms in the face of their potential transgression, it has also resulted in the reconceptualization of reproductive aging as biotechnologically alterable and the concomitant institutionalization of new norms for managing the "biological clock" in keeping with the temporal logic of broader cultural and socioeconomic structures. *Freezing Fertility* explores the dynamics between these two developments; it positions the construction of age-related infertility as itself politically relevant and therefore requiring critical reflection.

This project does not challenge the widely observed phenomenon that women's ability to conceive and birth children is finite and age contingent.[49] I advocate the widespread availability of information on female fertility and its age-related contingencies, especially given that significant contingents of women and men remain underinformed on these matters and overestimate the success rates of technologically assisted reproduction.[50] However, my main interest lies with *how* the relation between fertility and aging becomes legible as bodily truth in public discourses of egg freezing. In Gayatri Spivak's words, the aim is "not the exposure of error. It is constantly and persistently looking into how truths are produced."[51] By following their public manifestation in popular culture, online platforms, technological systems, and reproductive infrastructures, I examine egg freezing, associated models of female reproductive embodiment, and the figure of the frozen egg as material-discursive phenomena that both reflect and transform contemporary notions of what it means to age, and to be (in)fertile.

Fertility and the Frozen Egg

Egg freezing has introduced new ways in which we can become fertile throughout the life course. While late-20th-century technologies of IVF and egg donation have created possibilities of bearing children after the onset of age-related infertility, the 21st-century introduction of egg freezing offers a chance of not only birthing but also conceiving later in life with frozen eggs. Conversely, as a technology that is used to bypass reproductive aging, OC also uniquely implicates younger fertile women, who are confronted with the option of freezing eggs to anticipate future infertility at increasingly early ages. The possibility of egg freezing thus produces emergent modes of being fertile—beyond the fertile/infertile binary—now that age-related infertility may be lived prior to its arrival and its onset need not signal the end of the reproductive life span.

As a technology that is not directed at having children in the present but at "preserving fertility," egg freezing—unlike conventional IVF—separates the attainment of a technologically mediated form of fertility from the attainment of a pregnancy or live birth. This separation facilitates a reflection on how fertility operates in the absence of (attempted) childbearing. Sarah Franklin has described how IVF is used not only to help people have children but also to provide a "resolution to the uncertainty created by infertility" and a means to counteract future regret because one has "tried everything."[52] This observation is particularly pertinent in the treatment logic of egg freezing, which similarly provides a treatment to resolve uncertainty about infertility—albeit a future infertility—and requires action at present in order to avoid the potential future regret of not having frozen (more) eggs. In this way, the possibility of egg freezing renders these concerns about uncertain fertility and retrospective regret—commonly associated with IVF—relevant to and treatable for a new group of people, who need neither experience a current desire for a child nor have an infertility diagnosis.

Egg freezing is, unusually, an infertility treatment for fertile people. The indication for treatment is not the experience of infertility as such but the anticipation of the arrival of infertility in the future.[53] The World Health Organization defines the arrival of infertility as "the failure to achieve a clinical pregnancy after 12 months or more of regular unprotected sexual intercourse."[54] With the advent of reproductive technologies like IVF and IUI (intra-uterine insemination), infertility has shifted from being a condition that is necessarily manifest in the continued absence of pregnancy to being an indication for treatment, which, as the literature on IVF has described, may also function as an injunction of "having to try" treatment.[55] In the context of IVF, infertility may then arrive twice: first, an infertility that becomes an indication for ART treatment and, second, an infertility that is the outcome of a complex decision-making process about whether to access and when to stop this treatment. With the emergence of egg freezing, infertility may arrive a third time, earlier in life, as a future possibility that becomes an indication for anticipatory treatment in the present.

Freezing Fertility explores how fertility is rendered precarious earlier in the life course in relation to this possibility of freezing eggs in anticipation of future infertility. Precarious fertility functions as an alternative indication for infertility treatment, which arrives outside of the frame of the couple, and without attempted conception. I use the term "precarious" here both in the sense of uncertainty or "exposure to risk" and with reference to the older Latin "*precarius*"—derived from "*prex*," to pray—which denotes being "vulnerable to the will or decision of others," thereby signifying a sense of dependency.[56] Precariousness refers to the idea that the possibility of freezing one's eggs produces not only more treatment options but also a particular dynamic of epistemic uncertainty and agentic control over reproductive aging. In other words, egg freezing introduces ways of knowing fertility that create new uncertainties about reproductive risk and ways of controlling fertility that create new dependencies on others.

Following Judith Butler's reflection on precariousness,[57] the first, risk-based aspect of precarious fertility pertains to the discursive construction of female fertility in the context of egg freezing. Not simply referencing a biological reality, the notion of fertility in discourses of OC constitutes a public *mode of address* directed at a new group of women. Whereas the fertility industry was previously considered "irrelevant" to 85–90% of the population,[58] the possibility of egg freezing enlists a larger section of healthy women of reproductive age as potential candidates for treatment. Precarious fertility is the effect of discourses that, in lieu of symptoms that would be an indication for IVF, rationalize a fertility treatment aimed at people who do not currently experience infertility. If, for Butler, precariousness is a concept for thinking through the relationality of human subjectivity and the vulnerability to the constitutive address, the notion of precarious fertility likewise signals the sociality of becoming-(in)fertile through the address—and the importance of considering the public discourses of fertility to understand the reproductive politics of egg freezing.

Lauren Berlant describes precariousness as a "condition of dependency—as a legal term, *precarious* describes the situation wherein your tenancy on your land is in someone else's hands."[59] Following from this, the second aspect of precarious fertility references the new conditions of dependency that are produced to render fertility legible and manageable. On the one hand, egg freezing presents a new impetus to make fertility *legible* prior to the attempt to conceive. After the introduction of IVF, egg donation, and now egg freezing, an egg-based model of fertility has become dominant, in which the egg is the key locus of female fertility.[60] In order to know one's fertility, and decide whether to freeze eggs, one becomes dependent on third parties as these eggs are invisible without technical mediation, immeasurable without testing, obscure until extracted, and in perpetual decline since the time before birth.

On the other hand, precarious fertility signals the particular dependencies that emerge in the call to *manage* future infertility, including those that are required to freeze, to thaw, to acquire fertility. By extension, the egg freezing procedure itself operates through a logic in which fertility may, quite literally, be more assured by delivering it from the body, by entrusting it "in someone else's hands." So while egg freezing ostensibly makes people more fertile, the offer of preserving one's eggs can in fact intensify fertility precarity by making people vulnerable to pressures to maximize the future fitness of a fertility that is always already in decline. This transformation of fertility in the face of cryopreservation may be understood as exemplifying a broader sense of reproductive *bioprecarity*, which characterizes contemporary orientations towards the body—and biological substances like eggs—through a mutually reinforcing dynamic of intensified biotechnological dependency and speculative epistemic uncertainty.[61]

When fertility becomes legible with reference to the freezable and extractable egg, reproductive aging gains a cellular component. By dislodging the time of the egg from the time of the body, the possibility of OC complicates a clear, chronological, age-related trajectory from fertility to infertility. For example, if female fertility is understood as the ability to conceive with a chosen partner or donor, the presence of frozen eggs after the onset of age-related infertility gives rise to a state that can be characterized as neither fully fertile nor fully infertile, but rather as what we may call "postfertile." Likewise, when frozen eggs symbolize a timeless and "extended" fertility alongside the body's finite and aging fertility, the relation between fertility and infertility becomes further complicated. Postfertility, then, denotes the ambiguously in/fertile states that emerge when the possibility of egg freezing reconfigures the temporal logic of reproductive aging. This is not to say that categories of fertility and infertility have become obsolete— quite the contrary. Rather, precisely because notions of fertility and infertility can be mobilized for a variety of personal, political, and commercial ends, it is important to consider what is at stake when these categories are called into question, redefined, or reaffirmed in the context of OC.

Freezing Fertility aims to characterize *the postfertile condition* that emerges after the introduction of egg freezing. It explores fertility after its preservability has become commonplace, imaginable, and attainable, if out of reach for many. Postfertility signifies not so much a leaving behind of fertility but rather the conceptual and material flexibility of fertility enabled by new repro- and cryotechnologies. Specifically its postness references a preoccupation with "what comes after," with the futurity of fertility—a futurity that can easily reframe embodied fertility as always already in the process of being lost. More broadly, the "post" of postfertility points to the importance of temporal orientations—such as anticipation, retrospection, suspension, and acceleration—through which constructions of (non)reproductive futures and (in)fertile pasts come to bear on the present moment. In relation to these temporal orientations, egg freezing allows experiences of fertility and infertility to exist alongside one another in new ways as the frozen egg brings the concern and treatability of infertility earlier into the life course and extends new forms of emergent fertilities beyond the onset of age-related infertility.

In *Freezing Fertility*, I explore how the possibility of egg freezing is not just relevant for the increasing but still limited number of women who freeze their eggs but rather is so interesting because it destabilizes fertility—as concept, as practice, as finite—at large. The postfertile condition emerging with egg freezing, as a *condition*, refers to states of (non) reproductive embodiment shared by the wider public, beyond the people who consider or choose OC. Accordingly, this study analyzes public discourses, which engage this broader audience, that reconstruct what it means to be (in)fertile in the face of the possibility of cryopreservation. It also engages with the social structures that provide the conditions of emergence for these newly politicized and commercialized modes of becoming fertile. At stake here are not only fundamental changes to the meaning of fertility but a destabilization of some of the central tenets of aging and reproduction through which gendered organizations of social life are naturalized and themselves reproduced.

In the other, medical sense of the word, the *condition* of postfertility references its proximity to biomedicalization, as frozen eggs have instigated public renegotiations of when and whether (in)fertility becomes a medical condition that requires technological intervention. This is not only relevant for a new group of (potential) patients; the strict regulation as well as the slick promotion of egg freezing also articulate norms about the differential timing and desirability of childbearing for different groups of people—whether they naturalize age limits to pregnancy or normalize new technologized forms of reproductive life course management.

The postfertile condition does not start with oocyte cryopreservation; 20th-century reproductive technologies like the contraceptive pill, IVF, and egg donation have all radically redefined the temporal relationship between fertility and infertility. Nevertheless, by analyzing a reproductive choice that is uniquely oriented towards reproductive aging and future age-related infertility, *Freezing Fertility* gives insight into the particular types of postfertility that emerge when frozen eggs allow the relation between fertility and aging to become modifiable, contingent, and mediated in novel ways. In doing so, oocyte cryopreservation instigates a broader reshaping of the gender politics of aging as frozen eggs travel across time and space, across bodies and borders, with far-reaching effects.

Aging and the Frozen Egg

As the frozen egg shifts clinical possibilities and cultural ideas pertaining to the timing of fertility, aging—and particularly female reproductive aging—becomes politicized in new ways. If biopolitics describes the power, as Foucault famously suggested, to "make live and let die,"[62] the work of "mak[ing] live" relates quite literally to new reproductive technologies like egg freezing, which bring questions of (dis)allowing its attendant technologized forms of reproduction into the realm of politics. Yet the biopolitics of egg freezing is not only generative; it not only "makes live" but reorients the finitude of "let[ting] die" by keeping the eggs in a frozen, deathless state. Kowal and Radin theorize this point as the "cryopolitics" that emerges with contemporary efforts to augment life by making live and *not* letting die. Cryobiology, they argue, gives rise to a duality of a "latent life" oriented towards future potential and an "incomplete death," the deferral of which becomes subject to agentic control.[63] Likewise, frozen eggs can embody a latent fertility and an incomplete arrival of infertility at different times in the life cycle; reproductive aging is thereby not simply a given "fact of life" but is reconstituted in the realms of discourse, regulation, and industry. As the frozen eggs exist alongside the lived time of the body, it is then not just life and death, but the remaking of aging that is central to the cryopolitics of egg freezing.

The possibility of remaking reproductive aging with frozen eggs emerges at a time when growing biomedical and "cosmeceutical" industries cater to a general "will to youth"—Michelle Smirnova's term for "a civic duty of the aging female to pursue eternal youth"—that shapes many aspects of social life, including the lived experience and popular understanding of the body.[64] Contemporary examples are numerous, whether we consider a highly gendered market in anti-aging cosmetics (worth $1.15 billion in the United States alone), the medicalization of midlife, or the double standards of representing aging in popular culture.[65] Gender is a key organizing factor in contemporary biopolitics of aging, which, Brett Neilson argues, pertains to both the disciplinary effects of knowledge production about aging and the control exerted through the nation-state and the market logic of global capitalism, in which aging is increasingly understood as an individual risk rather than a collective responsibility.⁶⁶ This intersection of gender and age is at the heart of the particular reproductive politics emerging with egg freezing.

In order to understand the intersection of gender and aging as organizing principles within the promiscuous prefixing of the bio-, cryo-, and repropolitics, this study takes as its starting point the construction of gendered age normativities that inform contemporary egg freezing practices and their reconfiguration of life, latency, and reproduction.⁶⁷ Through this lens, the discursive production of reproductive aging and age-related infertility in the context of OC does not simply reflect a biological reality but emerges in relation to historically specific norms of aging and organizing time.

Age normativities specific to women have historically been predicated on reproductive changes in the female body.⁶⁸ With the establishment of gynecology and the concomitant pathologization of the many "diseases of women," mid-19th-century Western medicine fostered the institutionalization of a gender-specific history of naturalizing age-appropriate acts—such as when to have a partner and when to reproduce—with reference to (non)reproductive physical phenomena such as menstruation, childbearing, and menopause.⁶⁹ The anticipation and arrival of age-related infertility is a contemporary equivalent of a body-based moment in the female life span that becomes a reference point in validating or resisting a set of age- and gender-specific norms governing when to have children, when (in)fertility may be assumed, when infertility ought to be anticipated, when medical interventions are appropriate, and how the passage of time may be recognized in the body. In OC discourses, age normativities may be expressed in mediatized medical advice on when to pick Mr. Good Enough over Mr. Right, women's public accounts of the anxiety experienced at turning 35, and the proposition to offer egg freezing as a graduation gift, to name but a few examples that I will discuss in this study.

In the context of egg freezing, such age norms emerge in relation to broader, historically specific cultural organizations of time that Elizabeth Freeman defines as "chrononormativities." The term refers to the "hidden rhythms" of "schedules, calendars, time zones" that "seem natural to those whom they privilege." These rhythms, she argues, function as "technique[s] by which institutional forces come to seem like somatic facts."⁷⁰ Freeman's definition of chrononormativity as "the use of time to organize individual human bodies toward maximum productivity" points to an industrialized organization of time, which was first standardized in 19th-century England (1847) and temporalized the gender division into the "separate spheres" system.[71] In contrast with an industrialized time of standardized scheduling, women's space of the home was idealized within a discourse of domesticity that "validated a set of feelings—love, security, harmony . . . motherly instincts—in part by figuring them as timeless."[72] This domestic maternal space was associated with a cyclicality of a feminine "corporealized time" attendant to the "human tides," which was rhetorically opposed to the "linear time of history" and wage time of industrial capitalism.[73] What emerged was a cultural logic in which a nonlinear time seen to belong to the female reproductive body lay at the foundation of the reification of the gender binary in distinct "spheres" that became separated not only in space but in the particular chrononormativities that organized their temporal schemes.

The naturalization of this feminized chrononormativity was challenged in the 20th century not only by women's increased participation in the industrialized time of the public sphere and wage labor but also by the entrance of industrialized temporal schedules into the female reproductive body, primarily through the advent of reproductive technologies offering increased agency over the timing of menstruation and maternity. Hormonal contraceptives allowed the introduction of alternative temporal schemes into the cyclical rhythms of menstruation. Through precisely timed hormonal stimulation, *in vitro* fertilization techniques decoupled attempts at childbearing from cyclical ovulatory patterns and synchronized them with specific time schedules, such as those of the fertility clinic.[74] These developments did not necessarily entail a conceptual severing of femininity and fertility from cyclical rhythms. In fact, as Nelly Oudshoorn argues, they can reinforce a notion of "natural cycles" in contradistinction with these interventions.[75] Nevertheless, these reproductive technologies did posit the timing of menstruation and ovulation as manipulable by synthetic hormones and allowed for the popular reconceptualization of childbearing within linear temporalities as "family planning." In this way, the temporal regulation of the female reproductive body in relation to the chrononormativities implicit in standardized treatment protocols, mass-produced hormone strips, and clinical time schedules exemplifies Freeman's definition of chrononormativity as, this time more literally, becoming recognizable as "somatic facts."[76]

With this increased technologically mediated agency over the timing of childbearing, the end of the female reproductive life span gained cultural significance as a temporal limit to "family planning." Friese and colleagues describe the public concern with a female reproductive "deadline" following the increasing availability of contraceptive and abortion services, which centered on the notion that "the public domain, organized around paid labor, interferes and competes with a woman's fertile years."[77] The widespread preoccupation with this deadline—often referred to as the "biological clock"—also emerged in relation to the idea that age-related infertility is "the price women pay" for increased participation in paid labor, politics, and higher education.[78] Adopted in the neoconservative political climate of the 1980s, the female "biological clock" was popularized as a "temporal signifier of inter-gender difference" that naturalized a proximity between the female body and the family with reference to the temporality of women's bodies—particularly so in the face of a changed social order that permitted, and required, more participation of women in the workplace.[79] This coincided with the publication of influential scientific studies arguing that contemporary and historical data demonstrate that "female fecundity [is] a function of age."[80] The popularization of such findings, along with the advent of new reproductive technologies like IVF, displaced the common conceptualization of menopause as the end of the reproductive life span and menstruation as an affirmation of fertility in favor of an understanding of "ovarian reserve" and the age of the eggs as determinants of reproductive capacity.[81] This shift entails a move away from the easily observable and cyclical indicator of presumed fertility in menses to a more elusive notion of the age of the eggs that may be assessed through medical interventions like hormonal blood tests or ovarian ultrasound scans—or deduced from one's age in years since birth.

Rather than a cyclical conceptualization of women's reproductive embodiment, the dominant presentation of the temporality of female fertility in egg freezing discourses is characterized by a life-long decline of egg quantity and quality. The female reproductive body does not adopt an idealized position outside of standardized time, but becomes itself synonymous with clock time in tropes of "ticking ovaries" and the "biological clock." In this linear loss model of reproductive aging, eggs may themselves begin to function as measurements of time. As eggs may be "banked" as a means of "fertility insurance," they somatize an economy of time, in which time is understood to be quantifiable and delimited—a "'thing' that can be 'spent,' 'saved,' and 'lost'; indeed, it is frequently 'invested.'"[82] Alongside the more familiar family planning, these egg-based conceptualizations of female reproductive aging facilitate the popularization of "fertility planning," which references practices of timing not only when to have children but also when to have the *ability* to have children.

If the end of the female reproductive life span is then located in egg quality and quantity, the possibility of fertility planning with frozen eggs destabilizes the very previously naturalized temporal limits that govern when women can be considered fertile. It is therefore no surprise that the introduction of egg freezing has once more rekindled cultural negotiations over the relation between female reproductive aging and gendered chrononormativities. It is characteristic of the postfertile condition, with its temporal instability of in/fertility distinctions, that we may now witness cultural efforts to restabilize temporal limits to fertility that appeal to the notion of "normal reproductive years" to motivate bans or rejections of egg freezing.[83] Conversely, egg freezing is promoted precisely as a means to "extend fertility" and adjust these limits to the chrononormativities of labor arrangements or the "will to youth." In the context of egg freezing, the gender politics of aging thus pertains not only to norms associated with particular ages but also to the chrononormative temporal schemes in relation to which the time of female fertility may be understood, organized, and politicized.

The Egg's Journey: Outline

Freezing Fertility follows the journey of the egg in the OC process.[84] Each chapter addresses a step of the OC treatment, thereby reflecting the fact that egg freezing is not a single procedure but a set of consecutive interventions in which the egg undergoes various transformations. Immature eggs are stimulated in the ovaries; extracted eggs are cryopreserved and stored in the freezer; eggs may be thawed, fertilized, incubated, and implanted; frozen eggs also may become mobile, traveling between clinics and countries in portable freezers. Accordingly, the chapters focus on eggs in the body, their extraction for preservation, their frozen existence in the freezer, their incubation after fertilization, their subsequent return to the womb, and the implications of their unprecedented movement in global flows of eggs. By following the egg's journey in OC, I examine how the reproductive youth attributed to the egg propels it across time and space in trajectories that reflect economic, regulatory, and social power asymmetries, while also giving rise to a broader postfertile condition in which fertility and aging are repoliticized in ways that affect the public at large.

An interdisciplinary project, *Freezing Fertility* integrates insights from science and technology studies, medical sociology, cultural analysis, feminist theory, reproductive studies, and critical gerontology in order to analyze the discourses and practices of egg freezing. Rather than offering an exhaustive overview of one dimension of the OC practice, I offer a series of critical readings of cultural objects that are pertinent to understanding the situatedness and implications of egg freezing in relation to a broader gender politics of aging. Some of the selected objects, such as widely read newspapers and televised documentaries, are indicative of egg freezing's prominence in public debates and popular culture, while others, such as cellular images or informed-consent contracts, present a particular novel aspect of OC that distinguishes it from other reproductive technologies. My reading of these objects adopts a "cultural analysis" approach, which is an interdisciplinary research practice that employs diverse analytic lenses to offer detailed readings of case studies that are sensitive to the "interplay between the text and [its] context."[85] This approach allows me to situate critical readings of cultural objects within broader social frames, thereby positioning OC as a key technology for understanding new 21st-century biopolitical regimes of reproductive aging.

In order to examine how egg freezing is politicized in public discourses, chapter 1 analyzes coverage of OC in US, UK, and Dutch news media. It focuses on the time prior to the egg freezing procedure, when the eggs remain in the body, and considers how, and with what consequences, female fertility becomes precarious in the face of cryopreservation. New and old norms of reproductive timing become evident in criticisms and endorsements of egg freezing, in which categorizations of "lifestyle" versus "single" or "medical" versus "social" freezing play an important rhetorical role. The news coverage also features new subject positions for women who freeze their eggs, as their reproductive, relational, and life course decision making becomes subject to public scrutiny. Key elements in OC discourses are the trope of the "biological clock" and related egg-focused conceptualizations of reproductive aging, which shape both the need for and the nature of the reproductive choices associated with egg freezing. Drawing on these elements, the news coverage of OC reveals a gendered politics of aging, predicated on reproductive ability as the organizing principle for the temporal structuring of life, which both interpellates a contingent of women who may want to reproduce later in life and positions their reproductive decision making as a public concern.

Moving on to the decision to freeze one's eggs, the next chapter focuses on the new cultural and clinical practices of anticipating bodily futurity. The Dutch documentary *Eggs for Later* [86] gives insight into the anticipatory terms and affective states through which women's future age-related infertility is conceptualized in relation to the possibility of freezing eggs. The analysis draws attention to the contesting interpretations of egg freezing as either a postponement of motherhood or an extension of fertility—and proposes an alternative reading of OC as a means of transforming reproductive bioprecarity into biopreparedness for future infertility. At stake in these various conceptualizations of egg freezing is the reconfiguration of ideas and practices of what constitutes healthy embodiment, the reproductive process, and responsible aging. The analysis explores how egg freezing may function not only to (potentially) achieve future reproduction but also to resolve anticipatory anxiety by maintaining the futurity of potential motherhood.

Once extracted and frozen, the cryo-egg represents an emergent cultural entity that hitherto did not exist. Chapter 3 focuses on these disembodied, frozen eggs and the new modes of governing fertility emerging within broader reproductive bioeconomies. While the eggs remain in the freezer, discursive mediations of the cryopreserved cells become an important reference point in the reconceptualization of reproductive aging as distributed across bodies, freezers, and wider cryopolitical infrastructures. Reflecting the large capital investments in fertility preservation, the figure of the visible and quantifiable frozen egg also plays a key role in the treatment rationales and calculative practices presented by fertility companies. By tracing these developments, this chapter explores the relation between fertility accumulation and capital accumulation. With an analysis of the framing of frozen eggs in marketing efforts, treatment packages, and fertility insurance, the chapter moreover highlights how the mediated frozen egg plays a key role in the rationalization of OC as not just a single procedure but an ongoing process of technologized fertility management.

After the eggs are fertilized *in vitro*, it has to be decided which one(s) will be implanted in the womb in a process called "embryo selection." Time-lapse embryo imaging, a widely used method for embryo selection, analyzes the timing of embryonic development to predict the embryos' future viability. In keeping with this study's focus on aging, chapter 4 draws attention to the visualization and instrumentalization of embryonic aging in time-lapse embryo-imaging systems. Drawing on the politicized history of imaging prenatal life, it analyzes the cultural, political, and commercial significance of a new set of images of fertilized eggs—and their division into embryos—that circulate beyond the laboratory into the clinic, the intended parents' iPads, and their online social networks. What is at stake in the instrumentalization of embryonic aging in time-lapse systems is the creation of new risks and modes of value creation through the patenting of embryonic aging, the datafication of embryo selection, and the "packaging up" of treatment plans to include both egg freezing and time-lapse imaging. This method of embryo selection, then, may not just result in more or less "IVF success" but also affects the conceptualization and commercialization of aging at an embryonic level.

If selected, the egg—now embryo—proceeds to the next stage of its journey, in which it may be implanted into the intended mother's womb and a pregnancy may ensue. Focusing on this step, chapter 5 explores several new, technologically mediated ways of attaining fertility and motherhood with frozen eggs after the end of the reproductive life span, which both reflect and transform existing notions of "older motherhood." Since the emergence of donor-egg IVF in the late 20th century, older motherhood has become particularly politicized—whether as chrononormative transgression or as sign of successful aging. This chapter revisits these discussions and explores how younger women become newly implicated in the politicization of older motherhood when they freeze their eggs. Drawing on the stories of women who thawed their eggs, the analysis subsequently focuses on the social significance of conception in the context of OC and discusses how this technology allows fertility to be extended, but also to be lost in new ways. Egg freezing also opens up possibilities for new forms of posthumous conception and motherhood. Informed-consent forms institutionalize an encounter with one's own mortality and allow for the formation of intended kinship bonds beyond death. This chapter addresses these new configurations of fertility and motherhood by exploring how reproductive aging intersects with willfulness, kinship, and mortality.

Given that only a very limited percentage of cryopreserved oocytes result in live births, motherhood—older or not—is not a self-evident endpoint of either the egg's journey or this study on egg freezing. Consequently, chapter 6 zooms out to explore the alternative trajectories of frozen eggs in egg-donation networks for reproductive and research purposes. Once frozen, the eggs become as portable as the liquid nitrogen tanks that hold them; egg freezing is thus a key condition for the development of global flows of eggs. The US-based World Egg Bank ships frozen eggs to clinics worldwide and provides a case study for considering the implications of the transnational mobility of frozen eggs for reproductive egg donation. The analysis focuses on US-UK egg flows and discusses the regulations, matching practices, financial inducements, online platforms, and marketing strategies that are imported and exported along with the eggs. Such global flows of frozen eggs moreover emerge at a time when new developments in stem cell science revive the need for donor eggs. These stem cell technologies radically reconfigure the egg's relation to bodily time, and thereby raise questions about the relation between aging and reproductivity in new ways. They moreover provide a context in which to consider the potential rerouting of eggs frozen for one's own use into egg-donation networks, which is particularly pertinent given the fact that, so far, only a small percentage of women have returned to use their cryo-eggs. These developments in reproductive and research egg-donation practices allow me to highlight the significance of the frozen egg in a global biopolitics of aging. As the egg travels across bodies and geopolitical boundaries, as it is instrumentalized to halt, counteract, or regenerate age, OC's emergence radically transforms how the passage of time becomes meaningful, visible, and political in bodies and eggs alike.

1

Making Fertility Precarious

Egg Freezing and the Politicization of Reproductive Aging

Welcomed as liberation and dismissed as exploitation, the introduction of egg freezing has met with controversy and ambivalence, and is thus no exception to a longer tradition of politicized public responses to new reproductive technologies. The 20th century saw radical changes in the manipulation of reproduction through techno-scientific and biomedical means. Struggles for reproductive choice initially focused on avoiding pregnancy and birth, most prominently in relation to the introduction of the contraceptive pill and the legalization of abortion.[1] The achievement of conception and birth, by contrast, became newly politicized from the late 1970s onwards, with the introduction of reproductive technologies such as *in vitro* fertilization, egg donation, and gestational surrogacy. In the early decades of the 21st century, these approaches to avoiding and achieving reproduction are combined in egg freezing. This reproductive technology simultaneously represents both an active choice not to have children in the present and a commitment to future, possibly assisted, reproduction, thus calling into question easy distinctions between reproductive and nonreproductive behavior. Media discourses surrounding the introduction of egg freezing give insights into the significance of this technology for the public reconceptualization of the female reproductive body as the site of a gendered politics of aging.

Although egg freezing has often been described as a procedure for a small group of elite women who can afford the expensive procedure, this chapter emphasizes that the significance of egg freezing stretches far beyond the growing, but still limited, numbers of women who use this technology. As a relatively fringe procedure—in the United Kingdom, for example, OC comprises only 1.5% of IVF cycles—it nevertheless becomes so widely significant because the *possibility* of egg freezing is increasingly publicly recognized.[2] It is the widespread attention across print and screen media that makes OC relevant not only as a new clinical practice but as a cultural phenomenon that affects a much broader group of women and men.

The very possibility of freezing one's eggs—whether or not one would choose or be able to do so—shifts the meaning of fertility and reproductive aging. Public discourses on OC display a tension between the understanding of female reproductive aging as either immutable or adjustable. On the one hand, women's reproductive aging is framed as *foundational* to the formation of chrononormativities pertaining to idealized timings of when to have children, have a long-term partner, prioritize work or family formation—thereby renaturalizing them in the face of technological innovation. On the other hand, egg freezing may be presented as a technology that renders female fertility *adjustable* to meet broader social chrononormativities of wage time, education time, relationship time, and gendered ideologies of aging.

For example, in the Netherlands, the introduction of egg freezing for so-called social reasons was blocked by the Christian-Democrat-majority coalition government in order to maintain "natural" age limits to women's fertility, which were affirmed through a regulatory framework that did not permit using frozen eggs beyond 45 years. By contrast, US egg freezing insurance coverage through Fortune 500 companies, such as Apple and Facebook, has promoted OC as a means of extending fertility to the time when women are "ready"—whether the time of readiness is determined by relationship formation patterns, the temporal organization of careers, or other factors. In different national contexts, the introduction of egg freezing can thus provoke both the reaffirmation of age norms in the face of their potential transgression and the reconfiguration of reproductive aging as operating by a different temporal logic when eggs can be "frozen in time."

Both the British and the Dutch contexts are characterized by a high degree of national regulation of reproductive healthcare; yet egg freezing is regulated in strikingly different ways in the two countries. In 2009 the Amsterdam Academic Medical Centre (AMC) proposed to offer egg freezing not only to cancer patients but also to women who wished to anticipate age-related infertility.[3] A majority in the Dutch Parliament objected to the AMC's plan and a two-year highly mediatized public debate ensued, until "social" egg freezing was formally permitted in 2011.[4]

Although egg freezing had been allowed, the suggested maximum age for implanting the embryos was lowered from the 50 years the AMC had initially proposed to the customary 45-year age limit in conventional IVF.[5] The controversy surrounding the AMC's initiative, the public debate that ensued, and the subsequent implementation of OC reaffirmed reproductive aging limits in the face of the new possibilities associated with cryopreservation.

Twenty years prior, the United Kingdom had already drawn up egg freezing regulations in the 1990 Human Fertilisation and Embryology Act. At least 50 women froze their eggs during the nineties, but the Human Fertilisation and Embryology Authority (HFEA)—the national body licensing and monitoring UK fertility clinics—did not permit the use of these eggs for fear of chromosomal defects.[6] At the turn of the millennium, one of these women, Carolyn Neill, challenged the ban because she wanted to use the nine eggs she had frozen prior to having treatment for breast cancer. In response, the HFEA commissioned Dr. Sharon Paynter to write a report on the safety of egg freezing. Following her positive, albeit cautious, recommendations, the HFEA lifted the restrictions on using frozen eggs for fertilization and subsequent implantation.[7] The first British frozen egg baby, Emily Perry, was born in June 2002. Unlike the Dutch equivalent, the UK HFEA regulations make no distinction between "social" and "medical" egg freezing, and there are no national age limits prohibiting treatment after 45 years, although they do limit the storage of gametes to 10 years.[8]

In the relatively unregulated US fertility sector, egg freezing was also available from the early 2000s onwards. For example, CHA Fertility Los Angeles opened one of the first egg freezing clinics for fertility preservation in 2002.[9] Dedicated egg freezing companies—notably Extend Fertility—were founded as early as 2003.[10] Meanwhile, cryopreservation was also taken up to create the first US donor egg banks, such as the World Egg Bank (see chapter 6). In spite of this early availability of egg freezing, the American Society for Reproductive Medicine (ASRM) was cautious about the OC practice and issued a warning in 2004 that egg freezing should neither be recommended to healthy women nor "be marketed or offered as a means to defer reproductive aging."[11] When the ASRM lifted the experimental label almost a decade later, the announcement was often framed as an endorsement of elective egg freezing, even though they repeated their earlier statement that there were "not yet sufficient data to recommend oocyte cryopreservation for the sole purpose of circumventing reproductive aging in healthy women."[12] In 2018, they once more adjusted and declared so-called planned egg freezing for this purpose "ethically permissible."[13]

As OC was met with the public and political scrutiny characteristic of the introduction of new reproductive technologies, from donor-inseminated "virgin mothers" to IVF's "test tube babies," its news coverage is a key medium through which public understandings of fertility, egg freezing, and its users are shaped. For this reason, this chapter addresses OC coverage in newspapers to understand how public understandings of reproductive aging and female fertility are remade after the introduction of OC. The analysis focuses on three major national newspapers: the *Guardian* (UK), the *New York Times* (US), and the *Volkskrant* (NL), all of which have a relatively progressive orientation and include detailed articles on medical topics such as OC.[14] The news coverage also brings together various other public discourses on egg freezing, including parliamentary debates, medical expert advice, and patient narratives. From the reading of this corpus emerged several recurring narratives about women's motivations for egg freezing as well as specific dominant conceptualizations of female reproductive embodiment and aging. What is at stake in the OC newspaper coverage is, then, not so much the potential childbearing of a limited group of individuals who froze their eggs but the engagement of the wider public with popular narratives about fertility decline, reproductive choices, and the women who make them.[15]

Being effectively a prolonged IVF procedure, OC itself raised few objections when it was introduced. What stirred public discussions on egg freezing were women's motivations and considerations in choosing this procedure. This chapter therefore focuses on the ways in which OC's reproductive choice became politicized both through the categorization of women in binary oppositions of "social" vs. "medical" and "single" vs. "lifestyle" freezers and through the articulation of contemporary re-conceptualizations of female reproductive aging. With these oppositions emerge new subject positions related to reproductive identity through which age-related aspects of social life come under public and medical scrutiny. Key elements in this discourse are the trope of the "biological clock" and related egg-focused, decline-oriented understandings of reproductive aging, which reframe female fertility as being under perpetual threat and in need of intervention—whether medical or political. Media hypes surrounding OC marketing and fertility insurance moreover point to female reproductive aging as a lens onto a broader cultural renegotiation of the relation between production and reproduction as central axes of a wider social order. The news coverage of OC thereby reveals a contemporary reconceptualization of female reproductive aging as a public concern, predicated on the presentation of reproductive ability as the organizing principle for the temporal structuring of life, which not only interpellates (potentially) infertile women who desire to reproduce but also impacts the wider public.[16]

Having It All? Egg Freezing as Lifestyle Choice

Fertility clinics are gearing up to open their doors to fertile couples seeking treatment as a lifestyle choice rather than a medical necessity, experts said yesterday. . . . The shift reflects a rise in what some fertility specialists have called the "have it all generation" who do not want to compromise between career and family. "The great problem we've got now is you can't have your cake and eat it," said Dr Simon Fishel, director of the CARE Fertility centre at the Park hospital in Nottingham.[17]

Although small numbers of women facing cancer treatment had frozen their eggs since the turn of the millennium, initial public interest in egg freezing was sparked mainly by its availability to healthy women who might, as this *Guardian* article suggests, seek treatment as a "lifestyle choice" because they want to "have it all." At the heart of controversies surrounding OC's introduction were women's motivations for egg freezing—and the public negotiation of their validity. As divergent perspectives on egg freezing emerged, the subject of contention was not so much the OC technology itself but rather the situations in which women ought (not) to use it. And these discussions, in turn, revealed the instability of popular conceptualizations of fertility and reproductive aging in the face of cryopreservation.

In her discussion of reproductive technologies, Jana Sawicki argues that these "new technologies create new subjects—that is, fit mothers, unfit mothers, infertile women, and so forth."[18] What is likewise at stake in the case of OC is the construction of new subject positions for women who freeze their eggs, including the "lifestyle" freezer, the cancer patient, and the single woman who hopes to start a family with a future partner. These subject positions function as rhetorical tools in both critical and celebratory accounts of egg freezing and are indicative of a broader gender politics of reproductive aging and the social conservative and neoliberal discourses that underlie them.

Initial concerns about egg freezing were directed neither at those companies in the fertility sector who could stand to benefit from the influx of fertile women into the IVF clinic nor at the "changes to the conditions of life, work, childbearing, and child rearing" in late capitalism that rationalize later reproduction, and the concomitant demand for fertility preservation, among a growing group of women.[19] Instead, sceptical accounts of egg freezing revolved around reproductive aging. They expressed concerns about the technology introducing new possibilities of deprioritizing reproduction, encouraging postponement, and transgressing the temporal limits of the "normal reproductive years."

One central figure in the more sceptical presentations of OC was the "lifestyle" freezer who wants to "have it all." This section's opening quotation, which was taken from an article titled "Clinics Prepare for 'Lifestyle' Fertility Treatment," exemplifies the use of this popular phrase. It positions egg freezing as a technology for those who want to "have [their] cake and eat it," or for "the 'have it all generation' who do not want to compromise between career and family."[20] Even though gender is not specified in the "have it all generation," the article's focus on the novelty of female fertility preservation suggests that wanting to "have it all" in the face of fertility decline pertains more to women than to men.

Neither new nor unique to OC, the trope of "having it all" has been used as the defining feature of several postwar generations of women entering the labor force. Its perennial popularity signals a recurring public preoccupation with female fertility in the face of women's participation in the workplace. Writing about the backlash against feminism in the 1980s, feminist author Susan Faludi frequently returns to "the popular myth about the 'have it all' baby-boom women."[21] She discusses the

US news coverage of a supposed "trend of childlessness" described in headlines like "The Curse of the Career Woman" and "Having It All: Postponing Parenthood Exacts a Price."[22] The successful combination of family life and career was construed as "the myth of Supermom" that was debunked as mothers "recognized they can't have it all" while "'millions' of career women will 'pay a price for waiting.'"[23] Kelly Oliver likewise argues that the public concern with women "having it all" reflects "deep-seated anxieties about women's reproductive choices in an age of changing technologies."[24] It is therefore not surprising that the "having it all" trope framed the early public responses to egg freezing, as a new reproductive choice that was presumed particularly relevant—and affordable—to "career women."

As the phrase reemerged in the egg freezing debate, it gained a different temporal dimension; here "having it all" pertained less to the work-family combination per se. In Sample's quotation, the concern appears to be not necessarily with working mothers "having it all" but more with women of an age range associated with declining fertility who want to both focus on professional development and maintain the potential to have children. The combination in question is not so much career and family, but career and extended fertility. In the earlier concerns about working women "paying the price" of childlessness by deprioritizing reproduction for too long, fertility decline was used as a foundational biological fact to naturalize gendered differences in waged labor participation. The promise of egg freezing is that it will alter the very temporal limits to female fertility that underlie this logic. Sceptical responses to egg freezing suggested women may be using the technology to "suit their lifestyles and aspirations" and buy "time to enjoy an extended adolescence of vacations and cocktails or to single-mindedly climb the corporate ladder."[25] The implicit indulgence of "having it all" in the context of OC is, then, the stretching of a child-free but nonetheless fertile life course beyond established age ranges.

The potential of OC to threaten an understanding of reproductive aging as an immutable constant in the face of women's historically changing gender roles instigated a public reaffirmation of the temporal limits to female fertility. For example, Dutch CDA MP Janneke Schermers considered egg freezing to be "completely unnatural."[26] She objected to the possibility that "women who have their eggs frozen can have children at an age at which pregnancy is normally no longer possible."[27] Schermer's position demonstrates how egg freezing can trigger public assertions of the notion that there is a natural progression of the reproductive life span that may be threatened by the possibilities of this new technology. Indeed, in a poll among almost 20,000 Dutch people, the most prevalent argument against egg freezing did not pertain to health risks or to the medical treatment of healthy bodies but to the idea that women should reproduce during "normal reproductive years."[28] What is thus at stake in OC's public discourses is the cultural negotiation of the female reproductive aging process, and whether temporal limits to fertility could be considered as potentially alterable through these technologies, or immutable in spite of them.

Single Freezers and Absent Partners

Partly in response to the narrative that women are freezing their eggs to "have it all," an alternative prominent news story highlights instead that women undergo OC not because of their lifestyle or career but for lack of a partner. The foregrounding of the absent partner as motivating factor organizes an alternative subject position of the single woman freezing her eggs. For example, speaking against the notion that women put off childbearing for unspecified careers and "lifestyle reasons," Dr. Lockwood of the Midlands Fertility Services clinic[29] illustrates such a subject position:

> Often they've been in a relationship that they assumed was going to lead to marriage and motherhood—possibly for 10 years. Then at 37, 38, the boyfriend says, "I don't think fatherhood is for me." Or he meets someone else.[30]

The narrative of single women freezing their eggs in order to be able to reproduce with a partner in the future puts OC in a more positive light.[31] Women in this scenario are considered as having an active wish for a child, but as unable to get pregnant at present for want of the relationship required for the desired family set-up. Rather than a willful nonreproductive choice of women wanting to "have it all," egg freezing is here rationalized through the absence of the "right" male partner.[32]

In discourses favorable to egg freezing, the rhetorical function of this subject position follows from the presentation of OC as a solution to a reproductive desire that is externally thwarted, rather than a technology for deprioritizing reproduction to meet one's lifestyle preferences.

In another *Guardian* article, Dr. Lockwood argues that more needs to be done to "help those *forced* to delay getting pregnant."[33] In her accounts, she presents her patients in a sympathetic way by emphasizing their age-appropriate reproductive intent and its contravention by external factors; women's nonreproductivity happens *to* them, rather than *because* of them. Egg freezing is, in other words, not a sign of a woman unduly postponing reproduction. Instead, Lockwood presents it as the outcome of a boyfriend making nonreproductive decisions, and leaving the relationship—rather than the woman or the couple doing so together. The subject position of the single egg freezer is here characterized as a result of circumstance; age and singlehood become part of the plight for which egg freezing can provide the solution. The focus lies not on a potential subversion of the timing of motherhood but on OC's role in maintaining the possibility of a normative genetically related family model in the face of female reproductive aging. Childlessness is presented as a consequence of women's unfortunately incorrect assumptions concerning marriage and motherhood in their thirties. This framing absolves them from the judgment visited on women who use OC for "lifestyle reasons." Instead, she highlights that, for some women, potential childlessness worsens already painful situations, and egg freezing provides a potential solution when the timelines of relationship formation do not match those of embodied reproductive aging.

Contrasted with the woman who is single by circumstance, the subject position of the "lifestyle freezer" bears a different relation to the absent partner; here women's behavior is identified as the cause of their nonreproductive situation:

> The IVF expert Dr Gedis Grudzinskas says it's [conception] more difficult after the age of 27: "When women have got used to having a lot of freedom to run their lives as they wish, they do not want to hear that they may not be able to conceive. They perhaps need to compromise, find Mr Good Enough and have a family earlier."[34] Surveys of older mothers show half say they delayed because they had not met a suitable partner. Maybe

instead of waiting for Mr Right they ought to settle for Mr Good-Enough, if they want children.[35]

In the frame of lifestyle freezing, egg freezing is not presented as the solution to, but as the symptom of women delaying reproduction as a result of wrong partner choices. In contrast to the woman who is single by circumstance, the "lifestyle freezer" is at fault for not having a partner. Her singlehood is not attributed to an unwantedly broken or absent relationship but to being too critical of potential fathers or too passive about the pursuit of finding one. Singlehood, in the narrative of the lifestyle freezer recounted here, represents a youthful freedom that ought to be relinquished when women reach an age associated with declining fertility in order to have a family with a suitably available partner.[36]

In public statements on female reproduction by medical authorities, the subject of egg freezing thus becomes the occasion for including advice about age-related life decisions beyond matters directly related to health and medical treatment, such as relationship and career choices. In this process, the temporal limits to female fertility are once more reaffirmed as reference points for naturalizing existing age normativities of reproduction and relationship formation. Significantly, when articulated by IVF professionals, these age- and gender-specific ideas run the risk of becoming naturalized as neutral health perspectives—which pertain not only to the women freezing their eggs but to the public at large.

Social vs. Medical Freezing

The categorization of single and lifestyle freezers notwithstanding, the key opposition in egg freezing discourses is the binary between medical and social freezing—if only because it is an important principle in organizing access to OC.[37] Insurance coverage of egg freezing, for instance, is to a large extent contingent on whether egg freezing is considered to be medically motivated or not.[38] This division was also at the heart of the Dutch parliamentary debate on whether women with "social" motivations should be allowed to freeze their eggs in the way that women with "medical" motivations are. Such oppositional framings of egg freezing motivations provide insight into the gendered politics of reproductive aging underlying these divisions and discussions. For example, reporting on the political debate about the legalization of egg freezing, the *Volkskrant* writes,

> Today the Second Chamber debates egg freezing by "social indication." . . . Egg freezing already happens by medical indication, for example in women who have to undergo a cancer treatment that may damage fertility.[39]

In the "medical" versus "social" division, the cancer-related cases are contrasted with those of women without a serious diagnosis who wish to maintain a chance of having genetically related children as they grow older. Unlike its "lifestyle" equivalent, freezing by "medical indication" is not the subject of much controversy, and its use is generally deemed "legitimate."[40] Egg freezing simply becomes one optional step in a wider set of medical interventions that make up the treatment plan for diagnoses such as cancer. Fertility loss here gains a different meaning because it is not specifically caused by reproductive aging but by particular diagnoses or treatments.

Women's so-called social reasons for egg freezing reference the anticipation of future, age-related infertility due to, for example, decreased responsiveness of the ovaries to follicle-stimulating hormone (FSH) and luteinising hormone (LH) or reduced availability of viable eggs. Both "social" and "medical" motivations for OC anticipate physical difficulties in achieving future pregnancies at the time of the second phase of the procedure. The difference is whether these difficulties are caused by pathological or by age-related factors. The "medical" versus "social" binary opposition thus categorizes egg freezers by the reasons why they cannot have children at present, and, by extension, it positions the latter motivation as "nonmedical," thereby demedicalizing the age-related infertility that the procedure seeks to preemptively remedy.

The relative acceptance of medical egg freezing also points to the significance of aging norms in organizing reproductive healthcare. After all, the health concerns raised in arguments against IVF-assisted older motherhood—including later childbearing enabled by social egg freezing—are similar, if not worse in these cases.[41] Just as older age means a shorter remaining life expectancy, so serious disease and invasive treatment often entail a higher risk of the child losing a parent at an early age. The mother's health risks associated with pregnancy, labor, and postnatal healing may be higher at an older age, but may be equally challenging—if not more so—for a woman who is recovering from immuno-compromising treatments such as radiation or chemotherapy. The fact that these risks are widely accepted and taken in these difficult cases is a testimony to the significance ascribed to maintaining fertility during "normal reproductive years," even in circumstances that pose concerns not unlike those raised against older motherhood.

The seemingly commonsense opposition between "medical" and "social" egg freezing polarizes a situation that is far more complex than this binary suggests. Besides cancer, there are many other situations that may prompt women to consider the procedure, such as expected compromised fertility following polycystic ovary syndrome (PCOS), Turner Syndrome, or a family history of early menopause.[42] Egg freezing is increasingly practiced for patients with diagnoses such as endometriosis, which can affect fertility, or multiple sclerosis (MS), which may be treated with fertility-compromising stem cell therapies.[43] Egg freezing is also frequently used to tackle complications in IVF procedures, for example, when men cannot produce sperm or when women undergo several cycles of egg retrieval and "batch" the eggs together to do fertilization and incubation.[44] It may also function as an ethical technology to avoid concerns about freezing or creating embryos for people or institutions who believe life begins at conception. OC moreover facilitates egg donation by removing the need to synchronize two women's hormonal cycles or even their reproductive life spans. It also enables intergenerational egg donation, which may benefit women with daughters who suffer from diseases that will compromise their fertility when they grow up. Transgender men may want to freeze their eggs to leave options open for future reproduction as they transition. Women whose occupations may compromise their fertility, for example, those who take drugs such as anabolic steroids or work with harmful chemicals or radiation, may wish to use OC as a precaution. The variety of these possible scenarios illustrates the reductionism of a binary between social and medical reasons, as well as the potential pitfalls of regulating the procedure on the basis of this division.

The opposition of the "medical-social" indication is not unique to OC but also organizes other controversial medical interventions in female reproductive healthcare, including elective caesarean sections, hospitalization for childbirth, and the institutionalization of donor insemination.[45] Stoop and colleagues note that the term "social" is rarely used as an indication for medical treatments generally; it rather references a "nonmedical" and "deliberate choice" in cases like "social abortion, social sex selection or a social Caesarean section."[46] It is striking that these instances pertain to women's reproductive choices; the explicit "social" nature of the indication for treatment often appears to be associated with the role of female agency in accessing reproductive healthcare. Another instance is the distinction of "social" and "medical" indications for contraceptives, which was in widespread use during their 1950s introduction and reflects the morally controversial nature of their prescription. Once the use of contraceptives became popularized, this distinction fell out of use.[47] "Social" versus "medical" oppositions likewise organize public discourses on abortion, e.g., in the distinction between "social indication models" that permit "abortion when the woman can claim social or economic distress" and "medical indication models" that allow "abortion only in cases in which the physical or mental health of the woman is in danger."[48] These cases illustrate how the explicit characterization of a "social indication" for a treatment is itself indicative of the controversial nature of its accessibility at the patient's request—particularly so when that patient is a woman seeking to access reproductive healthcare.

The historical continuity of the "medical" versus "social" opposition in motivating the use of egg freezing and other (once) contentious reproductive technologies is also reflected in the representations of the women who use them. The single and lifestyle subject positions structuring OC's news coverage are reminiscent of the rhetoric used in historical abortion discourses, in which motherly and self-indulgent women were presented as opposites. Sociologist Annulla Linders analyzes the "opposite solutions" to regulating abortion in the US and Swedish contexts. She points to a distinction between stock narratives of the 1920s Swedish "exhausted mother" and the 19th-century US "frivolous wife" petitioning for an abortion. The popular trope of the "exhausted mother" of "eight to ten" children, whose pregnancy would threaten the welfare of the family, shifted the Swedish abortion debate in favor of legalization. As was the case for the single woman in OC, this trope counteracted accusations of "selfishness" by emphasizing that the problem was "not that she did not *want* to become a mother, but instead that she was effectively prevented from becoming one" by her circumstances.[49] In the stock narratives of the single freezer and the exhausted mother, OC and abortion are constructed as interventions that evidence prioritizing motherhood.

By contrast, the "frivolous wife" seeking abortions held strong cultural currency in the criminalization of abortion in the United States. Here women were criticized for wanting to "rid themselves of the care and responsibility of maternity," while being motivated by "self-indulgence," "extravagance," and a "fashionable life."[50] Reminiscent of the socially motivated "lifestyle freezers" whose use of OC suggests a deprioritization of motherhood and a "having your cake and eating it" attitude, the stereotype of the frivolous, carefree woman appears to be a persistent feature in negative portrayals of women using (non)reproductive technologies. For example, the continued newsworthiness of such reproductive frivolity as social provocation is evidenced in the media hype surrounding the promotion of OC at fashionable "cocktail parties" that target career women and "bring together fertility doctors, . . . financing information and cocktails."[51] In short, the binary stock narratives of frivolous and blameless women have functioned as key rhetorical tools in a number of reproductive struggles; their continuation in OC discourses points to a contemporary reproductive politics that is hinged on a public renegotiation of female fertility and its extendability.

In the context of OC's medical-social divide, the invocation of stark oppositions between women facing cancer treatment and others with "social" reasons for choosing OC—whether unspecified or described as "suit[ing] their lifestyles and aspirations"—can function as a rhetorical move to trivialize the motivations of women in the latter category by positioning them as fortunate and healthy by comparison.[52] In this move, reproductive aging and future infertility are demedicalized as "social" indications. Yet public discourses of female reproductive health—which are the subject of the following section—nevertheless frequently present healthy women's bodies in more perilous terms of continual decline. Contradicting the frivolous connotations of "lifestyle" motivations, articles on egg freezing emphasize that fertility cannot be taken for granted, especially not as women age. It is thus not uncommon to read statements in articles on egg freezing that posit female reproductive aging as a serious medical concern. For example, in a *Guardian* feature titled

"Mother Nature," clinical director Charles Kingsland comments that "the passage of time can quickly take away a woman's fertility and she should always bear in mind her fitness for fertility."[53] Assertions such as this one once again bring age-related infertility to public awareness and posit it as a serious health concern. In other words, although the "social" classification demedicalizes women's reasons for egg freezing, public discussions of egg freezing themselves play a crucial role in remedicalizing female fertility.

No Exit: Representing the Biological Clock and Reproductive Aging

Egg freezing emerges in the wake of widespread news coverage on older motherhood, whether of glowing celebrities having children in their fifties, demographic trends towards later childbearing, or sensationalist cases of women setting new records with technologically enabled pregnancies later in life. As has been the case before when IVF, and particularly donor eggs, enabled older and postmenopausal motherhood, egg freezing once more brings the timing of reproduction into the public eye. Now shifting not only the ages of childbearing but also those of conception, the understanding of OC as a practice that could extend women's reproductive age range once more raises questions about the appropriate ages for having children or freezing eggs.[54] In the face of these developments, the newspaper coverage of OC reveals a public renegotiation of the meaning of female fertility and the demarcation of "normal reproductive years." The media framings of age-related fertility loss, which this section explores, draw heavily on the "biological clock" trope and fertility statistics in ways that highlight the politicization of reproductive aging in the context of OC.

The Biological Clock

The biological clock is, of course, one of the key concepts in popular constructions of female fertility and in OC's media coverage. Although the term is used with reference to any bodily temporal regulatory system—circadian, hormonal, etc.—in contemporary news discourses, the biological clock has become virtually synonymous with women's reproductive aging. As a *clock*, it positions fertility decline as clockwork: as grounded in measurable facts and as a shared conceptual reference point for understanding gendered time. And as a clock that is *biological*, it frames fertility decline as a biological fact that particularly lends itself to naturalizing contemporary reproductive chrononormativities.

This rhetorical function of the biological clock can be traced back to at least the 1970s, when the term first started to be used as a marker of fertility decline. Medical historian Jenna Healey describes the biological clock's origin story and locates its starting point in Richard Cohen's 1978 *Washington Post* article "The Clock Is Ticking for the Career Woman."[55] In this article, Cohen describes the "Composite Woman": a representative woman he construed out of a group of women he had recently spoken to. Notwithstanding his dubious disavowal of sexism (he later wrote, "These were not male chauvinist pigs. These were men like me"), he depicts her as follows:

> There she is entering the restaurant. She's the pretty one. Dark hair. Medium height. Nicely dressed. Now she is taking off her coat. Nice figure. . . . The job is just wonderful. She is feeling just wonderful. It is wonderful being her age, which is something between 27 and 35.[56]

Yet in spite of her wonderful life, there is "something wrong." The Composite Woman eventually confesses to him, "I want a baby." Whether or not she is in a relationship, "there is always," Cohen suggests, "a feeling that the clock is ticking. A decision will have to be made. A decision that will stick forever."[57]

This notion of a biological clock struck a chord and became shorthand for a cautionary tale about women "postponing" having children amid the emergence of contraceptives, the rise of feminist movements, and women's increasing participation in the labor market. Media scholar Moira Wiegel traces the growing popularity of this term in public discourses and shows how the biological clock was used to naturalize a supposed universality of age-related reproductive desires amid a time of widespread, gendered social change.[58] Counterbalancing this social change, Cohen implied, was the immutable bodily truth of the Composite Woman's biological clock:

There was something about their situation that showed, more or less, that this is where liberation ends. This is where a woman is a woman—biologically, physiologically, uncontrovertably [sic] different.[59]

What the biological clock pointed to was a bodily reification of traditional gender roles, a biological limit to "liberation." Importantly, this recourse to gendered difference as a limit to social change is not a given from birth, or characteristic of adulthood, but is contingent on reproductive aging.

In the context of egg freezing, this trope of the biological clock, and its relation to social change, reemerges as a widespread, age-related concern. The biological clock here references a particular time frame in the female life span, typically starting in the early or mid-thirties, that is characterized by a sense of urgency. Rather than an ordinary clock that tells time, the biological clock here figures as an alarm clock going off at a certain age or as a timer counting down the years. For example, a *Guardian* article discusses egg freezing with reference to "this woman—who has always assumed that eventually a baby or two would come along—[who] finds herself single with her biological clock running down quite fast."[60] As this quotation suggests, the biological clock trope organizes popular narratives about women who live contentedly and subsequently become urgently aware of their reproductive ability—whether in the form of positive desires for children or negative fears of infertility—at the age at which their clock ostensibly starts ticking.

Specific ages may be identified as signaling a life course transition associated with the biological clock. For example, *Guardian* journalist Tahmima Anam both observes and reiterates the public problematization of female fertility when she describes her experience of reproductive aging: "Lately my eyes have been alighting on newspaper articles decrying the end of my fertile days, and the number 35 flashes before me like a blinking NO EXIT sign."[61] Significantly, Anam explains how the truth claims about fertility decline in media discourses affected her anxious attachments to both specific ages and her own reproductive embodiment. The biological clock is here associated with a particular age range that signals a departure from a time of idealized youth and the onset of a concern with the prospect of impending reproductive failure. The header of this article reads, "Anam felt 'footloose and fancy-free.' Then she hit 33—and baby-panic kicked in. Is freezing her eggs the answer?" As the article suggests, a sudden awareness of the impending end of her fertility jolted Anam out of the supposed carelessness of young adulthood to a life course determined by the pressure of the biological clock.

Strikingly, the references to the biological clock are accompanied by accounts of fear, stress, and worry. Newspaper reports on egg freezing cite stories of women who "were very worried by the ticking of the biological clock around the age of 34, 35 or 36."[62] One article notes that "doctors at Mount Sinai School of Medicine in New York interviewed 20 women with an average age of nearly 39 who had chosen to have their eggs frozen. Half said they felt pressured by their biological clocks."[63] Another describes a fertility doctor's observation about such pressure: "Many women worry about meeting the right guy because 'they hear that biological clock ticking loudly,' he says. That ticking is a stress factor in their lives."[64] Beyond a bodily phenomenon of decreased pregnancy chances, the term of the biological clock thus denotes—and produces—an age-specific affective experience of female fertility as, almost by definition, potentially imperiled and precarious in nature.

The possibility—and newsworthiness—of egg freezing provides the occasion to both reaffirm and reinvent the biological clock trope. As was the case in Cohen's 1970s article, popular concern with the biological clock reiterates a highly gendered narrative about tensions between "the workplace" and reproductive aging concerns. For example, the article "Born in the Nick of Time" argues that

> despite all the advances in technology and the workplace, that ticking clock is still there and if you don't have its existence at the back of your mind, you may miss the chance to have a family.[65]

Using the second-person mode of address, the text's warning about reproductive aging is directed at the readers. The option of not having children is construed as a loss, as a "chance" that one may "miss"—rather than a valid alternative—resulting from not paying attention to the biological clock. Having children earlier is proposed as the resolution to the supposed conflict between advances in the workplace—i.e., women working—and the "ticking clock." Beyond a straightforward pronatalist message aimed at working women, the article posits a particular affective experience of reproductive aging. In order not to miss out, it is suggested, the time pressure associated with the biological clock must be lived through an ongoing awareness "at the back of your mind" of a body that is ruled by "that ticking clock." Such recommendations betray a gendered temporal organization of the life span, which requires not only correct reproductive timing but also a continued awareness of the precariousness and finitude of fertility.

Infertile Numbers

Fertility statistics play a central role in this public articulation of female fertility and its temporal limits. Constituting a quantitative counterpart to the biological clock, they are ubiquitous in egg freezing coverage. In order to explain the relevance of egg freezing, articles frequently include a passage such as the following:

> A 30-year-old woman stands a 22% chance of getting pregnant in any given month. By 35, that drops to 18%. By 40, it's 5%. By 45 you're down to 1%. By 25, women have lost 80% of the eggs they were born with. By 35 that has dropped to a 95% loss.[66]

The predominance of quantitative data positions statements like this one as factual information, inviting little critical reflection from readers. However, precisely because it appears as objective data, it is important to consider the rhetorical effects of this quantified framing of reproductive aging, and its role in rendering fertility precarious.

These numbers convey the message to the readership that an objective, scientific understanding of the female reproductive system is characterized by an urgency about decreasing functionality. In this quotation, the diminishing chances of pregnancy per month appear slim to begin with, given that there is just over a one in five likelihood of pregnancy at a life stage normally associated with fertility. However, these are fairly optimistic numbers if translated into accumulative chances of pregnancy per year: the 30-year-old would have a 95% chance, compared to 91% for the 35-year-old and 54% for the woman trying to conceive at 40.[67] By instead presenting monthly chances with dwindling numbers in shortening sentences, the cited text conveys an understanding of female fertility as characterized by low likelihood of pregnancy and progressive decline from a relatively early age onwards.

The sense of loss is intensified where the eggs are concerned. Already at the age of 25, the text suggests, an overwhelming majority of a woman's eggs are lost, and this decline will accelerate over time. While diminishing ovarian reserves are indeed a key cause of age-related infertility, such representations of available egg percentages suggest that their loss is inherently problematic. However, egg loss is a normal process in fertile women. Given that a woman who has no or a small number of children will experience on average 450–480 menstrual cycles in her lifetime, even if she matured a healthy viable egg every month and was optimally fertile, she would lose a majority of the millions of eggs she was born with. The 25-year-old's loss of 80% of her immature eggs does not necessarily signify a loss of fertility, just as a girl's loss of 60% of her eggs by the time she hits puberty does not signal anything but normal physiological development.[68]

The focus on the loss of immature eggs suggests a conceptualization of the female reproductive body as characterized by decline throughout the life span. Understood in these terms, a woman is born in decline, with her body continuously failing to retain the eggs. The female reproductive system—whether fertile or infertile—is framed in terms of a negative economy of egg loss, in which the loss of eggs corresponds to the loss of time before "missing the chance" of having a family. It is this loss that is key to the reframing of female fertility as fundamentally a precarious condition.

In her analysis of medical metaphors of female reproductive embodiment in *The Woman in the Body*, Emily Martin contends that the nonpregnant fertile state, and its expression in menstruation, is understood "in terms of a purpose [conception] that has failed."[69] In newspaper reporting on egg freezing—and particularly in the narrative framing of declining fertility rates—it is not menstruation but egg loss and reproductive aging that are conceptualized as failure. In keeping with the understanding of menstruation as failed reproduction, the cited figures on age-related infertility conceptualize the female body, and its eggs in particular, as oriented towards the moment of reproduction. Yet here it is not so much the nonpregnant state that Martin highlights, but the body's being in time—or aging—that is understood in terms of a fail-ure to retain the continued possibility of conception. The newspapers' presentation of information on declining fertility rates and diminishing ovarian reserves suggests a collective diagnosis of failure—not the loss of blood, but the loss of eggs, and the reproductive potential they embody, is conceptualized as women's bodies' foundational failure.

What is at stake in this information is the establishment of new norms for the timing of fertility preservation. Whereas information on age-related fertility in newspapers previously primarily pertained to questions of timing childbearing, now it also provides the rationaliza-tion for deciding whether and when to freeze one's eggs. For example, the article "Have Your Eggs Frozen While You're Still Young, Scientists Advise Women" reports that women who freeze their eggs are typi-cally aged 37–39, but "flaws that accumulate in eggs over time lead to a rapid decrease in fertility over the age of 35."[70] Through the newspapers' inclusion of medical discourses, whether articulated through expert in-terviews or statistical information, the body becomes recognizable on its terms. In the absence of easily observable signs of the onset of age-related infertility, this type of reporting rationalizes the timing of egg freezing at particular ages. In keeping with Jana Sawicki's argument that "[ARTs'] control is not secured primarily through violence or coercion, but rather by producing new norms of motherhood . . . and by offering women specific kinds of solutions to problems they face,"[71] the emer-gence of OC instills new norms about when one may assume oneself to be fertile and what solutions are prudent in the face of the potential loss of fertility. When fertility loss points not so much to a decreased ability to conceive and get pregnant but to a decline in the IVF success rates associated with eggs frozen at a particular age, OC may become a rational choice—and fertility decline an actionable concern—much earlier in the life course.

More detailed statistical accounts of the temporal limits to female fer-tility are frequently included to explain the logic of the procedure:

> With age, women's eggs accumulate genetic damage which causes fertil-ity to fall rapidly after 35. Older eggs result in poorer quality embryos which are more likely to be miscarried. By 40, the average miscarriage rate reaches 40%.[72]

Although it is important that people are informed about their bodies' capacities and the likelihood of conceiving at different points in their lives, it is equally significant to address the implications of the rhetoric of failure in which this information is couched. This article equates aging with accumulating genetic damage, rapidly falling fertility, poor-quality embryos, and miscarriage. In the absence of specific data, these descriptors communicate a sense of urgency and rapid decline. Where a number is mentioned, the 40% suggests a problem, even though the reader has not been informed of the percentage of miscarriages that occur at other ages, variations in the population, or a specification of what counts as miscarriage. The citation nevertheless reads as a progression, in which the passing of years from 35 to 40 signals increasingly intensifying reproductive failure: from "genetic damage" in the gametes to the evocative notion of miscarriage. The article refers to the eggs', rather than the woman's, age. Taking up a central role, the older eggs appear to "result" in poorer-quality embryos through a process in which sperm, and its quality or age, or the bodies from which these gametes are derived, play no mentionable role.

Although these statistics are disseminated in the context of egg freezing, their framing of fertility pertains to all women—irrespective of their interest in OC. The description of 30-year-olds as having a 22% chance of getting pregnant every month, for example, has particular rhetorical effects. The exact percentage both suggests a precise, calculable conceptualization of fertility and requires a statistical literacy to assess the limitations of such precision in population averages. The inclusion of these numbers conveys that it is important to know the details about fertility decline in order to make informed reproductive decisions. Yet when one becomes knowledgeable about these figures, their limitations for predicting one's own specific fertility become apparent. In this way, fertility statistics produce a *dynamic of knowing and not knowing*. It is this dynamic that is itself productive of a precariousness of fertility—as not only in decline but as by definition unknowable save through further interventions. This precarious fertility provides a driver for the rising popularity of fertility testing—even if it is not a very reliable predictor—and egg freezing—even though its success rates are limited. And these biotechnological resolutions may themselves, as we shall see, be institutionalized in ways that produce new forms of fertility precarity.

Cocktail Parties and Health Perks: Institutionalizing Infertility

So far we have seen how sceptical responses to the introduction of egg freezing were linked to a public concern about reproductive aging. Stories about women who freeze their eggs were important rhetorical instruments in public rejections of the potential shift of reproductive aging limits enabled by OC. The subject position of the lifestyle freezer was invoked to emphasize women's agency in changing the previously fixed limits to reproductive aging to suit their lifestyles or career ambitions. This figure played a key role in the social conservative project that appealed to the supposed naturalness of age-related limits to conception to oppose, or limit access to, egg freezing. Often in response to this negative framing of women, an alternative narrative highlights the singlehood of the majority of women freezing their eggs, whether with reference to a broken relationship or to unwanted singlehood. This framing of egg freezers highlights women's social circumstances in order to raise understanding for their decision to cryopreserve their eggs. And indeed, most academic studies of egg freezing confirm that the majority of women freeze their eggs because they are not with a (suitable) partner.[73]

More recent media coverage on OC has also broadened the focus on the market forces and structural conditions driving the growing popularity of egg freezing. As various UK and US fertility companies are heavily marketing egg freezing, news media may adopt or critically reflect on these marketing narratives, thereby bringing them into a wider public conversation about female fertility. This section highlights the gender politics of reproductive aging that emerges in the institutionalization of (in)fertility through the widespread promotion of egg freezing—often to a younger target audience—and its coverage in news media.

In the summer of 2018, a "fertility van" appeared on the streets of New York City. With pleasing pastel aesthetics, the yellow-and-white van sought to create a pop-up wellness boutique experience for passersby to discuss fertility and egg freezing. A chalkboard next to the van said, "The fertility facts you need!" and inside, quotations in picture frames encouraged women to "understand your fertility today, so you can set the stage for tomorrow" and "own your future." The fertility company running the pop-up, Kindbody, also offered the option of undertaking a free fertility test in the van. The test measured women's antimullerian hormone (AMH), which Kindbody presented as determining the "number of eggs in your ovaries."[74] Although the predictive value of such tests for pregnancy rates has been seriously questioned by the medical community,[75] the results—irrespective of their accuracy—provide an individualized indicator for an otherwise rather opaque and precaritized fertility. And, in doing so, the tests can function as an ideal promotional tool. Good results mean that now is the perfect time to freeze your eggs while they are still healthy and plenty; below-average results mean that now is equally a great time to freeze your eggs before you lose them all.

Interest in the van was overwhelming; the 100 appointments available in the pop-up van were booked up in 20 minutes. The company behind the project is run by Gina Bartasi, who, in her previous role at Eggbanxx, also organized egg freezing cocktail parties at "swanky hotels," which similarly moved egg freezing information events away from the clinical and baby-focused setting of the fertility clinic.[76] These parties—not unlike the van—sought to lower the barrier for younger women to learn about egg freezing and fertility decline.

Of course, in the van and at the parties, the lines between education and marketing are blurred. Reminiscent of cosmetics campaigns suggesting that "you're worth it," Kindbody's marketing strategy of stating that "you deserve the facts" imparts a set of supposedly neutral truth claims as a means of encouraging a neoliberalized quasi-feminist mode of self-empowerment. Marketers often appeal to notions of deservingness in their slogans, especially when promoting "indulgent products," such as higher-calorie or higher-end products. Examples include "You deserve a break today" (McDonald's), "You deserve a car this good" (General Motors), and "Because you're worth it" (L'Oréal).[77] This notion of "deservingness" is also often used at the introduction stage of a productive cycle for "consumers who are new to the product" and "capitalize[s] on a person's motive to get what they deserve," which, in this case, means to become informed.[78]

The information on offer in this instance leaves little doubt that female fertility requires technologized management and that egg freezing is a rational, proactive, and empowering reproductive choice to make. On its website, Kindbody exemplifies this logic with the following list of "facts:"

We are born with all the eggs we will ever have
The quality and quantity of our eggs declines [sic] with age
There are ways to measure your ovarian reserve
Freezing eggs is the way of the future
Freezing eggs is like freezing time
You'll never be more fertile than you are today
Freezing eggs doesn't affect your ability to get pregnant naturally
Using frozen eggs is safe
Egg freezing works[79]

It is striking that, in this list, fertility is reframed as deficient and in decline from birth onwards. This framing of fertility as subject to continued slippage ("you'll never be more fertile than today") invokes a specter of loss and scarcity that drives the popularization of new forms of biotechnological dependency, which is presented as "safe" and "work[ing]" in spite of OC's limited success rates and potential side effects. Barbey's analysis of US egg freezing websites confirms that this message of time running out is widespread and, he argues, both "appear[s] crafted to cause alarm" and suggests that it is normal for women to "feel out of control" prior to using this technology.[80]
Promotional initiatives such as vans and parties received ample news coverage, including in the *Guardian* and the *New York Times*. "Egg-freezing cocktail parties . . . held in New York by profit-driven clinics" were presented as examples of the "commodification of fertility" and were positioned in the wider context of a "rolling back of reproductive rights" in the United States.[81] Several articles criticized "cocktail part[ies]" where women "learn how to freeze your eggs" and "companies like EggBanxx [that] host egg freezing–themed cocktail parties" for promoting a solution to reproductive aging that "isn't going to work for all women" and is "anything but foolproof."[82] As opposed to the accusatory frame of the "have it all" freezer, here it is not women but fertility companies that become the subject of contention for promoting a frivolity and an "enthusiasm" that are "epitomized by information sessions rebranded as 'egg freezing parties.'"[83]
Yet what is at stake in these developments is not only the potential failure of the frozen eggs to produce babies but also the popularization of new narratives about fertility that target ever younger women for IVF

treatment. Rather than focusing on the lifestyle freezers, these news reports draw attention to the lifestyle marketing of egg freezing that touts
"the procedure as a breezy, accessible and eminently sensible lifestyle
choice for the youngest members of the millennial generation."[84] As egg
freezing companies are unabashedly announcing that they "are now targeting women in their 20s and early 30s," while younger women and
their fertility clinics declare that fertility "begins to wane as early as one's
20s," fertility becomes precarious at increasingly early ages. Clinics that
previously served women at the "older end of the childbearing years" are
now planning "national advertising campaign[s] encompassing radio,
television, print and social media" to convey the message that fertility
is finite to ever-younger women.[85] The emergence of the narrative of an
ever-reducing female fertility illustrates how the popular redefinition of
reproductive aging is at the heart of the growth agenda of this part of
the fertility sector.

Insuring Precarious Fertility

This institutionalization of the precariousness of fertility is nowhere
as publicly contested as in the discussions surrounding corporate egg
freezing insurance. When Facebook and Apple announced in 2014 that
they would cover egg freezing for their employees, a media hype quickly
ensued. Lisa Campo-Engelstein and colleagues' media analysis of OC
confirmed that the introduction of workplace fertility benefits prompted
a remarkably significant increase in the US news coverage of egg freezing. Their study suggests that this media coverage painted "a simplistic
and rosy picture that more options, especially reproductive options or
financially neutral options, automatically enhance women's autonomy."
In line with this, they note that their media outlets framed corporate
fertility insurance as a resolution to the prohibitive costs of OC and the
companies offering these benefits as "heroes that offer a 'life-altering
benefit: paying for employees to freeze their eggs.'"[86]

However, both the newspapers selected here and Campo-Engelstein's
sample also found widespread concern about how this so-called perk
would intensify employers' influence on female employees' reproductive autonomy and decision making. The *Guardian* health editor Sarah
Boseley, for example, wondered whether Apple and Facebook "acting

MAKING FERTILITY PRECARIOUS | 53

as caring employers in offering egg-freezing" will make women "feel under some sort of psychological pressure to carry on working, rather than trying for a family when they might have, because they have eggs in store?"[87] *Guardian* editor Harriet Minter put it more strongly, suggesting that the message is, "Work through your most fertile years and when you can't have kids anymore, use the eggs we froze for you as a perk."[88] The *New York Times* similarly proposed that while the benefit may be a "highly welcome surprise" to women planning to freeze their eggs, "workplaces could be seen as paying women to put off childbearing. Women who choose to have babies earlier could be stigmatized as uncommitted to their careers."[89]

Here egg freezing was not presented as serving carefree or career women, but instead became a threat to reproductive autonomy in the face of corporate control. As a health "perk," commentators argued, egg freezing could function as an implicit mechanism to discourage reproduction. The tension between career and reproductive aging here resurfaced not in an accusatory tone that chastised women for "having it all" but as a criticism of the corporate management of female employees' reproductive aging processes through fertility-preservation programs. What is, then, at stake in these fertility-preservation programs is not simply women's use of these schemes or not, but the institutionalization and corporate endorsement of a precarious model of female fertility as at once fundamentally deficient and technologically salvageable through biotechnological cryopreservation.[90]

I read the media attention to corporate fertility insurance as another iteration of the tension between the professional and the private that also emerged in the mediatized oppositions between career-minded and single freezers. It is this tension that gets renegotiated when egg freezing (potentially) changes the temporal limits to female fertility. This tension is important, and is so frequently invoked in public discourses on egg freezing, because it points to a more fundamental renegotiation of the relation between production and reproduction—and specifically the temporality of this relation—as a central axis in the wider social order.

Reproduction vs. Production: Redirecting Accumulation

The opposition between reproduction and production has long been regarded as the "constitutive institutional separation" of capitalism. Political philosopher Nancy Fraser discusses the importance of this separation in the regime of "financialised capitalism" that characterizes the contemporary moment. One of its key elements is a move from the Fordist family wage to the ideal of the two-earner family. This shift is accompanied by the "steep rise in the number of hours of paid work now required to support a household," which effectively entails an obligation to "shift time and energies once devoted to reproduction to 'productive'" (i.e. paid) work." As a result of the combination of increased working hours and cuts to public services, Fraser argues, "The financialized capitalist regime is squeezing social reproduction to the breaking point."[91] Indeed, in a survey into the reasons why young American adults are having fewer children, the scarcity of money and time and the concomitant need to outsource care make up the top five motivations:

Child care is too expensive (64%)
Want more time for the children I have (54%)
Worried about the economy (49%)
Can't afford more children (44%)
Waited because of financial instability (43%).[92]

Here the socioprecarity characteristic of financialized capitalism drives both trends of later childbearing and associated concerns with age-related female reproductive bioprecarity.

In light of these developments, Fraser contends that egg freezing is simply another coping mechanism used by time-poor women in contexts characterized by high female labor participation, limited parental leave, and a society's "love affair with technology." In such contexts, egg freezing can function as a techno-fix aimed at resolving the tension between reproduction and production in capitalism. In other words, OC becomes symptomatic of a social organization in which women are required to "shoehorn social reproduction responsibilities into the interstices and crevices of lives that capital insists must be dedicated first and foremost to accumulation."[93] In a similar vein, Mwenza Blell characterizes this social organization as one in which "many people are afraid to risk having children (or as many children as we would like) because of precarity and because (as people said to me) you might never be productive enough again, which means not able to work from early morning until 10 or 11pm every day with a child."[94]

In this process, egg freezing not only offers a resolution to the scarcity dynamic between production and reproduction but also collapses them by bringing fertility itself into the realm of capital accumulation. First, egg freezing produces new means of accumulation in the fertility industry through the creation of novel business models and the widespread promotion to fertile women as a key target group for IVF. In a largely privatized fertility sector, egg freezing presents expansion possibilities by commercializing not only the creation of babies but also fertility itself through the accumulation of frozen eggs as a proxy for reproductive youth and extendable fertility.

Second, the biomedical management of reproductive aging enters the realm of production through the popularization of fertility insurance. The critique of corporate fertility insurance, as we have seen, has primarily focused on the possibility of employers influencing employees' reproductive decision making with egg freezing coverage.[95] This possibility, of course, is at least in part newsworthy for further collapsing reproduction into the realm of production, i.e., the workplace itself. Yet what also happens in this process is that egg freezing and fertility-preservation insurance offers a new means of wealth accumulation for employers, insurers, lenders, and dedicated egg freezing companies. In other words, the expansion of infertility treatment to the fertile population also enables the expansion of IVF provision to a broader set of organizations, which recognize and reinforce the idea that assisted reproduction has become relevant for a much larger group of their employees or customers. In this way, financialized capitalism, and its associated socioprecarious arrangements that render employees reliant on their employers to attain health insurance, thus also provide the context for intensifying reproductive bioprecarity by normalizing and rationalizing egg freezing through the offer of corporate fertility benefits.

This institutionalization of the egg freezing "perk" by employers, the marketing thereof by specialized fertility benefits companies, and the media hypes that surround it all contribute to a wider public discourse that positions female fertility as precarious and in need of preservation, protection, and investment. Symptomatic of a broader neoliberalization of reproduction, fertility—and its extension across time—thus becomes a site of proactive investment for women themselves, employers, and fertility companies. Underlying this neoliberal model of egg freezing is an approach to reproductive aging as malleable, investable, and subject to market logic.[96]

This particular framing of egg freezing, which brings fertility into the realm of capital accumulation, contrasts with the abovementioned, more social-conservative problematization of OC as a type of "luxury medicine" and "lifestyle choice" for carefree and career-minded women. The rejection of women "having it all" precisely insists on the opposite movement in the relation between reproduction and production: not the collapse of one into the other but an insistence on their continued, gendered separation is key to maintaining the existing social order. The upholding of women's reproductive aging as a given, biological fact naturalizes a host of gendered chrononormativities pertaining to the prioritization of reproduction over production at different points in the life course. This conservative, sceptical approach to egg freezing relies on a model of reproductive aging that is, or ought to remain, fixed and unalterable as a gendered site of naturalness.

So we see, on the one hand, a social-conservative discourse that positions childbearing as a goal in women's lives that must be attained within natural aging limits and, on the other hand, a more neoliberal trend that frames egg freezing as a potentially empowering choice to invest in one's future self and change the existing age limits to conception. What they have in common is the mobilization of a precarious framing of fertility to rationalize the promotion or rejection of egg freezing.

Here fertility's precariousness reflects not simply a bodily reality or the result of a new form of biotechnological control over the timing of reproductive aging. It is, perhaps more importantly, the usefulness of a conceptualization of female fertility as defined by its ongoing precarious decline that lends itself to a gender politics of reproductive aging that suits both neoconservative and neoliberal agendas. Reproductive aging may be mobilized either to accumulate capital and promote proactive self-investment or to naturalize gendered differences in chrononormative arrangements of the life course. Whether it functions as a motivation to promote technological interventions or earlier childbearing, the precarious framing of female fertility is a foundational and influential element of egg freezing news coverage that affects not only the women who freeze their eggs but the wider readership.

Conclusion

Whether through statistics of fertility decline, stock narratives about the biological clock, or subject positions for women freezing their eggs, the news coverage of OC expresses the public negotiation of when and how fertility becomes precarious. Whereas female fertility has long been subject to public scrutiny, particularly since the introduction of the contraceptive pill and assisted reproductive technologies, egg freezing repoliticizes age-related (in)fertility by suggesting new ways of exerting agency over reproductive aging. It is now not only the timing of childbearing that is of concern but also an intermediate stage of timing egg freezing. Given that most women learn about egg freezing through media outlets,[97] the newspapers do not simply describe a situation or opinion but constitute a public mode of address through which fertility becomes legible. They play a key role in interpellating a particular contingent of women by marking various ages in the twenties and thirties—particularly 35—as the onset of female reproductive decline and as a time when singlehood becomes problematic and childlessness becomes a risk of "missing out." The time when fertility becomes precarious is characterized by heightened uncertainty and implicit—or explicit—calls to mitigate the sense of concern by freezing eggs, having children, or becoming informed.

In these public discourses, egg freezing becomes meaningful through oppositions between "social" and "medical" motivations and between stock narratives of the single woman who prioritizes motherhood but is looking for Mr. Right and the "lifestyle" freezer who deprioritizes motherhood and wants to "have it all." As a set of subject positions is developed in relation to these oppositions, women's life choices come under medical and public scrutiny, whether these are related to romantic or professional commitments or to other priorities that are not direct expressions of reproductive health. These subject positions moreover function as important rhetorical tools in framing OC in negative or positive terms as a technology that could, respectively, exacerbate an existing trend of delayed motherhood or provide a chance to avoid unwanted childlessness.

Whereas the popularity of the biological clock trope signaled women's changing social roles in the 1970s, the contemporary biological clock becomes relevant once more as the notion of reproductive aging itself is being reconceptualized and repoliticized after the introduction of egg freezing. Reproductive technologies such as IVF have prompted widespread reflection on the status of "the biological" as no longer fixed and foundational, but itself denaturalized in the face of technological manipulation.[98] Likewise, the introduction of egg freezing has raised questions about the (not so) foundational status of reproductive aging. Should reproductive aging continue to be conceptualized as a given, biological reality that is immutable in the face of techno-social change or has reproductive aging become a manipulable phenomenon now that eggs can be frozen?

The former position was upheld in the public response to egg freezing in the Netherlands, where OC posed a potential transgression to accepted reproductive age limits. The Dutch reinforcement of the 45-year age cap for using frozen eggs shows how legal limits may reaffirm a biological limit—whether to liberation or otherwise—*in spite of* it no longer being biologically inevitable.[99] Conversely, the OC coverage also presents claims to "turning back" or "reversing" the biological clock. Corporate fertility-preservation insurance highlighted how, in a neoliberal logic of self-investment, egg freezing can be framed as a means of overcoming bodily limits—whether in one's private or professional life. Here a celebration of the abolishment of women's "limit to liberation" through corporate benefits also renders fertility precarious by affirming its ongoing decline and universalizing financial and clinical dependencies to counteract it. These dependencies at once exclude women along established lines of social inequality and enlist other women to subject themselves to a new cultural logic of self-investment, which, as I discuss below, is fraught with potential conflicts of interest from which various third parties stand to benefit.

The introduction of egg freezing has thus triggered both the *reaffirmation* of existing reproductive aging norms against the threat of their transgression with OC and the *reconfiguration* of reproductive aging as operating by a different rationale when eggs may be "frozen in time." Both the confirmation of "normal reproductive years" and the redefinition of fertility as extending later into life position female fertility as unreliable and subject to loss at an unknown and inopportune moment. Whether as false promise, unnatural transgression, or pragmatic solution, egg freezing operates at the tension between the simultaneous rejection and suggested inevitability of the future nonreproductive body that is invoked in OC's newspaper coverage. Egg freezing is, then, not simply a solution to a preexisting issue of female fertility decline, but its introduction provides the occasion for a public reconceptualization of reproductive aging as profoundly precarious—and thereby in need of social or medical management.

At the heart of the following chapters, then, is the question of what power relations are reproduced in the resultant contemporary management of female reproductive aging.

2

Freezing in Anticipation

Fertility Planning with Eggs for Later

I've been feeling pretty alone lately. Because everybody
around me is having children. And I don't even have a relationship. Haven't had one for five years. I just feel that I, that
soon it won't be possible anymore because I am now 35. That
perhaps I will never have children.
—Marieke Schellart, *Eggs for Later*

Facing the camera with teary eyes, documentary maker Marieke Schellart gives an affectively charged account of the key concerns of her film
Eggs for Later (2010) in its opening minutes. With a close-up shot framing her face, she addresses us directly, as if confiding to a friend. Creating
intimacy in this way, Schellart's confessional opening statement lays out
her motivations for freezing her eggs. Rather than simply wanting to
have a child, she conveys a complex set of concerns about the future loss
of fertility, the finality of "never" having children, and the pressure of
time running out because "soon it won't be possible anymore."

Eggs for Later gives an account of the new ways in which fertility is
lived—and infertility anticipated—after the introduction of egg freezing.
After earlier technologies such as IVF turned diagnosed infertility into
a public concern that could be mitigated by medical innovations, egg
freezing is the first ART to enable the biomedicalization of anticipated
potential infertility. For the first time, future infertility becomes a medical concern over which agency may be exerted in the present.

Signaling a broader biomedical and cultural preoccupation with
bodily futurity, Vincanne Adams and colleagues argue that the state of
anticipation is one defining quality of the current moment. Anticipation,
they suggest, "pervades the ways we think about, feel and address our
contemporary problems."[1] What is at stake for them is the production

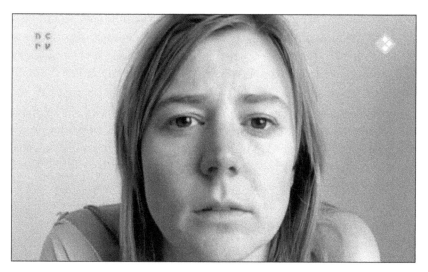

Figure 2.1. Schellart's opening statement.

of "regimes of anticipation" organized by "a particular self-evident 'fu-turism' in which our 'presents' are necessarily understood as contingent upon an ever-changing astral future that may or may not be known for certain, but still must be acted on nonetheless." In a neoliberal context, a heightened awareness of predictable but nevertheless uncertain futures gives rise to a "politics of temporality," which is characterized by an individualized moral injunction to anticipate individualized future perils and decline as a sign of responsible citizenship.[2]

In this chapter, I zoom in on the specific ways in which the anticipation of bodily futurity functions in relation to egg freezing. I do so with a reading of *Eggs for Later*, which provides a case study for analyzing the affective and discursive dimensions of the egg freezing process. The documentary is at once a highly mediated account of one woman freezing her eggs and a widely circulated cultural object. It follows Schellart's 18-month journey towards freezing her eggs, moving from a general concern with future fertility and her consideration of OC as a remedy to the hormonal stimulation and surgical extraction of her eggs. Her story is particularly significant for understanding the early introduction of egg freezing because, according to the Amsterdam Medical Centre (AMC), Schellart was the first woman in the Netherlands known to opt for elective egg freezing.[3] In her documentary she was thus able to capture the early public and private resistances to the novel technology prior to OC's legalization in 2011 and its subsequent wider acceptance. *Eggs for Later* stages both the promotion of egg freezing in US news reports and medical discourses and the disapproval of OC Schellart encountered among her local friends, family, and members of Parliament. Because OC was not yet allowed in the Dutch context at the time of filming, she traveled to Belgium to undergo the procedure. Reaching international audiences, *Eggs for Later* was televised in nine countries and screened at international film festivals worldwide.

Given its subject matter, dissemination and documentation of a specifically relevant historical moment, *Eggs for Later* offers a compelling case study for analyzing the particular complexities of anticipating bodily futurity with the aid of OC technology. In line with Lauren Berlant's assertion that the case study "took aesthetic form in [the] documentary [genre]," Schellart's film is itself a montage of cases that give insight into the discursive and affective dimensions of egg freezing.[4] I explore what futures of in/fertility and non/parenthood the film invokes in relation to egg freezing and what their discursive and embodied effects are on the documentary's lived present. In other words, this chapter analyzes the discursive construction of the promise of OC, consisting of both the reproductive futures that are invoked in its name and the particular understanding of egg freezing as an agentic anticipatory strategy to achieve them. What is at stake in this analysis is the potential of the various modes of anticipating bodily futurity with OC to reconfigure ideas and practices of what constitutes healthy embodiment, the reproductive act, and responsible aging.

Beyond her own story, Schellart's autobiographical documentary also provides insight into the broader discourses informing the public reception of egg freezing as a new technology for reproductive decision making. Rather than taking age-related reproductive limits as a biological given, I read *Eggs for Later* to understand how featured medical, political, and personal discourses shape the affective states and anticipatory terms through which women's (in)fertility and reproductive aging are conceptualized. The documentary gives insight into the emergence of new reproductive normativities concerning when, whether, and why to freeze one's eggs by relating a story in which egg freezing functions as an endpoint in its own right—irrespective of future live births—as a resolution of the anticipatory injunctions that are produced in public discourses of OC.[5]

From Assumed Fertility to Anticipated Infertility

The possibility of freezing one's eggs presents a new means of antici-pating reproductive finitude. With the introduction of egg freezing, reproductive aging can be refigured as a variable over which agency may be exerted, rather than only an unalterable biological given. With this possibility emerges the medicalization of the condition that OC can anticipate and treat: potential future infertility. Lauren Martin has argued that this process of medicalization erases the "normal" fertile life stage, leaving us with two pathologies: "anticipated infertility and infertility."[6] It is, however, important to address that a stage of "assumed fertility" continues to exist. In fact, the transition from "assumed fer-tility" to "anticipated infertility" is a highly significant moment in contemporary gendered cultures of aging, in which fertility becomes precarious and warrants anticipatory action.

Eggs for Later gives insight into the cultural negotiation of the tim-ing of this transition from assumed fertility to anticipated infertility and portrays two approaches to this process. In the first, egg freezing offers a last-minute option for women who wish to have children in the future, but are approaching the prospective end of their reproductive life span. The second approach encourages proactive egg freezing for women at earlier ages to preserve optimal fertility for later use. In both approaches, the anticipation of future infertility gains an embodied dimension.

Last-Minute Freezing

Exemplifying the first approach, Schellart's opening statement, which also opened this chapter, conveys a deep concern that "soon it won't be possible anymore." Her tense facial expression and teary eyes express the sense of anxiety she experiences in anticipating potential infertil-ity and future childlessness. In the absence of any clinical symptoms, she interprets her chronological age as a confrontation with reproduc-tive finitude. She positions herself as at risk of age-related infertility "because [she] is now 35." Her reference to this age is indicative of how 35 in particular is charged with cultural codes of reproductive finitude. Thirty-five is commonly used as the starting age for the medical cate-gory of "advanced maternal age" and, according to Budds and colleagues' media analysis, news outlets frequently present this age as the time when women start becoming "too old" for motherhood.[7] The cultural significance ascribed to 35 shows how age-specific conventions organize the time frame within which possible (non)reproductive futures must be anticipated. Beyond simply referencing a biological phenomenon, *Eggs for Later* gives insight into the personal and cultural negotiation of timing when fertility becomes precarious.

Schellart's concern with prospective infertility at the age of 35 fits in a broader social trend in which women freeze their eggs at a time when their fertility is expected to decline. Given that the age of women choosing OC averages around 38 years, egg freezing is usually a last-minute option before age-related fertility further reduces chances of conception.[8] Because freezing at this time is "suboptimal from a clinical point of view," medical professionals have advised women to "freeze their eggs while they are still young." Bioethicists have likewise raised concerns about egg freezing at later ages as a practice that gives false hope.[9] However, Schellart's documentary suggests that the motivation for OC follows not simply from a consideration of success rates but from complex affective, anticipatory approaches to future age-related infertility.

Beyond the focus on a specific age, the temporal norms governing when potential future infertility should be anticipated are also relational in nature. In *Eggs for Later*, Schellart imagines her future in accordance with a normative life course progression from singlehood to partnership to reproduction. She describes herself as "falling behind" because she has not progressed through these stages at the same pace as "everybody around [her]." Similarly, her ideas about reproductive timing are shaped in relation to her mother, who figures in the documentary's frequent intermezzos of childhood home video footage during which Schellart's voiceover muses on future motherhood. As the statements that her mother in these images is "eight years younger" and her feeling of "falling behind" her friends suggest, the timing of Schellart's experience of anticipated infertility and reproductive desire is both relationally shaped and strongly contingent on the "repronormative" temporal schemes of life course progression.[10] In other words, Schellart's anxiety about age-related infertility and hope for motherhood later in life are intimately bound up with normative and social models of life course progression that become urgently recognizable against the threat of their transgression.

The timing of the movement from assumed fertility to anticipated infertility is frequently naturalized with reference to the popular narrative of the "biological clock" I discussed in the previous chapter, in which a particular age signals a sudden departure from the carelessness of young adulthood to a life course characterized by concern about the impending finitude of fertility.[11] One scene visualizes this transition of the biological clock particularly clearly. It shows fast cuts of a younger Schellart dancing at music festivals, followed by a shift to a long, slow, contemplative horizontal pan across the Amsterdam night-time city skyline. The accompanying voiceover states,

> I could do what I wanted. I went to parties, festivals, and traveled far. Long live freedom. I did not think about children. That was something for later. But now that it is later, I am confronted with shocking numbers. One in three women is infertile by the time she is 40, and one in five women born in the seventies will remain childless. Maybe I will be that one woman.

Here the onset of the biological clock signifies a transition in which happiness moves away from the present of youthful experience towards a concern with an imagined reproductive future ahead. Coinciding with a move from assumed fertility to anticipated infertility, the biological clock marks the onset of an anticipatory concern that, for Schellart, can find its resolution in having children or freezing eggs.

This scene frames Schellart's experiences of infertility and childlessness as widespread threats that affect an entire generation. Indeed, in an interview about the documentary, Schellart stated that she did her "best to make it universal: a story of my generation."[12] Yet Schellart's lived experience of fertility and use of OC reveal a highly specific social and economic reality, more so than a generalizable story. For one thing, Schellart's consideration of egg freezing reflects her ability to pay for the procedure's high costs, which would be prohibitive for most women. The biographical account she offers to explain her situation, which includes an extended period of higher education and traveling the world, reflects a specific middle-class life course progression. This is in line with the fact that highly educated, middle-class, white women living in urban settings are significantly more likely to have a first child at later ages or to remain childless.[13] The documentary's presentation of Schellart's story, and the particular crisis of infertility it foregrounds, moreover align with the representational history of US IVF, which Lisa Harris describes as one in which the "infertility of privileged professional white women was understood to be a crisis while the infertility of poor women and women of color was not, at least as defined by the mainstream media."[14] Both the particular type of reproductive conundrum Schellart is confronted with and its representation in *Eggs for Later* thus point to the gender, class, and race specificity of her story.

The rhetorical function of positioning Schellart's story in relation to the "shocking numbers" of her generation is that it primes the viewer to attach a similar affect of anticipatory concern to these fertility statistics. Providing the terms through which reproductive futures may be understood—desirable fertility-parenthood and undesirable infertility-childlessness—the documentary frames the population data with Schellart's particular sentiments. It thereby suggests that the "story of [her] generation" is not only characterized by a certain prevalence of childlessness and age-related infertility but also by the affective experiences of reproductive desire and anticipatory anxiety about nonreproductive futures.

For Schellart, the value differentiation between reproductive and nonreproductive futures—combined with their attainability as a matter of risk—has the effect of producing anxiety about future infertility. Sara Ahmed comments on this effect by exploring "an intimacy between anxiety and hope. In having hope we *become* anxious, because hope involves wanting something that might or might not happen."[15] Adams and colleagues understand this anxiety for the future as foundational to anticipatory regimes:

> The anticipatory regime cannot generate its outcomes without arousing a "sense" of the simultaneous uncertainty *and* inevitability of the future, usually manifest as entanglements of fear and hope.[16]

In *Eggs for Later*, such entanglements of hope and fear are tied to reproductive and nonreproductive futures. The tension emerging from the value differentiation between these two parallel invoked futures thus increases anticipatory anxiety by positioning the subject in a speculative relation to a desirable reproductive and an undesirable nonreproductive outcome. Affirming this value differentiation, Schellart frequently references anticipated infertility, but the documentary does not visualize its accompanying futures in the way that it invokes potential future parenthood and pregnancy throughout—future nonreproduction remains an invisible threat.

A consideration of alternative (non)reproductive futures in a more favorable light could counteract anxiety about future infertility in the manner of Ahmed's politics of the hap, which "would be affirming the possibilities of life in whatever happens; we would be opening up possibilities that are negated by the very demand that we live our lives in the right way."[17] Regimes of anticipation function in the opposite way: they create anxiety by dividing the future into a value-differentiated binary, the positive side of which is suggested to be attainable through biomedicalized anticipatory action in the present. Schellart's case draws attention to the age-specificity of anticipatory regimes; speculative futures become pertinent at specific moments in the life course, imagined in relation to tropes like the biological clock and cultural associations of particular ages—like 35—with reproductive decline.

Preserving Peak Fertility

Whereas Schellart's case is an example of a "last-minute" approach to egg freezing because "soon it won't be possible anymore," OC can also be motivated as a method of preserving optimum fertility at a much younger age. This second approach is featured in the documentary when Schellart first encounters egg freezing at home in bed, watching a US Fox News report on her laptop:

> Another health story that may be important to a lot of women: women putting their eggs on ice. It is a controversial procedure for women who want to have children, but are worried that their biological clocks will run out before they can get pregnant.

Dr. Sherman Silber is interviewed as part of the report:

> We could freeze a 20-year-old's eggs and 20 years later we could thaw them, do IVF with them, and she'd have the pregnancy rate of a 20-year-old.

In keeping with Catherine Waldby's observation that news media are one of the key means by which people become familiar with egg freezing,[18] the documentary's inclusion of US and Belgian news reports stages their international reach and influence in making OC meaningful to the wider public. The anchor states that OC is relevant to a large group of women who are concerned about their biological clock. Although she does not specify the age frame for this concern, the interviewed doctor indicates that egg freezing could be relevant for women as young as 20. Silber's scenario is similarly evoked by other medics, including inventor of the contraceptive pill Carl Djerassi, who imagines a future in which young women freeze their eggs and get sterilized to fully divorce reproduction from the contingencies of sex and aging.[19] Gillian Lockwood, whose patient Helen Perry gave birth to the first British frozen-egg baby, envisions egg freezing as parents' ideal graduation gift to their daughters.[20]

Rather than a biological clock that begins ticking in the fourth decade, age-related infertility is here positioned as a condition that can be anticipated with OC from early adulthood onwards.[21] Replacing "assumed fertility" with "anticipated infertility" at ages well before the prospective infertility, news reports such as these can function as a way of disseminating regimes of anticipation that "interpellate, situate, attract and mobilize" an increasingly large group of healthy women by engaging them with the risks presented or implied—even if these were not a prior concern.[22] Rather than simply reflecting a biological reality, these discursive mediations of an egg-based model of female fertility constitute a public mode of address directed at a new group of potential patients.

In this approach to egg freezing, fertility becomes precarious not because age-related infertility is imminent but because the optimum time window for egg freezing may expire soon. The US-based Extend Fertility, which opened the first egg-freezing-only clinic in New York in 2016, exemplifies this treatment logic when it explains that "the younger you are, the better" because "you'll be able to produce and freeze more eggs in one cycle" and more will be of high quality. Extend Fertility advises women under 30 to freeze "about 'one year's fertility'—or 12 eggs," while women freezing after that age should aim for up to 24 or more eggs, which will probably require more than one cycle.[23] Prelude Fertility, a $200 million US start-up aimed at mainstreaming and promoting egg freezing to women "during their peak fertility years," similarly suggests that "if you are in your 20s or early 30s, there is no better time than now to bank your eggs and sperm. They are stretchy and full of reproductive life force, just like you! . . . The more you keep your options open, the less you need to worry."[24]

This way of "understanding your fertility" exemplifies the notion of precarious fertility. It is framed in a discourse of empowerment and care, yet has a persuasive power by suggesting that to know one's fertility is to know its uncertainty and to mitigate this uncertainty is to engage with the possibility of medical intervention. For example, population-based fertility loss statistics raise questions about one's own ovarian reserve. *In vivo* eggs, swaddled in the opaque body, remain obscure until they are measured by ultrasound or blood tests. As Prelude's slogan "you'd worry less if you didn't have to guess" suggests, fertility testing can be promoted as a means to shift an affective orientation to bodily futurity.[25] Once a test is taken, an above-average outcome can be framed as an encouragement to proactively preserve optimum "peak fertility," while a below-average outcome may provide the rationale for a "last-minute" freezing option. Extracted eggs, as mentioned above, are framed as a collective that require a minimum of 12 or 24 eggs for a good chance of having a child—a logic that may provoke a second or third freezing cycle.[26] In these ways, fertility becomes precarious through constructions of uncertainty and decline, which function as conditions for calls to individual, proactive reproductive control. This emphasis on control and empowerment in which the language of egg freezing is often couched, in turn, obscures the new interdependencies and the incremental logic of the treatment pathways produced as their effect.

Having said that, however, implicit in Silber's suggestion that reproductive foresight and anticipatory action could offer his 40-year-old patient "the pregnancy rate of a 20-year-old" is not so much an injunction for all young women to freeze their eggs. Rather, it reconfigures the reproductive life span, and future reproductive health, as variables over which women can exert agency, instead of being a given, if uncertain, "fact of life." Consequently, with the possibility of circumventing age-related infertility may emerge an increased individual responsibility for "fertility planning" to maintain reproductive ability within culturally variable age ranges. Minimizing future risk of infertility could function as an extension of "the obligation to 'stay informed' about possible futures [which] has become mandatory for good citizenship and morality, engendering alertness and vigilance as normative affective states."[27] Medical and popular risk information surrounding OC may thus function as an implicit injunction to stay informed, and equally as an obligation to live the future in the present body, an imperative to feel the future in the flesh.

The embodied dimension of this injunction becomes evident in *Eggs for Later* when Schellart explains to her parents that

> instead of all of us dying at 50, you also live to 80. But that belly, well, doesn't, you know. And people become much more healthy and everything. That's why medical technologies are developed, right? To prolong lives, and to prolong fertility, in my case.

Reasoning from an analogy between mortality and reproductive finitude, Schellart proposes the extension of the reproductive life span with frozen eggs as a goal comparable to the extension of the human life span. Schellart's understanding of biomedicine references a popular narrative that reads an increase in the average human life span as an affirmation of a telos of medical progress. Lafontaine argues that the extension of life is not only the quintessential symbol of modernity and progress but "the supreme value of postmortal society" that validates "re-engineering" the body.[28] OC likewise entails a bodily re-engineering motivated by supplanting this supreme value to an extension of the reproductive life span.

Schellart's statement also conveys the concurrent resignification of her body in the face of that goal. Disavowed as "that" belly, the reproductive system is discursively split off from the rest of the body as a site of reproductive finitude—a sign of halted evolution in the face of overall increased longevity. In line with Rosalind Gill's characterization of contemporary concern for the body as always "requiring constant monitoring, discipline and remodelling (and consumer spending)," Schellart's belly is "at the risk of failing."[29] In this way, as was the case for amniocentesis and the codeterminate "tentative pregnancy" that resulted from the redistribution of pregnancy risk,[30] egg freezing is another example of how the introduction of new reproductive technologies can impact the perceived risk of preexisting embodied experiences. The anticipatory

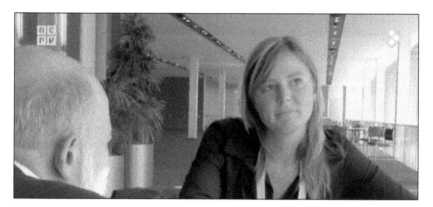

Figure 2.2. Silber and Schellart discuss fertility preservation.

injunction of OC affirms the precariousness of a fertility that is at risk in the absence of biomedical interventions.

Exemplifying the age-specificity of the anticipatory imperative associated with "that belly," when Schellart interviews Silber later in the documentary, he advises her, "I think if you are 35, or even 30, I think it is a very good balance to have an entire ovary frozen and then an entire ovary intact. Come to the US and let us freeze your ovary." In this statement Silber proposes ovary freezing as a new way to enable a balanced, healthy embodiment. The "balanced" body, according to Silber's advice, not only functions well at present but is also preserved well for continued future functionality.

This perspective on healthy reproductive aging can be positioned within a broader trend of "healthy ageing," which is "conceptualised in terms of body maintenance and [forms] a central feature of consumer societies," with an expanding range of markets accommodating a sense of agency over signs of aging, whether through plastic surgery, anti-aging cosmetics, or hormonal treatments.[31] Appealing to neoliberal qualities of autonomy and self-regulation, Silber's approach similarly suggests that women can achieve "balanced" reproductive aging with the aid of the right procedures. Implicitly, Silber suggests that *not* freezing eggs may signal a lack of self-regulation in securing a fertile future.

Yet Schellart's documentary equally points to a counternarrative represented by the featured Dutch politicians, Schellart's GP, and her father, who all advise against egg freezing as a solution to her concerns about future infertility. Schellart's juxtaposition of sources from different national and ideological contexts in *Eggs for Later* reflects a complex situation in which OC is both encouraged and denied. The documentary thus stages how distinctly different discourses are similarly accessible and relevant from the potential patient's point of view. US Fox News, Dutch news reports, and online Belgian newspaper articles are equally accessible from her home. And each propels the narrative forward by introducing OC, wrongly suggesting its availability in the Netherlands, and offering Belgium as an alternative. Their juxtaposition highlights the tension that emerges from the concurrent dissemination of risk narratives on age-related infertility and a widespread discomfort with employing egg freezing to mitigate it. The anticipatory impetus of exerting agency over future infertility with OC is thus in conflict with the Dutch governmental and institutional foreclosure of doing so, leaving Schellart in a situation that she characterizes as "pretty intense for a 36-year-old." OC holds the promise of an antidote to prospective infertility, but in doing so it reinstates a dependence on, among other things, external medical interventions and government regulations that control their accessibility.

Alongside the biomedical manipulation of physical temporality in the extracted frozen eggs, one of the major temporal shifts that emerges in the context of oocyte cryopreservation is thus a set of discursive effects that position the body as a site of anticipation and potential failure. Egg freezing can function, respectively, to maintain a notion of "peak fertility" or to avert impending age-related infertility. These different rationales for egg freezing are linked to new norms about when fertility may be assumed and when "fertility planning" requires active intervention in reproductive aging. The combination of the public framing of fertility as precarious, the promise of OC as a means to mitigate it, and a cultural context in which aging means life-long decline that must be managed and counteracted from early adulthood onwards results in a body of futurity—in which the present is lived through anticipation of the future.

Reproductive Orientations and the Future Family

In Schellart's body of futurity, lived fertility becomes precarious in relation to a *reproductive orientation* towards future childbearing. Just as

Sara Ahmed has argued for sexual orientation, Schellart's reproductive orientation entails a constitutive "tending towards" objects of desire, where "toward" marks "a space and time that is almost, but not quite, available in the present."[32] *Eggs for Later* tells the story of Schellart's anticipatory reproductive orientation towards the future family. Yet it is not anticipation alone but also its proximity to retrospection that animates the reproductive futures central to Schellart's motivation to freeze her eggs. Her documentary reveals the dynamics between anticipation and retrospection in the formation of reproductive orientations.

Eggs for Later invokes Schellart's desired reproductive future with a retrospective reflection on home video footage of her childhood, which is interspersed throughout the film and is used for its opening and closing scenes. "This is me," are Schellart's first words in *Eggs for Later* as we see a baby and, soon after, a toddler in the characteristically blurry aesthetic of 1970s home video. The film closes with similar footage of a young Schellart "frozen in time" by the camera. Through the use of montage and voiceover, Schellart employs the "mediated memories" of these home videos to imagine a desired reproductive future and, in doing so, articulate a visual argument in favor of egg freezing.[33]

The home video footage frequently functions as the visual counterpart to the voiceover's musings on future motherhood, as is the case when Schellart reflects on a conversation with her friend Olaf about the age limits to using her frozen eggs. Schellart tells him that she would consider using her frozen eggs up until she was 48. Subsequently, home videos of a summer holiday appear as Schellart's voiceover contemplates future motherhood:

> My mother was 27 when she had me. That is eight years younger than I am now. I enjoyed having young parents. What would it be like for my child if I freeze my eggs? Would I be a good mother, even if I was a bit older? I think it is more important that you are young at heart, and full of life. But the most important thing is that my child is wanted and that I will give it attention and love.

The home video footage shows a sunny day with Schellart's parents walking arm in arm, holding a baby. A guitar strums gently in the background. At the mention of "my child," Schellart appears as a toddler

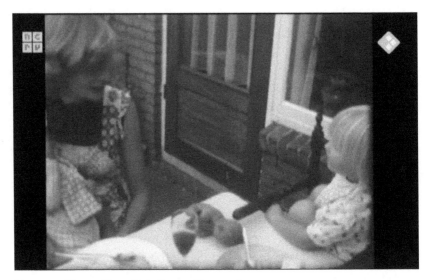

Figure 2.3. Home video of Schellart and her mother.

sitting at a table and the "good mother" coincides with a pan to the left that reveals her mother talking to the child. The voiceover's "attention and love" coincides with a final shot of a young Schellart holding on to her mother as they swim in a lake.

In this way, Schellart's voiceover reframes the home video from a personal memory to an image of an anticipated reproductive future that could be enabled by egg freezing. The voiceover first identifies Schellart as the child she used to be in the home movies and subsequently positions her in the mother's place, thereby presenting the prospect of her own future motherhood. Likewise, Schellart's younger self becomes a visual reference to her own hypothetical child. By narrativizing and presenting the home videos as a future ideal, Schellart transforms what Annette Kuhn calls "memory work" into anticipation work.[34] As "dual instruments for constructing and remembering family life,"[35] these home videos thus attain a third function as instruments for anticipating future family life.

Schellart's approach to anticipating the future family exemplifies queer theorist Lee Edelman's concept of "reproductive futurism," with which he criticizes a "mandate of futurism" that seeks to affirm a social order by mobilizing "fantasies [that] reproduce the past, through displacement, in the form of the future."[36] The documentary's use of the 1970s home videos reflects the "home mode," a mode of media production that "articulates generational continuity over time" and provides "a format for communicating family legends and stories."[37] In keeping with this "home mode," Schellart presents the traditional family structure of her childhood as a fantasy of a potential reproductive future, thereby affirming the significance of her continued fertility.

In doing so, she moreover employs the videos to normalize the use of OC technology to "extend" her fertility and maintain the familial kinship connection. The home videos' quaint, outdated aesthetics are the antithesis of the fears about futuristic technologized reproduction with frozen eggs. They function as familiar low-tech cultural referents through which OC—as a novel high-tech practice, choice, and biotechnology— may become normalized; they visualize the work of memory in making sense of unfamiliar technologies and anticipating uncertain futures.

Schellart's depiction of an idealized future by means of the ambiguous figure of the remembered self and hypothetical future child is a testimony to the significance Edelman ascribes to the child "as disciplinary image of the Imaginary past or as site of a projective identification with an always impossible future."[38] Yet in Schellart's case, the potential impossibility of reproducing this future follows not from the transgression of reproductive norms of (hetero)sexuality that Edelman identifies but from a threatened normativity of reproductive aging.

This age-normative framework becomes explicit in her friend Olaf's disapproval of childbearing at an age at which the resulting generational difference would resemble "child-grandparent relations," reflecting a widely held standpoint by the Dutch that women should not have children beyond their "normal reproductive years."[39] "Parents will become increasingly older with these kinds of technologies. You could have a child when you are 50," Olaf says. "If you are 50 . . . then you will be 80 when that child is 30. I don't think you can do that to your child." In the name of the future child, Olaf validates his view of acceptable ages for using frozen eggs.

Schellart counters Olaf's disapproval in the documentary by visualizing this future child in an idealized family setting. Operating at the meeting ground of the politics of reproduction and representation, the home videos respond to this criticism by erasing Schellart's future age-related transgression from view and visualizing older motherhood with images of her 27-year-old mother instead. They show the parents running around and swimming with their children, illustrating the vitality Schellart associates with young parents—and then reinterprets as a more age-neutral parental love and attention. The voiceover refigures aging as primarily a question of "being young at heart" and "full of life," rather than a matter of time passed since birth or a concern with mistaken (grand)parental kinship assumptions.

By using historical images of desirable parenthood as depictions of the future, Schellart suggests that what matters more is not the specificity of historical time or age, but a dehistoricized familial continuity that underpins her reproductive orientation. Writing about the temporality of the family, Sara Ahmed theorizes the concept of orientation as a means of exposing "how life gets directed through the very requirement that we follow what is already given to us," by imagining "one's futurity in terms of reaching certain points along a life course."[40] In *Eggs for Later*, Schellart not only visualizes her reproductive orientation in keeping with Ahmed's assertion, but she employs the home videos as themselves a reproductive technology that keeps the continuity of the family line intact. Through this visual "anticipation work," she maintains her position as a future mother in the social order of the family. By bringing together several means of freezing time—in the filming of the documentary, in the frozen eggs, and in the montage of the home videos—Schellart reorients time to maintain the seemingly ahistorical continuity of the family structure's reproduction in the face of the time constraints of reproductive aging and repronormative temporal schemes.

While Edelman focuses his critique on the heteronormativity inherent in reproductive futurism, Schellart's case shows that its politics of anticipation also has a chrononormative component. Although Schellart upholds her childhood's traditional family ideal, she also evokes OC as a way of shifting repronormative temporal schemes by advocating using her eggs at an age that her friend considers to be too old. With these home videos, Schellart depicts the retrospective origins of her reproductive orientation towards the future child, which animates both her anxiety about age-related infertility and her desire to freeze a "couple of good eggs." The documentary thus functions analogously to egg freezing by manipulating time to maintain the futurity of motherhood, whether by reframing home videos of the familial past into an image of reproductive futurity, rendering aging and nonreproduction invisible, or presenting egg freezing as a means to ensure familial continuity by extending fertility. It is therefore not anticipation as such but its proximity to retrospection that positions an idealized familial past both as a normative reference point against which continued fertility becomes precarious and as a vehicle to reimagine the temporal logic of reproductive timing with the possibility of egg freezing.

Extending Fertility and Postponing Motherhood

Eggs for Later reveals how the notion that women can exert agency over age-related reproductive ability results in new discourses on how to *account* for the choice of egg freezing. Although, for Schellart, OC represents a means for fulfilling her reproductive orientation, others position egg freezing as a technology that only deters or delays childbearing. These conflicting interpretations of the nature of egg freezing as a reproductive or nonreproductive technology are at the heart of the public debates on fertility preservation. In *Eggs for Later,* and the broader discourses the documentary references, three different interpretations of OC may be distinguished—as extending fertility, postponing motherhood, and preparation for future infertility—each of which implies different understandings of what entails a reproductive act. This section addresses how these conflicting interpretations of OC correspond to opposing views on whether this technology helps or hampers the pursuit of having a child, which are at the heart of the politicization of egg freezing.

In the documentary, these conflicting interpretations of OC are expressed when Schellart first tells her parents that she wants to freeze her eggs:

> FATHER: Oh. Well, yeah, that is also a possibility. But I actually think that you are putting off the problem. You have not really taken a decision. You have not really taken action to solve the problem. What do you want? Really, you are postponing business. . . . It seems to me that the primary issue is for you to decide whether you want a partner or you don't want a partner. . . .

MOTHER: No, but Marieke has already said that.

FATHER: And then, once you have a partner, you can see whether a child will come or not. But now you have to work on that first issue and take a decision.

MOTHER: No but she has already done that. . . . Marieke sees herself with a partner and also with a child. But because there isn't much time, . . . it is nice that by the time she has her partner, she still has a couple of good eggs. . . .

MS: Well, yes, and I don't see it as postponement; I see it as extension.

At the father's mention of postponement, the documentary cuts to the mother's alert turn of head, thereby emphasizing this term as a point of contention. Schellart likewise responds to his idea and suggests that extension is a more apt description of egg freezing than postponement.

Rather than a neutral term, "postponement" is widely used to describe women's nonreproductive decision making at culturally specific ages during which motherhood may be expected. Dutch news media strongly associated the notion of postponement with egg freezing, to the extent that women freezing their eggs were referred to as "postponement mothers."[41] Medical experts sceptical of egg freezing dismissed it as "a false insurance policy" that promotes delayed childbearing in spite of limited success rates.[42] Dutch political parties like the Christian Democrats (CDA) opposed the 2009 initiative to introduce "social" egg freezing by referencing postponement, suggesting that egg freezing encourages an undesirable passivity in pursuing motherhood by "women who are waiting for a suitable partner."[43] Schellart's father's stance can be related to these positions, as he similarly reads OC as a passive option of "not really taking action" and warns his daughter about the health risks and limited success rates of egg freezing.

This OC-specific focus on postponement echoes existing debates on older motherhood. Shaw and Giles note in their media analysis of UK debates of older motherhood that the notion of postponement reinforces the "optimum age" for motherhood, which potentially marginalizes mothers outside of that age frame.[44] Budds and colleagues contend that this marginalization follows from the criticism that women "choosing" older motherhood are not "taking full advantage of their biological window of opportunity" for conception and not making the "right" decision in timing childbirth.[45] Kelhä likewise argues that, as an effect of the public perception of age-related reproductive risks, the timing of motherhood is part of civilized "self-regulation."[46] In this context, the risk of postponing motherhood with OC as "false insurance" points to a potentially flawed self-regulation that may result in involuntary nonreproduction or a later reproduction that transgresses risk-informed age norms.

Whereas "postponement" positions OC as a way of delaying motherhood, the alternative "extension" presents OC as a means for achieving motherhood. The term is widely used in fertility clinics' marketing materials to promote egg freezing—markedly by the abovementioned Extend Fertility company. The term "extension" suggests that OC enables, rather than delays, motherhood by improving fertility prospects in the future. Schellart, similarly, argues for OC as an enabling technology, a way of prolonging her fertility, which allows her to extend the time she has to find a partner to reproduce with. Within this logic, egg freezing is not reproductive risk behavior; rather, the choice of *not* extending fertility with OC could point to lacking self-regulation in securing a fertile future.

These two readings of OC present a conflict between more conventional and newly technologized methods of anticipating age-related infertility. The former approach, as voiced by Schellart's father, suggests that a woman either foregoes (further) reproduction or attempts to conceive with a partner. The father does not recognize egg freezing as a valid step towards having children but only as "putting off the problem." For Schellart, by contrast, egg freezing does represent a step towards reproduction—one that enables future motherhood.

Schellart thus accounts for her choice of egg freezing by positioning it as a reproductive act. Because Schellart wants to have children with a partner and given that the presence of this person is posited in the future, her commitment lies with the creation of a future family, as distinguished from a current desire for childbearing and motherhood. In her case, OC is a reproductive commitment she can make without a partner, in anticipation of this imagined future. While elective OC represents a decision not to have children in the immediate future, it can nevertheless be read as the first step of an IVF fertility treatment that would more unambiguously be recognized as a reproductive act if it did not involve the period of cryostorage. Schellart's framing of egg freezing as an extension of fertility presents it as enabling reproduction, while her father emphasizes the procedure's nonreproductive results.

When egg freezing is interpreted as a reproductive act, the reproductive process itself becomes differently extended over time. With the introduction of embryo freezing in IVF, the duration between fertilization and embryo implantation has become manipulable, stretching the reproductive process to encompass years rather than the conventional nine months. With OC emerges a new temporal separation between the egg extraction and fertilization that hitherto could not be lengthened. For Schellart, the consequent lack of a need for a partner or donor at the start of the reproductive process represents the option to be proactive in her procreative desires. For her father, who does not view OC as a reproductive act, finding a partner remains the first step to "really [take] action to solve the problem."

Yet what constitutes "the problem" differs in the two approaches. In the postponement frame, the main concern is the absence of the desired child. Postponement implies the activity of putting something off that could happen in the present, whereas for many women, current reproduction may not be perceived as an option or desire. To describe women who would like to have children at some point in the future but not at present as postponing misreads their intention as necessarily aiming for immediate conception and childbearing.

By contrast, Schellart's understanding of OC as extension suggests a concern with the temporality of fertility as much as with having children as such. From the opening statement emerges a set of interrelated concerns about the prospective decreased ability to reproduce ("soon it won't be possible anymore"), the finality of childlessness ("perhaps I will never have children"), and the pressure of "time running out." When understood as an extension of fertility, egg freezing mitigates these concerns by allowing Schellart to lengthen her imagined reproductive life span, even if the frozen eggs are fallible. Notwithstanding her doctor's warning that he cannot guarantee they will result in a pregnancy later on, the cryopreserved eggs enable Schellart to reconceptualize her reproductive life span by prolonging the period within which the possibility of future motherhood is maintained. When 35-year-old Schellart and her mother discuss her biological clock, they estimate she will be infertile in "three or four years." With egg freezing, Schellart tells her friend

Olaf that she would consider using her eggs until she is 48. Regardless of OC's success or Schellart's actual reproductive ability, she thus extends the imagined age frame of fertility by roughly a decade. Throughout this period, egg freezing can thus function to maintain an imagined future motherhood, which may be distinguished from the desire to be a mother at present. The extended reproductive time frame thus alleviates the anticipatory anxiety that "soon it won't be possible anymore."

Egg Freezing as Biopreparation

Besides postponement and extension, I propose a third way of conceptualizing OC, namely, as a mode of anticipation that Vincanne Adams and colleagues call "biopreparation." "Biopreparation" is a term more commonly used in public health contexts to refer to governmental efforts to ensure readiness in the event of disasters like biological warfare and emerging infectious diseases. Adams and colleagues argue that the preemptive logic of biopreparation similarly characterizes anticipatory biomedical interventions that promote a need of being prepared for one's future. DNA scans for genetic testing, menstrual blood preservation as a source of stem cells, and cord blood banking to benefit a newborn's future health are all examples, to which egg freezing may be added, of interventions that offer ways of being prepared in anticipation of potential future medical problems. Rather than preventing future health conditions from developing, biopreparation acts "in 'preparation for' the event . . . as if it were already here."[47] Here I propose a reading of biopreparation specific to the context of OC as a strategy of preparing for anticipated futures by preemptively "freezing" the present to preserve it for the arrival of "later."

OC approximates biopreparation more than preventative medicine because it does not in fact prevent age-related infertility. Rather, it starts infertility treatment on the fertile body in preparation for potential future infertility. Instead of treating diagnosed infertility, OC treats the precarious state of "anticipated infertility" and replaces it with a bioprepared sense of fertility, which preempts infertility's arrival by the halting of eggs' aging through cryopreservation. This approach is evident in Schellart's mother's recognition that her daughter's potential reproductive failure presents the need for securing "a couple of good eggs."

Fertility thus departs from the medical definition of the physical ability to conceive within one year of unprotected heterosexual intercourse towards an egg-based model. Rather than an ability, the bioprepared fertility that OC offers is conceived as the possession of "good eggs" that prepare women for the future loss of embodied eggs.

In *Eggs for Later*, the presentation of this process of achieving bioprepared fertility through OC mirrors the conventional reproductive process. At the start of OC's alternative reproductive trajectory, Schellart draws a circle on her belly for each daily hormonal injection shot, resulting in a row of eight numbered circles that look like a visual reminder of the eggs developing inside. The sideways mirror image of her belly bloated by ovarian stimulation suggests a visual anticipation of future pregnancy. At the end of the hormonal treatment, Schellart jokingly suggests that if she were to have sex, she might "get, I don't know, octuplets or something," invoking the eight eggs drawn on her belly. During the egg extraction, her facial expressions are pained and her legs are in stirrups, as if in a mini-delivery. Instead of her birthing a child, this presentation of OC suggests that she has gestated and given birth to her eggs: the materialization of her continued, ageless fertility. This mirroring of the reproduction process enacts both the possible future pregnancy and the experience of OC as a reproductive process in its own right that, irrespective of a live birth, produces the continuation of maternal futurity.

The mirroring of future reproduction gains a more literal meaning when Schellart films herself cupping her naked tummy in a mirror framed by photos of young children. The mirror image allows Schellart to anticipate an imagined reproductive future through the image of her body. This scene shows how, rather than only an injunction to act, anticipation may also manifest as a kind of pleasurable hope: "If we hope for happiness, then we might be happy as long as we can retain this hope. . . . Hope anticipates a happiness to come."[48] Similarly, Schellart's mirror image of imagined pregnancy expresses a desire not only for attaining motherhood but for maintaining the continued possibility of future motherhood. Schellart's presentation of her belly signals that the day she will "never have children" has not yet arrived. Prolonging an anticipatory state in this way may be a goal in and of itself, to be distinguished from anticipating future conception and childbearing itself.

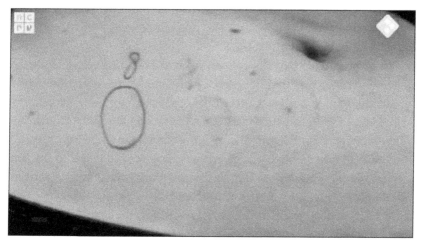

Figure 2.4. Eight injections in preparation of the egg extraction.

After the extraction procedure, as the documentary shows how the eggs are examined under microscopes and put in storage tanks, Schellart's voiceover says,

> There they go at last. My eggs. Strange that they are now outside of my body. They are so fragile, and so small. I want to know what happens to them and where they will be kept. Will I ever come to pick them up? The strange thing is that after all that effort, I somehow hope that I will never need them. But it does give me a comforting feeling to know that they are now here. Ten of my eggs are now safely stored, among thousands of embryos.

Soon after, the documentary concludes:

> After two treatments, I now have 20 eggs in Brussels. This gives me the feeling that my child has come closer. I know that there are no guarantees, but nevertheless my clock ticks a little less loudly.

Here Schellart's reproductivity becomes mediated through her affective orientation towards the extracted eggs. While the extraction provokes concern towards the "small" and "fragile" eggs that were once in her body, Schellart is less anxious about their future now that they are "safely stored." Responsibility for maintaining future fertility is now externalized to biomedicine and cryotechnology, rather than exclusively contained in her own body.

If the pregnant body "is conceived of as both protective container for the foetus and as [its] dangerous conductor,"[49] so similar ambiguity about the female body as "protective container" for the eggs emerges with OC technology, which introduces the freezer as a substitute host to human oocytes. In the anticipatory logic of OC, the freezer is an ageless alternative to the fallible ovaries, whose aging poses a threat to the continued viability of the eggs. If in bodies of futurity the anticipated risk is lived in the present, OC offers to preemptively expel the threat of losing eggs from the aging body. Conversely, it expels the threat of the aging body from the eggs, which are now "safely stored" in the freezer. In other words, if anticipated infertility is embodied in "that belly," which is preemptively disavowed as site of reproductive finitude, Schellart's story suggests that OC resolves this embodied failure through the exteriorization of "a couple of good eggs" as symbols of continued fertility.

Eggs for Later is, then, a story about the rise of anticipatory anxiety about future infertility and the resolution of that anxiety through the reorientation of reproductive time. The documentary's presentation of the move from assumed to anticipated infertility highlights that the possibility of egg freezing produces not only an affective resolution but also a rise of anticipatory anxiety when fertility becomes precarious. Apart from the more or less explicit calls to freeze one's eggs, the production of anxiety is established through the discursive framing of the disparate temporal logic governing the *in vivo* and *ex vivo* eggs. Eggs inside the body are comprehended through a metric of increasing loss that is intimately tied to aging. The unstimulated eggs inside the body are not quantified or tangible, and are subject to accelerating decline. Yet after extraction, Schellart's eggs no longer signify in a negative economy of loss. They become measurable and observable when the medical team counts the eggs during the extraction procedure ("I see ten nice follicles"; "We have the first egg!"). By returning for a second cycle, Schellart doubles the number of stored eggs from 10 to 20. Once distributed to the freezer, the eggs operate under an alternative temporal logic of frozen time and averted loss. The rise and resolution of anxious anticipation thus matches with the material-discursive acceleration of reproductive time in the embodied eggs and deceleration of reproductive time in the extracted eggs.

In the closing statement, Schellart's feeling that her child had come closer through the procedure is followed by the statement that "my clock ticks a little less loudly." Significantly positioned as the closing words of the documentary, the quieting of the anxiety associated with the biological clock is as much a result of the affective engagement with OC as the actual success of the procedure measured by future live births. Echoing this sentiment in an interview, Schellart looks back at the project and says that it brought her peace as she moved from fearing to facing her reproductive future: "Not just because my eggs are now in the freezer. The most important thing is that I faced my future for a year."[50] Both the documentary's closure and this statement validate OC as an endpoint in itself. In this way, the narrative closure of OC differs from that of IVF, which focuses on "hope fulfilment" and "dreams come true" in the "miracle baby."[51] Regardless of whether the eggs will be used, and whether children will be born from them, Schellart has already achieved what she needed through the promise of OC: the relief from anticipatory anxiety about infertility, the finality of childlessness, and the feeling of running out of time.

Conclusion

Precisely by presenting the outcome of Schellart's egg freezing experience as not primarily oriented towards the birth of a child but towards the resolution of anticipatory anxiety, *Eggs for Later* highlights how the promissory offer of egg freezing can interpellate and enlist a new group of fertile women as potential patients. Given that neither the desire for a child at present nor the arrival of infertility is a requirement for the procedure, egg freezing allows for a wide variety of potential indications that are not solely physical in nature but are linked to new temporal norms of "fertility planning." *Eggs for Later* stages some of the cultural negotiations of such new norms revolving around when, whether, and why to freeze one's eggs and anticipate future infertility.

If the figure of the freezable egg opens up the possibility of bypassing future infertility and reconfiguring the declining telos of reproductive aging, it equally provides the conditions of emergence of a precarious notion of a fertility whose finality becomes a responsibilized concern at earlier points in the life cycle. Schellart's documentary, and the medical and political discourses it features, portrayed two age-specific approaches to anticipating future infertility. One approach positioned egg freezing as a "last-minute" measure because "soon it won't be possible anymore." The other replaced "assumed fertility" with "anticipated infertility" at much earlier ages, thereby engaging a potentially larger group of healthy young women with future reproductive risks and suggesting OC as a means to proactively mitigate them. Both options adopted existing age-related affects and ideas about the onset of fertility decline as an indication for treatment. The earlier freezing moreover reflects a rationale of "peak time" fertility, materialized in extractable egg quality and quantity, which may be preserved through cryopreservation. A sense of *reproductive bioprecarity* could, then, follow not only from the threat of losing fertility at the prospective end of the reproductive life span but also from the possibility of losing peak fertility much earlier in life.

Discourses advocating OC that were featured in *Eggs for Later* made implicit injunctions to minimize risk in the face of anticipatory anxiety about future infertility. I proposed that the mitigation of this anticipatory anxiety through egg freezing can be read as an instance of biopreparation for potential future infertility. Biopreparation is an alternative to the conflicting conceptualizations of OC as an extension of the fertile life course or postponement of childbearing. The major effect of the treatment that Schellart documents in the film is the move from reproductive bioprecarity to biopreparedness as the anticipatory anxiety that opened the documentary shifts in its closing scenes to the sense of readiness for the future. The documentary's narrative closure is thus not the child or the lack thereof, but the silencing of the "ticking of the [biological] clock" by the freezing of reproductive time with OC. In this way, egg freezing can function as an engagement with bodily futurity that changes it from a threat, an incentive to action, to a futurity that has been taken care of. It absolves bodies of futurity from the responsibility of failure by mitigating anticipated risks in the present.

Whereas egg freezing functions in this documentary as narrative closure, Schellart's story represents only the first stage in the egg freezing procedure. If cryopreservation resolves anticipatory anxiety by opening up reproductive futurities and outsourcing reproductive aging to extracorporeal institutions, these very movements rekindle new forms of reproductive bioprecarity during the next stage in the OC procedure. After having been extracted from the body, the eggs are stored in the liquid nitrogen freezer, where they remain out of sight to the women who freeze them. Nevertheless, as will become clear next, the visual mediations of the extracted cells, the promise of their future reproductive value, and the ongoing financial obligations of treatment plans play a key role in bridging the distance between the body and the freezer. Schellart's documentary ends with a song, in which a female voice sings "I was freezing, freezing time" as the credits roll. This notion of freezing time, and its significance in the visualization and the marketing of egg freezing, is central to the next chapter.

3

Frozen Eggs and the Financialization of Fertility

Distributing Reproductive Aging in the
Reproductive-Industrial Complex

With the possibility of OC emerges a new cultural entity: the frozen egg. This egg is not swaddled in an ovarian follicle, swept into the fallopian tubes by engorged fimbriae, or surrounded by sperm in an *in vitro* scene of (imminent) fertilization. Rather, the frozen egg is a cell that exists, for the first time, outside of the female reproductive body while retaining its reproductive potential for prolonged periods of time. The cryopreservation of sperm and embryos has been routine practice for decades, and the viability of the human egg outside of the female body has been manifest in the birth of *in vitro* conceived children from the late 1970s onwards. Yet, combining the two, OC uniquely introduces the emergent cultural entity of the viable extracorporeal frozen egg, which is at the heart of this chapter.

Following the journey of the egg, previous chapters considered embodied and extractable eggs, which functioned as reference points for conceptualizing precaritized yet extendable fertilities. Once they are frozen, in the next step of OC, cryo-eggs enable a reconfiguration of reproductive aging as no longer only an embodied process but as distributed between the body and the freezer and beyond. As they remain in the dark of the liquid nitrogen tank, the eggs' visual and textual mediations are instrumental in the concomitant reimagination of reproductive aging and the relation between the cell and the self. The newly legible and quantifiable frozen egg also functions as a key metric in treatment rationales for egg freezing presented by fertility companies. This chapter considers how the frozen egg becomes both the basis for a distributed form of reproductive aging and a key metric in emergent political economies of fertility preservation.

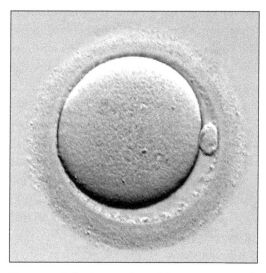

Figure 3.1. A fresh metaphase II human oocyte collected by follicle puncture after ovarian stimulation.
Courtesy of Lucinda Veeck Gosden.

Reproductive technologies are also often visual technologies, with
which the reproductive process may be visualized in new ways. OC is
no exception and gains a visual dimension through the photomicrography of extracted eggs.[1] After egg-extraction surgery, fertility clinics may
offer women a photograph of their egg(s).[2] Although such a photograph
shows a recently extracted egg before cryopreservation, it may also function as a visual referent for the frozen eggs once they are stored in the
freezer. The photograph is a registration of the microscopic examination of the extracted egg; it is a visual record of a procedure that takes
place in laboratories that normally remain closed to patients, which now
brings the egg into visibility for the woman from whom it was extracted,
her social networks, and the wider public. For example, one of the first
women to blog about freezing her eggs was offered such a photograph
by her clinic; using "Eggfreezer" as her online alias, she publicly shared
the image on the Blogspot website and added a reflection on her relation to the depicted frozen egg (quoted below). Linking constructions
of cellular exceptionalism and embodied fertility loss, the frozen egg
image references a contemporary moment in which the manipulation
of biological time changes what it means to age as much as culturally

specific ideas about aging change what it means to manipulate biological time. This chapter explores the relation between the cell and the self, which forms the basis for a distributed conceptualization of reproductive aging that exceeds bodily boundaries and incorporates wider, cryopolitical infrastructures.

This distribution of reproductive aging with frozen eggs is situated within broader commercial and clinical infrastructures constructed around the promise of fertility preservation. This chapter discusses how egg freezing has emerged in tandem with significant capital investments, new fertility start-ups, and specialized financial products, all of which provide interpretative frames for a reinvented and precarious notion of fertility and its futurities. The analysis draws attention to how the presentation of frozen eggs by fertility companies plays a key role in the treatment rationales and calculative practices of OC. For example, the framing of the frozen eggs can provide the terms for rationalizing particular treatment pathways and asking not only "Should I freeze my eggs?" but also "Have I frozen enough eggs?" What is at stake in these discursive mediations of the frozen egg is also a broader reconfiguration of the relation between capital and reproductive value in OC. With an analysis of the framing of frozen eggs in marketing efforts, treatment packages, and fertility insurance, this chapter highlights how the mediated frozen egg is crucial in the rationalization of OC not just as a single procedure but as an ongoing process of technologized fertility management.[3]

Between the Cell and the Self: Distributing Reproductive Aging

> Here is an actual egg from my retrieval. (the whole thing is the egg and the spot is the nucleus). Life is a pretty crazy thing. This egg was inside me (in a premature state) for 32 years—even before I took my own first breath as a newborn. Had I not had the retrieval, this egg would have just never developed and died off last month—just another one of the many millions that die off over a woman's lifetime. Instead, through modern medicine, it was able to be matured and extracted and it is now quite literally frozen in time alongside 27 others, potentially to be the starting building block of a future human being. And this egg is what is fully sufficient and necessary to make that human my biological child. This is the

tie—the everything and anything that is what a woman prefers when she wants "her own" biological baby. Whatever it is that she wants—what I want—it's in there. Part of me is in there.[4]

This is Eggfreezer's vivid description of her frozen egg, which is accompanied by a photograph of the (soon to be) cryopreserved cell. As the last in a series of 47 posts describing her experience of OC, this blog post—titled "Picture of My Frozen Egg"—presents the conclusion to her egg freezing process. Unlike the familiar generic cellular images of human eggs circulating in medical publications and popular culture, Eggfreezer's photographed cell attains a specific individuality as the egg that had been "inside [her] for 32 years" and the "building block of a future human being." At the meeting ground of the lived self and imagined child, the frozen egg—both as photographic imagery and as biogenetic substance—also figures as a materialization of a more relational kind of fertility that is distributed across the body and the freezer.

Highlighting the egg's individuality, Eggfreezer draws a direct connection between her egg and the potential child conceived from it by positioning the cell as "the starting building block of a future human being" that would be "fully sufficient and necessary to make that human my biological child." In line with earlier studies on IVF, in which patients describe images of embryos as the first visual encounter with their (potential) children, Eggfreezer stretches the visual recognition of the future child to an even earlier, preconception stage of development, in which the nucleus represents a visible genetic connection to an "'own' biological baby" and the cell itself, a "building block" from which this potential child may one day grow.[5]

Because sperm is, quite literally, not yet in the picture, the resultant primacy of the egg in imagining the reproductive process reverses the "preponderance of narratives describing the exceptionalness of the one sperm that gets to fertilize the egg."[6] In the familiar trope of the "sperm race," a multitude of male gametes compete, and the exceptional sperm that first reaches the single, ovulated egg becomes the genetic building block for the future child. Here, instead, Eggfreezer's egg emerges as the exceptional one among "the many millions," in the act of visualization rather than fertilization. The fact that the egg survived and has been extracted against the odds, as the one singled out of millions, imbues it with an individuality that finds its visual reflection in the photograph of the cell. The meeting of egg and eye, rather than egg and sperm, becomes the occasion for establishing this particular egg's exceptionalism as the "starting building block" for the potential future child. Only once it is removed from the body and rendered observable by the camera does this particular egg become recognizable as an individual entity onto which reproductive futures may be projected. In the transition from the opaque body to the transparent petri dish, from an aging to an arrested state, the photographed egg becomes exceptional in the visual encounter—as the one that continues to live out of the "millions that die off."

Providing a means to partake in the medical gaze, the photograph of the disembodied, extracted egg renders Eggfreezer's (interior) bodily self, and its reproductive potential, legible.[7] Given its ambiguous status as both extracted body tissue that may be considered "part of me" and "building block" of the potential future child, the photographed egg depicts a cell that simultaneously signals a corporeal past and a reproductive future, while staging a cellular temporal "latency," or life in suspended animation, in the face of bodily finitude.[8]

As counterpoint to the frozen egg as a symbol of anticipatory and unaging generativity, the body from which the egg originates is framed as a site of loss. Retrospectively recognizing this loss, Eggfreezer writes, "Had I not had the retrieval, this egg would have just never developed and died off last month."[9] After framing the image of the *in vitro* cryopreserved egg as a sign of its continued aliveness and future potential, Eggfreezer invokes an *in vivo* past of the egg in which it is "going to die" and would have been "already dead" at the time of writing. With the younger cryopreserved egg functioning as a foil for her aging body, Eggfreezer adopts a model of reproductive aging as mournful, in which the female body becomes the site of the incessant dying of "many millions" of eggs in a process that culminates in the finitude of age-related infertility. In this model, the salvaging of eggs and their preservation in the freezer entail a rescue from the aging body "through modern medicine."[10]

Eggfreezer thus positions OC as a life-or-death intervention to save the egg. The invoked imminent death of the photographed egg has the rhetorical effect of positioning the OC technology as a rescuing "helping hand" to the physical limitations of Eggfreezer's reproductive body. Sarah Franklin and Celia Roberts observe in *Born and Made* that the notion that IVF is simply "giving nature a helping hand"—just as Eggfreezer's egg was saved "through modern medicine"—is a trope so familiar that it is expressed in the term "*assisted* reproductive technologies." Yet the framing of OC as a helping hand to circumvent reproductive aging also positions the reproductive body itself as a risky environment for the egg.

As opposed to an understanding of her ovaries as the site where her eggs live, mature, and ovulate, Eggfreezer presents her body as the place where the eggs "die off." The liquid nitrogen tank, by contrast, figures as "a new type of body" in which the eggs do not die off as time passes; it substitutes the aging ovaries and maintains the eggs' viability.[11] The egg, captured in the frozen moment of the deathless portrait, is—at least conceptually—unthreatened by the transitory nature of organic life. That egg, which, more than any other cell, carries the significatory weight of the future, may be rescued from an aging body and frozen into an unchanging stillness that promises potential life.

Through this dynamic between the lived self and the cryopreserved cell, reproductive aging is profoundly reconceptualized; it now encompasses both the body and the egg in the freezer. Even after the egg's extraction, Eggfreezer describes it as "part of me." So while the vulnerability of the *in vivo* cell allows the aging body to be reimagined as a place of loss, the egg's frozen, resilient stillness *in vitro* may also provoke a reconceptualization of reproductive aging as incorporating the extracorporeal, cryopreserved cells. In Eggfreezer's case, the frozen egg, and its photographic depiction, offer an opportunity to reflect on the self in relation to this cell—as a body that once enveloped the egg, as a self genetically transferred to its nucleus, and as a self that remains bound to the egg even after its extraction.

This conceptualization of the frozen egg as a foundational element of fertility and reproductive aging resonates with the question Hannah Landecker asks in *Culturing Life*, her 20th-century history of tissue culture: how does biotechnology, and the interventions in cellular plasticity and temporality, change "what it is—what it means at any given moment—to be cellular living matter"?[12] Not unlike Landecker's tissue cultures, which introduce "systematic change into biological existence," the emergence of the frozen egg presents a systematic change in the way female gametes can exist and reproduce outside of the body. Providing the occasion for both visualizing the eggs and generating a new set of reproductive choices predicated on the *in vivo* and *in vitro* existence of these cells, egg freezing provides an emblematic case for examining what it means to be a cellular being when cryopreservation becomes widespread practice.[13]

Addressing the implications of cellular cryopreservation for reimagining aging, Landecker argues that "to be biological, alive, and cellular also means (at present) to be a potential 'age chimaera,' to be suspendable, interruptible, storable, and freezable in parts."[14] In other words, she suggests a reconceptualization of bodily aging as predicated on the technical possibility of altering the way in which its cellular components exist in time. If the photograph's frozen moment, which captures unaging eggs that "remain 32 forever," can be mobilized to frame the aging body as an environment in which eggs simply "d[ie] off" in a "really cruel decline," the meaning of reproductive aging may be extended to encompass a variety of processes within and without the body. Indeed, if, as previous chapters suggested, the egg becomes the quintessential locus of fertility, the frozen, extracted egg is not only the foil for an unsuitably aging body, but its freezability also suggests a chimaeric model of reproductive aging that encompasses both living and latent, intra- and extracorporeal elements.[15]

The *in vitro* egg functions as a key reference point for this new model of reproductive aging. Not unlike Suzanne Anker and Sarah Franklin's reading of IVF as a mirror that "over-determin[es] the viewer position of witnessing ourselves, our technology, our future, and our obligations to one another," the observable egg can function as a mirror onto the self that refracts multiple cellular and bodily temporalities of life.[16] In Eggfreezer's case, the photographed egg suspended in time stages an encounter with the latent temporality of the frozen cell, which she expressly identifies as "part of me." Situating aging at the meeting ground of the life cycle and the cell cycle, the extracted egg's photograph allows reproductive aging to become conceivable as a *distributed* process that encompasses both the latent state of the ageless egg and the body living in time.

With reference to Michelle Murphy's notion of "distributed reproduction" as "the ontological politics of embodied reproduction," distributed reproductive *aging* points to the dispersal of biological substances inside and outside the body, that comprise the multiple temporalities of reproductive aging in contemporary technologized models of reproduction.[17] In other words, distributed reproductive aging references the arrangement of different biological elements that are seen to exist differently in time, yet can partake of one another's vitality, latency, and reproductive potentiality.

Yet the distribution of reproductive aging does not only pertain to bodies and eggs but extends to wider infrastructures through which newly technologized modes of living and aging are selectively enabled and disenabled. Murphy writes that "distributed reproduction is the extensive sense of existing over time that stretches beyond bodies to include the uneven relations and infrastructures that shape what forms of life are supported to persist, thrive, and alter, and what forms of life are destroyed, injured, and constrained."[18] The reconfiguration of reproductive aging as incorporating frozen *ex vivo* cells must thus also be understood in relation to the material conditions and infrastructural relations that enable this distribution in the first place. In order to fully understand what is at stake in this process, it is crucial to consider the clinical and commercial infrastructures through which reproductive aging is distributed in what Sigrid Vertommen calls the "reproductive-industrial complex," which includes "a biomedical establishment—consisting of academic entrepreneurs, venture capitalists, biotech companies and pharmaceutical giants."[19] Beyond a conceptual question, the distribution and mediation of cryo-eggs provides a lens onto these infrastructural shifts in contemporary IVF and their embeddedness in structural economic stratifications and capitalist regimes of accumulation. The next section analyzes these reproductive infrastructures—and the calculative practices and treatment logics that organize OC within them—in order to examine how the accumulation of eggs and capital meet.

Oocyte Calculations: Financializing Reproductive Time

In *Staying with the Trouble*, Donna Haraway proposes that we should "make kin, not babies" as she takes her readers on a tour through a vibrant collection of multispecies kinning practices.[20] Although the increasing popularity of reproductive technologies is frequently criticized for investing in exactly the opposite of Haraway's adagio, egg freezing peculiarly aligns with her controversial tenet by predominantly producing eggs, rather than babies. Eggfreezer used photography and blog writing to make kin with her cryopreserved cells, thereby remaking reproductive aging into a more distributed notion in the process. Yet the clinical and commercial infrastructures of egg freezing are likewise integral to the kinning of fertile cells and fertile subjects that become newly separated with OC. Whether through marketing, treatment packages, or insurance arrangements, fertility companies play a central role in producing novel rationales for investing in frozen eggs, propelled by the specter—more so than the imminent creation—of a future child.

OC has emerged in the context of a growing fertility industry, large capital investments in egg freezing start-ups, widespread mergers and acquisitions of fertility clinics, and the platformization of reproductive care. Although egg freezing only accounts for a small percentage of IVF cycles—in the United States, only 3.7% are performed for oocyte banking even though the procedure is on offer in 97% of clinics—the relative annual increase of women freezing their eggs and the promise of future growth has attracted the interest of fertility and capital markets alike.[21] Existing IVF clinics have invested in practicing and promoting OC, and, particularly in the United States, specialized egg freezing start-ups have received hundreds of millions of dollars of venture capital and private equity. These investments materialize the promise of egg freezing as a growth technology that may be targeted at a wide group of younger, fertile women, who may or may not want to have children in the future—a far greater segment of the population than those currently accessing IVF. They also illustrate how processes of financialization play a central role in the organization of contemporary US IVF—and the propelling of a widespread mainstreaming of OC in particular. Given that fertility has become a new frontier for corporate investment, it is pertinent to consider how the institutional, clinical, and financial context of OC also plays a key role in setting the terms for what it means to "extend fertility."

Previous chapters have focused on the idea that fertility may be extended by moving eggs from the body to the freezer. Yet this movement to the freezer need not be limited to a single cycle. After the first cycle, in the absence of any immediate fertilization or pregnancy outcome, the question arises whether one has frozen enough eggs to achieve a sufficient degree of "fertility extension." Although OC is presented as a way to "turn back the biological clock," there is no consensus on the number of cycles or cryo-eggs one needs to freeze before the clock is indeed considered to be adequately adjusted. In the face of this uncertainty, particular quantities of frozen eggs may come to stand in for a reasonable chance to have a baby, or for a certain amount of reproductive time. Such mediations of the cryo-eggs as measures for extended fertility are particularly interesting to explore, as they provide the rationale for the number of cycles women are advised to undergo and, by extension, the extent to which egg freezing is a single anticipatory gesture or the basis for an ongoing technologized fertility management.

Eggs per Baby

The number of mature frozen eggs is a key measurement of a successful egg freezing cycle, which is linked to the likelihood that these eggs will result in a live birth. The American Society for Reproductive Medicine (ASRM), for example, advises women that frozen eggs do not "guarantee a future baby" because each egg only has a 2–12% success rate.[22] In IVF clinics, guidelines about how many "eggs per baby" are required provide an important metric in treatment rationales for OC. Shady Grove Fertility, one of the largest US fertility groups, for example, recommends that women under 38 should freeze 15 to 20 eggs. Because "a woman with normal ovarian reserve will produce, on average, 10 viable eggs per cycle, . . . she will need about two egg freezing cycles to produce enough eggs to better ensure the possibility of having a child in the future."[23] Likewise, CARE Fertility, the largest private fertility clinic in the United Kingdom, states that "ultimately, by collecting and freezing 20 eggs in total, we believe when you're ready to start your family we'll be able to give you your very best chance of success."[24]

Following these guidelines, each cycle can itself become an indication for a further cycle, depending on the number of eggs it yields. The guidelines suggest that multiple cycles are recommended for the majority of women, as most do not extract 20 eggs in a single cycle. This was the case for Schellart in *Eggs for Later*, who returned for a second cycle after freezing ten eggs from the first. Eggfreezer rejoiced about 32 eggs, assured that this number is a sufficient amount to store. As these two cases show, with OC practices emerge new norms about the number of eggs that are required for achieving a sense of bioprepared fertility.

Although commonsensical, this discursive framing of the eggs does more than provide guidelines for deciding on the number of OC cycles; it also positions eggs as the materialization of ongoing fertility. While the reproductive potential ascribed to the frozen eggs is reliant on the highly technologized context of IVF, they also become the reference point for understanding embodied, *in vivo*, fertility. For example, a common question people ask about egg freezing is whether fertility will be reduced if there are fewer eggs left in the ovaries after oocyte extraction.[25] In keeping with what Sarah Franklin has called the "analogic return," eggs that are situated in the IVF infrastructure thus become the basis for reconceptualizing embodied eggs, and the fertility they represent.[26] Much as assisted reproduction has become the model for the public understanding of the reproductive process more broadly,[27] so the measurability, quantification, and cumulative reproductive potential that characterize frozen eggs in OC has become the reference point for appraising fertility—both inside and outside of the body.

Oocyte Biotemporalities

As an alternative to the "egg per baby" metric, eggs can themselves become a measurement of time. "Freeze 12 eggs to freeze one year of fertility," the Extend Fertility network writes on its website. Conceding that there is no "magic number" to guarantee a future pregnancy, it suggests that "women 30 or younger can feel confident that freezing about one year's fertility—or 12 eggs—will have a high potential for creating at least one child if used later on." For women above 30—the vast majority of women seeking to circumvent age-related infertility—12 to 24 eggs are recommended.[28]

Fertility is here not just correlated to age but becomes measurable in units of fertile time condensed in the cryo-egg. The equation of 12 eggs with 12 months of fertility suggests that the time of the monthly ovulatory cycle is matched in the time represented by each frozen egg. If every extracted egg symbolizes a month of embodied fertility, superovulation becomes a temporal event, compressing the time of multiple unstimulated ovulatory cycles into a single, more efficient ART cycle. The simultaneous superovulation of many eggs in OC cycles is then not so much a future extension but a temporal *expansion* of fertility. When each gamete embodies a monthly chance of pregnancy, a single egg freezing cycle yielding 12 eggs could expand to a year of fertility. Whether or not this is in fact an accurate description, it presents a temporal logic in which extracted cryo-eggs materialize nuggets of reproductive time that can be accumulated in the freezer and transposed into the future. At a point in their lives that women describe as characterized by accelerated time,[29] such a temporal expansion can be a welcome proposition.

This treatment rationale, which proposes quantitative thresholds (such as 12 eggs) for achieving a sense of reproductive success, suggests a model of reproductive aging that is distributed along two divergent models of biotemporality ascribed to *in vivo* and *ex vivo* eggs. *In vivo* eggs, and the notion of the embodied ovarian reserve, collectively represent the accelerated linear time of fertility loss, which intensifies as the years pass. The extracted, *ex vivo* eggs embody the recursive time of fertility accumulation, which references both the ovulatory cycle that is materialized in the eggs and the future return of reproductive potentiality after their cryopreservation. Reproductive aging after cryopreservation is distributed across both of these divergent *in vivo* and *ex vivo* temporal trajectories. As the embodied eggs follow the tracks of downwards graphs, the accumulated cryo-eggs offset this trajectory by both symbolizing units of frozen fertile time and introducing a potential reproductive return at some future date.

Package Plans and Fertility Accumulation

These figurations of eggs as measurable reproductive potential or fertile time are particularly important when they function as the organizing principle for treatment and financial plans. Because a single cycle may not yield the recommended number of eggs, fertility clinics and companies commonly offer multicycle packages for egg freezing. Modeled after similar packages for IVF treatment, multicycle packages require an up-front payment for several cycles, but offer a significant discount for doing so. For example, some of the major UK fertility clinics, including the Lister Clinic, London Women's Clinic, and Bridge Centre, present three-cycle egg freezing packages at discounted rates of about 20%. As the multicycle package is presented as an instrument to make individual egg freezing cycles more affordable and potentially less stressful, they also provide a financial incentive to approach egg freezing as a longer-term, multicycle treatment course.

Frozen-egg guarantee packages, by contrast, present a different model of organizing IVF treatment by shifting from payment per cycle to payment for a certain quantity of eggs. One example of such an outcome-focused approach is the US Shady Grove Fertility's "Assure Fertility" package. This program offers qualified women a flat fee of $12,500 and $18,000 for its 20- or 30-egg packages, respectively, which allow up to four or six cycles to extract and freeze the specified number of eggs.[30] In effect, this means that the patient runs the risk of overpaying if a high number of eggs are extracted in the first cycles, but may also pay less than she otherwise would have done if more cycles are required to extract the desired number of eggs. The Extend Fertility network likewise offers

> to freeze at least one year of your current fertility—12 eggs or more—for an all-inclusive fee of $4,990. . . . If it takes more than one cycle to get 12 eggs, it's on us. You can do up to 4 cycles if you need to—but you probably won't![31]

UK-based CARE Fertility launched a similar program called "EGGsafe," which covers the cost of retrieving 20 eggs for up to four cycles. The program is open to women under 36. With this package, CARE proposes, "You have a realistic chance of producing enough eggs for storage to give you a high and realistic chance of having a baby when you are ready."[32] As this phrasing suggests, these packages have a clear rhetorical effect of affirming the number of eggs upon which realistic chances of having a baby are contingent. Even for women who do not opt in to the packages, but choose the conventional "fee for service," these packages present 12, 20, or 30 eggs as referents for what constitutes "reproductive success" in the context of egg freezing. In so doing, they raise expectations that multiple OC cycles will be necessary to achieve a reasonable chance of a future live birth.

Although these arrangements are modeled after multicycle and guarantee IVF packages that have been around since the 1990s, when they are used for egg freezing rather than IVF cycles, a new dynamic of "reproductive success" emerges, which aims at achieving fertility rather than a live birth. Currently on offer in over a third of US clinics, IVF guarantee packages charge a higher fee in return for a refund in case there is no so-called take-home baby at the end of treatment.[33] These arrangements may reduce anxiety and increase access to repeat IVF cycles but have also been criticized as offering contingent fees for medical treatments and stacking the odds against patients by selecting only those with the best chances of having successful treatment.[34] Rather than a "take-home baby," reproductive success in OC packages is a matter of degree reflected in the quantity of frozen eggs.[35] Instead of a succession of IVF cycles, each of which represents a clear chance at successfully concluding treatment, the egg freezing process becomes an *ongoing course of fertility accumulation*, the endpoint of which is organized by new and rather flexible norms for the number of extracted eggs required for achieving a sense of reproductive success.[36]

A Calculus of Fertility: Reproductive Success and Multicycle Norms

As the abovementioned packages show, there is significant variation in the number of eggs that clinics recommend freezing. Achieving "reproductive success" is, then, a much less stable notion when success is measured in eggs rather than in babies. Especially given the relatively recent popularization of egg freezing, the limited information about the number of babies born from frozen eggs, and the considerable variation between women's bodies, clinics' guidelines for the number of eggs per desired child are by necessity an approximation. In determining this number, there is a tension between lowering the chances of future pregnancy with lower guideline numbers and increasing the risk of overtreatment by increasing them. Amid uncertainty about required egg numbers, it is clear that the recommended egg quantity increases with women's age and given that, at present, most women freeze their eggs in their late thirties, most women freezing their eggs will not yield the recommended number of eggs in one cycle.[37] Indeed, according to a survey on OC in the United States, the average woman who freezes her eggs returns for another cycle.[38]

When the reproductive value of the cryo-eggs is coupled with a particular quantity that becomes contractualized as reproductive success, the egg freezing decision is framed in an economic logic of cost per cycle or per egg—such as $5000 for 12 eggs. This foregrounds egg quantity and cost efficiency as the key levers in decisions about repeat cycles, rather than a primary focus on, for example, gauging medical risk, time investment, or emotional response to treatment. What is, then, at stake in the first phase of egg freezing is the emergence of a *calculus of fertility* in which expected success rates and egg quantities form the basis of a treatment rationale for determining the degree of "reproductive success" associated with the eggs in the freezer.

Precisely because there is no clear outcome of a live birth or lack thereof, the goalpost for reproductive success can become contingent on the fertility clinic's standards or new norms in egg freezing discourses. It is this uncertainty of the goalposts that makes drawing attention to the advertised treatment rationales so pertinent. The difference between a recommended 12 or 30 eggs to complete the first phase of an egg freezing course would typically translate into a difference of several treatment cycles and increased treatment costs running in the thousands. Because egg freezing is a practice that is marketed as a means for women to be proactive and motivated by a sense of being informed about fertility, there is potential for conflicts of interest as fertility companies at once offer this information, determine guideline numbers for pricing packages, and deliver the treatments themselves.

Although guaranteed "take-home baby" and multicycle IVF packages frequently result in patients paying more than they otherwise would, those who overpay because the treatment worked early on still report positive experiences because of the popular conceptualization of children as "priceless" and irreducible to market value.[39] If no child is born, the money-back arrangement mitigates the financial loss and offers people the means to pursue other options with the refund. In other words, these packages present a dynamic in which reproductive success is worth the financial investment, while the financial loss of reproductive failures is limited in comparison with a nonrefundable single-cycle payment.[40]

In egg freezing packages, where eggs instead of babies represent the treatment outcome, a different dynamic of pricelessness emerges. The cryo-eggs' pricelessness follows from their "promissory" value as vital elements for creating future children as well as what Waldby calls their "singularity" as a means to establish a genetic kinship link to this potential offspring.[41] Bringing together monetary and reproductive value in new ways, the cryo-eggs both promise a priceless future return and presently embody a reproductivity that is preserved while embodied fertility declines.

The pricelessness of frozen eggs also relates to the affects associated with the procedure in egg freezing discourses—including peace of mind, empowerment, and a sense of being in control. Much as the London Women's Clinic offers discounted three-cycle IVF packages and states that patients feel "more relaxed" from the outset because "they know that they have further opportunities for pregnancy," so the egg freezing packages cater to an affective result of relaxation, empowerment, and assurance associated with the potential and perceived fertility extensions enabled by frozen eggs. The very names of packages like "Assure 20" and "EggSAFE" foreground the sense of safety, security, and reassurance associated with the frozen eggs. In keeping with Schellart's sense that her biological clock ticked a little less loudly after she froze 20 eggs, the egg freezing treatment and financial packages position 12, 20, or 30 eggs as the reproductive achievement that functions as a reassuring endpoint for treatment. The priceless value of the eggs, then, follows from the way in which they are understood to turn the uncertainty associated with precarious fertility into a more assured bioprepared fertility. Yet precisely in this move, this unstable and changing referent of reproductive success can equally function to extend anticipatory anxiety beyond the first egg freezing cycle by setting up a multicycle norm through an egg-based calculus of fertility.

Financing Fertility

Because egg freezing packages have a relatively high up-front cost, they are frequently offered alongside fertility loans. This is not unique to OC practices; the distribution of consumer credit through clinics is widespread throughout the fertility industry. In the United States, almost 50% of fertility clinics mention credit on their websites, often through third-party fertility lenders, such as CapexMD, IntegraMed, and Prosper.[42] Reflecting a national context characterized by a fee-for-service economy of healthcare and higher treatment fees, 70% of women using fertility treatment in the United States accrued debt. Almost half of these women incurred over $10,000 in debt, and younger women (25 to 34) borrowed significantly more than their seniors.[43]

In the United Kingdom, where medical loans are much less prevalent due to the general health coverage of the NHS, fertility financing companies have only begun to appear more recently, in the 2010s. At the time of writing, Access Fertility, incorporated in 2013, offers multicycle and guarantee packages for 33 major UK clinics—including CARE, GCRM, and Bourn Hall—and Fertility Finance, incorporated in 2016, provides loans to pay for these packages. These two main players in UK fertility financing overlap with the US fertility sector, as clinicians from major US clinics hold majority shares in these companies. So while fertility lenders' websites typically emphasize the intention to help or understand intended parents' financial stress,[44] fertility loans offered through clinics also regularly double as investment opportunities for physicians, as is the case for major lenders, including the abovementioned CapexMD (US) and Access Fertility (UK).[45]

Fertility lenders may present financing as a "win-win situation" for patients and clinics that make treatment and package deals more accessible to intended parents, while also improving the clinics' cash flow.[46] In the case of multicycle and guarantee treatment packages in particular, clinics can increase revenue by requiring advance payment for future treatments and attracting more patients while lenders benefit from the interest paid over the loans required to meet the associated high up-front cost. In the particular type of reproductive-financial decision making that is required in package arrangements, the availability of loans runs the risk of encouraging overtreatment or overpayment.[47] Legal scholars have raised concerns about the potential conflict of interest arising from arrangements between clinics and lenders, given the specificity of the power and trust relation between doctors and patients and the potential financial incentives for prescribing both particular treatments and the means to finance them.[48] So while they may be valuable to people struggling to afford treatment, fertility loans can also change the dynamics between financial and reproductive decision making for patients and professionals alike.

High up-front costs present a different consideration for women who are interested in egg freezing. The group of potential egg freezers is quite

large; in one survey among over a thousand women, almost a third indicated that they would consider freezing their eggs. Yet what kept them
from doing so was, at least in part, the high treatment costs of egg freezing.[49] This is understandable; the total costs for an egg freezing cycle run
in the thousands in the United Kingdom and the Netherlands and av-
eraged $16,000 in the United States in 2017. The frozen eggs moreover
require annual storage fees that vary from €40 in the Netherlands to an
average of $1100 in New York City.[50] Traditionally, fertility clinics have
offered high-priced IVF treatments to a relatively low volume of patients
at rates that exceed 30% of the US average household income. Predictably,
highly educated, white, and middle-class people are overrepresented in
this group—even when treatment costs are covered by insurance.[51]

Likewise, the uptake of egg freezing is skewed towards this particular
group of women. June Carbone and Naomi Cahn propose that this reflects differences not only in access to wealth but also in education and
career opportunities, relationship patterns, and understandings about
the trade-offs between "work and family, fathers and mothers, single
and dual-parenting." As egg freezing reorients highly educated women
to "match the cycles of the male-oriented workplace they have won the
right to enter," Carbone and Cahn argue that it has the potential to exacerbate existing class differences in timing reproduction.[52] It likewise
reproduces other social stratifications; although economically privileged
people of all racial, ethnic, and national origins can and do freeze their
eggs, those more likely to possess the means to afford treatment or loans
remain "over-determined by the racial, class and opportunity structures
established over the previous centuries of slavery, genocide and colo-
nization."[53] Strikingly, however, unlike the reproductive stratifications
produced by more unambiguously conceptive technologies, egg freezing practices may reflect social inequalities that promote elite, affluent
childbearing, but in practice only a relatively limited number of children are born from frozen eggs as few women return to use them and
most cryo-eggs won't result in a live birth. The status of OC as at once
a reproductive and a nonreproductive technology thus complicates the
relation between access to this particular technology and its reproductive outcomes.

While access to egg freezing is largely determined by, and indeed reinforces, existing class and racial inequalities, the capital investments

in egg freezing reflect an effort to address a larger group of women as egg freezing candidates—including those who cannot (easily) afford the procedure and who are younger.[54] Because costs are a key barrier to treatment for these groups, which neither seek to get pregnant at present nor necessarily experience the urgency of a perceived "fertility cliff," it is not surprising that programs aimed at broadening the appeal of egg freezing are regularly offered in conjunction with offers of lower treatment costs as well as payment plans and fertility loans. This is particularly evident in the specialized financing that is at the forefront of three major egg freezing start-ups in the United States—Extend Fertility, Progyny, and Prelude—which seek to turn fertility preservation into a mainstream procedure.

Mainstreaming Fertility Preservation

Representing an alternative model for organizing fertility care, the three egg freezing start-ups function as integrated fertility companies that bring together different services on their online platforms. Rather than fertility clinics offering the OC procedure, these egg freezing start-ups amalgamate geographically dispersed clinical, financial, and communication services under one recognizable brand name, which becomes the point of contact for the (potential) patient.

These fertility start-ups have all received significant capital investment, as the increasing number of women freezing their eggs year on year suggested potential for future growth.[55] Buoyed by millions of dollars of private-equity and venture-capital investments, specialized egg freezing start-ups have emerged and scaled up rapidly, thereby changing the landscape of US IVF. Prelude Fertility, for example, is a major new player focused on egg freezing; it was founded in 2016 with the aid of a $200 million investment from Lee Equity. With its investment, Prelude bought dozens of IVF clinics across the country and became the second largest US fertility company within a year.[56] Extend Fertility has operated for a decade through its network of IVF clinics and, in 2016, opened the world's first egg-freezing-only clinic in New York.[57] This business is backed by private equity from North Peak Capital and received a further $15 million in 2019 from Regal Healthcare Capital Partners. Progyny, which sells fertility benefits covering egg freezing to employers, secured almost $100 million in equity to grow its corporate fertility benefit business, a process that has been aided by a strategic alliance with Mercer, the world's largest HR company.[58] Progyny subsequently became the first fertility benefits company to go public, as it started trading on the NASDAQ Stock Exchange under the ticker symbol "PGNY" in 2019. Symptomatic of a wider financialization of fertility, the funding attracted for these companies highlights that capital investment is a driving factor in the expansion and promotion of egg freezing.[59]

Online platforms provide a key means for these fertility start-ups to reach out to a larger group of potential patients as well as wider affiliated clinical networks. A case in point, Prelude used its equity investment to build a nationwide fertility network and concentrate its marketing efforts through its online presence—and this is exactly what the equity investors had in mind when they funded the company. Lee Equity was interested in the growth potential of IVF, in part because of the rising age of first-time mothers, some of whom would experience difficulty conceiving, but also because fertility "awareness" could function as a means to further broaden the demand for IVF-based treatments. Collins Ward, a partner at Lee Equity, says that the "biggest surprise" he encountered in the fertility industry was the "low awareness of fertility services." So the investment in Prelude was coupled with the "significant costs" of a big marketing push intended to, in Ward's words, "speak to younger patients and younger Americans who live in social and digital media." It is this drive to "increase awareness" that bears the promise of "a sizable upside in years to come" by proactively appealing to a new group of potential patients, who are themselves encouraged to be proactive about fertility.[60] Now comprising a nationwide network, Prelude's mission "to educate a generation of women of childbearing age about their fertility" and its "commitment to improving fertility awareness, and providing a proactive approach to family building" has a widespread reach.[61] This shows how the discursive framing of fertility as proactively extendable and capital investments in egg freezing mutually reinforce one another.

This platformized approach to promoting egg freezing combines presenting aesthetically pleasing fertility information that outlines the conditions for fertile women's self-referral with specific payment plans. Extend Fertility's online platform, for example, links detailed information about fertility decline with financial plans that allow women to purchase egg freezing from $101 a month, which is described as "a price that makes sense at this point in their lives."[62] Likewise, Prelude provides fertility and treatment information on its online platform and offers egg freezing payment plans that may be purchased from $99 a month, stating that "finances won't stand in your way."[63] Rather than the conventional fee-for-service approach to IVF, Prelude offers a long-term plan that lowers patients' initial financial investment, but extends the time of financial transaction with the fertility company. It thus sets up an ongoing financial engagement that mirrors an ongoing engagement with reproductive potential across the fertile and infertile life stages. Progyny instead promotes egg freezing through employer insurance packages, which have been adopted by a growing number of Fortune 500 companies.[64] Developed from a merger with Fertility Authority, the largest US online fertility portal with one million monthly visitors, Progyny's insurance services are intertwined with its online communication portfolio, consisting of its website, online concierge services, and mobile apps.

The shared message of these companies is that young women should be encouraged to be "proactive" in managing their fertility in the face of the progressive loss of their embodied eggs' reproductive potential. This notion of being "proactive" is at the core of these companies' missions. Prelude describes itself as "a comprehensive fertility company with a focus on providing proactive fertility care," a focus that is reflected in its slogan: "It's time to take charge of your fertility."[65] Likewise, Extend Fertility presents itself as "the first service in the country to focus exclusively on women who want to proactively preserve their fertility options," and CEO Gina Bartasi defines Progyny as a "leading digital healthcare company combining data and science to provide the first end-to-end, proactive fertility solution for employers."[66] The emphasis on proactive fertility care suggests a contradistinction with the existing—by implication reactive—model, in which clinics treat people who would like to have children, but experience infertility or other barriers to reproduction. By contrast, in the proactive model of fertility care, female fertility requires active, technologized management earlier in life in order to enable the possibility of having children later on.

The Debt Financing of Egg Freezing

When coupled with financing plans, this emphasis on proactive, earlier freezing expresses a treatment rationale in which it is better not to save up and freeze eggs later, but to do so now at "a price that makes sense" and preserve youthful reproductive potential sooner.[67] As the means to enable proactive freezing, fertility financing thus plays a key role in expanding the assisted reproduction market to include the fertility management of healthy, presumably fertile women. Fertility loans are presented as a form of financial support that increases access to egg freezing—albeit by making the people who can least afford it pay more over time.[68] By promoting both a "proactive" treatment rationale and fertility financing, this debt financing of egg freezing thus creates value through a double temporal movement of anticipation and deferral; it combines treating future infertility in the present and paying for present treatment in the future.

By means of this double movement of anticipation and deferral, egg freezing is not only a technology that extends infertility treatment to the fertile population; it also transforms fertility treatment into an *ongoing* relation of value exchange between women and fertility companies. Both through its future-oriented treatment rationale and its debt financing, egg freezing aligns neatly with the key premise of "relationship marketing": that "the real purpose of a business is to create and sustain mutually beneficial relationships."[69] Because it requires the financial and physical investment of an egg-extraction cycle at present, but defers potential fertilization and implantation procedures to the future, egg freezing particularly facilitates building a long-term relationship between the patient and the fertility clinic.

In relationship marketing, "the cement that binds successful relationships is the two-way flow of value."[70] The abovementioned egg freezing arrangements establish such a two-way flow of value between women and fertility companies through the figure of the egg. They require ongoing loan and storage payments to assure the eggs' continued preservation. In turn, the patient receives the priceless reproductive value ascribed to the cryo-eggs. As debt becomes itself a source of revenue for fertility companies and lenders, value is created through an exchange of financial and reproductive risk: as patients shift the risk of future infertility to the clinic through egg cryopreservation, clinics and lenders transfer the risk of nonpayment to patients through interest rates and fees.[71] In this dynamic exchange, fertility lending thus aligns companies' capital accumulation with patients' fertility accumulation.

However, because the cryo-eggs' value is not directly legible to the patient, the eggs are a rather adaptable referent for reproductive value. In the absence of a live birth to signify reproductive success, it is the discursive framing of the cryo-eggs as materializations of continued fertility, potential children, or a halted biological clock that renders them valuable. Egg freezing companies play a key role in discursively mediating the cryo-eggs by setting the terms for the exchange between capital and reproductive value in treatment and financial arrangements. If the exchange of capital and reproductive value couples the ongoing financial investment in the cryo-eggs with a symbolic investment in their continued reproductive value, egg freezing becomes a condition of emergence for a *capitalist reconfiguration* of reproductive aging, in which value exchange lies at the foundation of the postfertile relation between the cell and self.

Streamlining Fertility

The mainstreaming of egg freezing as a technology for ongoing, proactive fertility management in these networks is part of a broader development of *streamlining* treatments into pre-set pathways towards future reproduction. More than only a treatment to circumvent potential future infertility, egg freezing here functions as one element in fertility treatment packages that cover the entire reproductive process "from beginning to end." Egg freezing then becomes an entry point into a long-term, technologically managed reproductive trajectory across the life course.

Branded packages bundle a set of treatments under a single, binding rationality that both discursively constructs and offers to mitigate the precariousness of fertility from early adulthood onwards. For example, the Prelude Method bundles "freezing sperm and eggs when you are fertile, making embryos when you are ready, genetically sequencing parents and embryos to reduce the frequency of congenital illness, and transferring one at a time to reduce multiple pregnancies."[72] This method presents an alternative to the "menuization" of IVF, which has been controversial for requiring patients to decide whether they should include additional "add-on" treatments—such as genetic screening—in their IVF cycle. Instead, the Prelude Method proposes a streamlined approach to fertility management that combines egg freezing with a predefined treatment trajectory that spans an extended time during the reproductive life course and beyond. In this classic attempt at medicalization, egg freezing plays a pivotal role in a wider project of recruiting healthy people to undergo an IVF cycle and genetically screen their embryos. The financial-clinical rationale of the Prelude Method encourages an ongoing exchange of value in order to achieve a notion of risk-reduced fertility and reproduction.

The Prelude Method follows the vision of Martin Varsavsky, a serial entrepreneur who made his fortune with real estate, biotechnology, and telecom companies such as FON, self-reportedly the world's largest WiFi network, with 21 million hotspots across the globe. Branching out to fertility technologies, Varsavsky secured $200 million in investments to launch Prelude in 2016. He seeks to mainstream infertility treatment by appealing to the fertile population and convincing them to preserve their gametes and screen their embryos. Accordingly, Prelude is marketed as a "fertility company" rather than an infertility clinic. In this fertility company, reproductive technologies are not a treatment for infertility but "a complementary strategy to starting a family by having sex."[73] Just as US people generally *have* babies in clinics rather than at home, Varsavsky proposed at a technology conference in 2015, people should *make* children in clinics rather than in bed. He makes the case that, compared to the Prelude Method, relying only on sex to conceive runs increased risks of future infertility, medical abortions, miscarriage, and congenital diseases.[74] The Prelude Method is thus presented as a safer alternative to avoid such risks and "have a healthy baby when you are ready."[75]

As opposed to a binary between fertile and infertile states, the Prelude Method suggests a more postfertile approach in which these categories overlap:

As opposed to people who solely rely on sex to make babies, people who rely on both sex and Prelude have a much greater chance of achieving their parental goals of having healthy babies when they are ready. Prelude uses the technology available to infertile people, on fertile people. At Prelude we believe that something as important as having a baby, and equally important, a healthy baby, should not be left to chance.[76]

Varsavsky's words point to a shift away from distinct reproductive categories that separate out those who need fertility treatment and those who do not. Rather, the Prelude model points to a parallel shift that Kaushik Sunder Rajan described in the context of postgenomics: "a reconfiguration of subject categories away from normality and pathology and toward variability and risk, thereby placing *every* individual within a probability calculus as a potential target for therapeutic intervention."[77]

Varsavsky specifically positions age as the driving force behind this shift. He suggests that the Prelude Method is

an alternative that only occasionally would be necessary if millennials had their children at the same age as baby boomers had theirs. By stretching youth into our 40s, we've squeezed maternity out of the equation. A large segment of women is ending up with no children, or just one or two, when they wanted more. Or, because of advanced maternal and paternal age, they are having babies with significant health problems.[78]

Varsavsky thus proposes a shift towards a situation in which social constructions of "youth" and an incongruent biological "advanced maternal and paternal age" have begun to overlap. This shift motivates the new treatment rationale he proposes, in which reproductive technologies are no longer solely indicated for infertile people but also for a large, if class-specific, segment of a generational cohort whose continued fertility has become precarious in the face of changing trends of later reproduction.

The narrative of rising involuntary infertility provides the motivation for a shift towards a more speculative model of reproductive care that is universally indicated and organized around a self-investment logic. In this model, potential future childbearing requires ongoing reproductive risk management—with screened ovaries and frozen eggs—at a time that is altogether divorced from the moment in which a pregnancy is desired. With the move of serial entrepreneurs into the fertility industry, and the significant private equity investment raised for egg freezing, the very understanding of fertility becomes itself entrepreneurialized as the site of ongoing personal investment into reproductive futures.

Fertility Insurance

Yet this neoliberal self-investment logic, which marries reproductive and financial decision making, is not altogether individualized; it is also increasingly embedded in the organization of labor. Progyny's egg freezing benefit packages, which integrate reproductive and productive labor, illustrate this point. Not unlike Prelude, Progyny streamlines egg freezing into a long-term treatment package with its SMART™ (Science and Member-Driven Assisted Reproductive Technology) Cycle. This package covers consultations, tests, and infertility treatments, such as egg freezing, intra-cytoplasmic sperm injection (ICSI), assisted hatching, and genetic selection technologies (PGS) for single embryo transfer. Progyny describes its bundled coverage as

> the first end-to-end proactive fertility solution for both large, self-insured employers, as well as today's informed consumer looking to manage their reproductive health, reduce their time to pregnancy, reduce cost and improve outcomes.[79]

Akin to the Prelude Method, this approach similarly streamlines egg freezing into a more extensive treatment trajectory. Yet instead of a monthly payment package sold directly to women, Progyny arranges fertility benefits through their employers. The management of female reproductive risk is thus not only a matter of self-investment but is further expanded to include corporate investment in employees' continued fertility.

Progyny's SMART packages thus streamline egg freezing into a long-term, highly technologized treatment plan driven by a proactive rationale. On the one hand, this occurs through the coverage of future treatments, including "add-on" treatments like assisted hatching and genetic embryo screening (PGS).[80] On the other, Progyny's various online communication services provide the basis for conveying a treatment logic through which egg freezing makes sense as a form of investment on the part of both employer and employee. Self-identified as a digital health company, Progyny emphasizes online communication as an important part of its services, which include a "concierge fertility benefit" for remote treatment advice to people covered by the insurance, fertility education initiatives, podcasts, and mobile apps. In 2018, it moreover launched an app in collaboration with wellness technology company Happify Health to help people "manage their emotions in a way that supports their fertility objectives (with a goal of shortening the path to pregnancy)."[81] The particular logic of relying on reproductive technologies to both slow down reproductive aging and, later on, speed up "the path to pregnancy" thus becomes part of the discursive framing of egg freezing through Progyny's streamlined package of clinical, financial, and communication services.

When Facebook and Apple first started offering egg freezing insurance benefits in 2014, this move prompted widespread journalistic and scholarly discussions. Although some welcomed the initiative to broaden access to egg freezing technologies to the women working in these organizations, many commentators raised concerns about the covertly coercive nature of this benefit, which could be framed as an encouragement to delay having children and may send out a signal that career success and motherhood are incompatible. Questions have moreover been raised about whether these benefits cover all female employees equally, whether they would set new standards that require women to alter their bodies to fit into a workplace ideal, and whether they would jeopardize support for other policies, including enhanced salaries, family leave, childcare subsidies, holiday time, and general healthcare coverage.[82]

While the discussions about these benefits focused on the possibility that companies may be implicitly encouraging their female employees to delay having children, the rationales suggested to these companies rely on a more indirect logic of return on investment. Many companies offer the egg freezing benefits not in isolation but as part of relatively generous fertility and family benefits, often including parental leave, childcare services, and a "baby bonus." Even though this does not rule out that the addition of egg freezing could be an antinatalist measure in certain business cultures, it does suggest that cryopreservation and parental benefits are not, in principle or even in practice, mutually exclusive.[83]

Rather than necessarily discouraging employees' reproduction as such, these insurance packages encourage the abovementioned *proac-*

tive model of reproduction. Progyny makes the case for fertility benefits to companies by suggesting that this proactive approach to managing fertility will provide employers with better returns on investment (ROI) than the reactive model of IVF. The SMART Cycle, they suggest, proposes an alternative to a reactive model in which people undergo IVF treatment only when they are diagnosed as infertile and subsequently transfer multiple embryos at once to increase chances of a live birth per cycle. Progyny argues that this is not beneficial to employers, because they first risk paying for absenteeism associated with infertility and repeated IVF cycles. Subsequently, the higher percentages of multiple pregnancies associated with this approach could result in elevated costs of high-risk maternity care, multiples, and neonatal care (NICU) for employers, even if they did not pay for the original fertility treatment.

So instead Progyny suggests that its SMART Cycle offers a proactive alternative that uses younger, frozen eggs and implants fewer embryos after genetic testing. This, Progyny proposes, provides better return on investment because it limits the abovementioned costs associated with reactive IVF treatment. Furthermore, the company advises that the SMART cycle is a "retention tool" for HR departments and helps PR by fostering a company's "family friendly" and innovative image.[84] Within this ROI-driven treatment rationale, egg freezing is positioned as a sensible first step towards a more cost-efficient method of technologized reproduction for employees. With the introduction of OC workplace benefits, fertility thus becomes enlisted in the calculative practices of corporate insurance and human resource management, as well as the financial investment logics that underlie them. Therefore, the shift represented by egg freezing benefits is not so much a discouragement of reproduction altogether as an institutionalization of a proactive, technologized approach to fertility management, which is rationalized as a means of maximizing both reproductive and financial return on investment.

Beyond simply another perk, egg freezing benefits represent a broader, infrastructural shift both in the rationale for fertility treatment and in the organization of assisted reproduction. In 2019, Progyny served 80 self-insured employers across 20 industries, including three of the top 10 Fortune 500 companies, and its fertility benefits covered 1.4 million employees.[85] Its network spanned 800 fertility specialists across the United States.[86] Thus broadening its reach to more potential patients, this online, platformized organization of fertility treatment centralizes the discursive framing of egg freezing as, on the one hand, a tool for employees to self-invest in future fertility to both extend and speed up the time to pregnancy and, on the other, a tool for employers to increase ROI on health benefits. Egg freezing is thus at the heart of a "shift from current reactive treatments . . . to the proactive management of lifelong reproductive potential,"[87] which is reinforced through the employer and the online, platformized fertility company alike. Significantly, the notion of fertility itself is rethought through capital logic as the financial investment rationales for the employers underpin the suggested reproductive investment rationales for their patient-employees.

Conclusion

The emergence of the frozen egg as an entity that can exist outside of a woman's body, yet maintains its reproductive potential, poses new ways of imagining what it means to be fertile. In her account of undergoing the OC procedure, blogger Eggfreezer offers insight into the implications of the egg's temporal latency for the conceptualization of reproductive aging. The photographed frozen egg, and her textual framing of this image, convey that the eggs rendered visible in OC may be seen both as individualized "building blocks" of the potential future child and as a means to distribute reproductive embodiment across bodies and freezers. These cryopreserved cells also play a central role in the marketing and education efforts, treatment rationales, and calculative practices presented by fertility companies. When cryo-eggs become a metric for calculating chances of future reproduction, egg freezing is reframed as not necessarily a one-off intervention but rather a first step in a longer-term technologized reproductive trajectory.

Eggfreezer's presentation of her frozen egg highlights its potentiality, individuality, and temporal plasticity, while also framing it as the antidote to a decline narrative of embodied reproductive aging—it stays 32 forever in the freezer and the photograph. Rather than a supportive environment, Eggfreezer's body is positioned as a problematically aging vessel for the egg, to which the liquid nitrogen freezer is an ageless alternative. However, because Eggfreezer also reads the egg as "part of me," the cryopreserved cell's image also functions as the means to agentically reconfigure and reconceptualize reproductive aging as encompassing both cell and self. In this process, the egg's temporal plasticity becomes the basis for an engagement with finitude and a reflexive reconsideration of reproductive aging as a distributed process.

The precariousness of fertility characteristic of egg freezing discourses is, then, not only relevant to the initial stage of treatment but repeated in the *incremental steps* of fertility preservation. After the choice for egg freezing has been made, fertility can be rendered precarious once more after the first cycle. In the marketing of egg freezing by major fertility networks, the discursive framing of frozen eggs as measurements of reproductive time or reproductive potential is the foundation for treatment rationales that set up multicycle norms for OC treatment. The concomitant doubling or tripling of expenses may be mitigated by multicycle payment plans or guarantee plans. Because there is no current cultural or clinical consensus on the quantity or quality of eggs required for achieving a form of bioprepared fertility, patients are vulnerable to the potential conflicts of interest that may emerge in the absence of a clear marker of reproductive success. Situated in a reproductive-industrial complex in which increased treatment cycles benefit not only clinics but also third-party lenders, digital health networks, investors, and pharmaceutical companies, the choice to freeze one's eggs ought not to be conceptualized as simply an individual consideration, or only reflecting a set of social and demographic changes. Rather, it is important to also analyze how specific discursive mediations and clinical infrastructures provide the conditions for navigating the new reproductive and financial decisions that emerge with egg freezing.

In the context of US egg freezing, the financial products such as subscription, loan, and guarantee plans are presented as a means to democratize access to treatment, yet, in doing so, they set up a dynamic of investment and indebtedness in the process of preserving fertility. Characteristic of financialization, this brings debt relations to the heart of fertility preservation and sets up additional sources of OC-related revenue through financial products, while enabling more spending on treatment cycles. Fertility insurance displaces the promissory value and speculative investment associated with egg freezing to the level of the employer and thereby integrates the (financial) management of fertility into the realm of labor. In turn, equity investments in egg freez-ing start-ups have significantly reshaped the reproductive-industrial complex—through new mergers and acquisitions, network formations, online marketing, and financial products. The financialization of fer-tility, in this context, references the significant financial investments in a future in which ever more women freeze their eggs, the role of equity investments in establishing the clinical and commercial infra-structures through which egg freezing becomes accessible, the calcula-tive practices underlying dominant treatment rationales, and the role of financial products in shaping both the stories and the streamlining of fertility preservation.

This chapter's analysis of the framing and distribution of frozen eggs highlights how OC can function as an entrance point into a techno-logically mediated reproductive life course. It points to a shift in the presentation of egg freezing as not simply an intervention to extend fer-tility but rather a technology for ongoing fertility management. As noted above, these egg freezing practices enlist potential patients both before and after they become infertile. Unlike reproductive technologies that seek to achieve immediate conception and childbearing, egg freezing enables the construction of different material-discursive iterations of fertility throughout the life course. In this way, the biomedicalization of both infertility and fertility begins to overlap. Critics have pointed out how each stage of the (post)reproductive female life course has become biomedicalized and requires ongoing intervention, whether through the contraceptive pill, assisted reproductive technologies, or hormonal re-placement treatment. With egg freezing, these different phases of the biomedicalization of fertility start to overlap with one another: women may now physically and financially invest in simultaneously preventing conception with contraceptive pharmaceuticals and ensuring contin-ued fertility with egg freezing. This ongoing technologized reproductive management of women's bodies is indicative of an emergent postfertile condition, in which one can be at once too fertile and not fertile enough. As egg freezing practices expand the target group for assisted reproduc-tion, so embryo selection technologies expand the IVF cycle with ad-ditional steps and investments. One such embryo selection technology, which is linked to egg freezing and the instrumentalization of reproduc-tive time, is at the heart of the next chapter.

4

Aging Embryos and Viable Rhythms

The Visualization and Commercialization
of Time-Lapse Embryo Selection

On June 11, 2013, a baby named Eva was born in Glasgow. Nine months prior, the embryo from which Eva grew had been selected for implantation into her mother's womb with the aid of time-lapse embryo imaging. This technology films IVF embryos while they grow in the incubator and uses the visual information to predict which ones are most likely to result in a live birth. Eva's birth made national headlines because she was the first baby to be born after the use of a particular time-lapse system called "Early Embryo Viability Assessment" (Eeva).[1] The media coverage followed a press release by Auxogyn, the company that produced the Eeva system, which emphasized the visual nature of this technology by including a video of Eva's embryo in the press release.[2] Framed by logos and the caption of "Baby Eva," the video shows a black-and-white image of the fertilized egg, which divides several times before the green-lettered word "HIGH" appears above it, referring to the embryo's predicted viability.

Auxogyn lauded time-lapse embryo imaging as "the most important breakthrough in IVF in recent decades."[3] In an earlier *BBC News* report on a different time-lapse system called the EmbryoScope, Dr. Simon Fishel of CARE, the largest UK fertility group, similarly claimed, "In the 35 years I have been in this field, this is probably the most exciting and significant development that can be of value to all patients seeking IVF."[4] Although many questions have since been raised about its efficacy, time-lapse embryo imaging has changed the face of IVF by introducing a new set of images, risks, and investments that revolve around the fertilized egg and early embryonic aging.

In the egg freezing procedure, embryo selection is the next step after the cryo-eggs are thawed and fertilized. The resulting embryos are put in

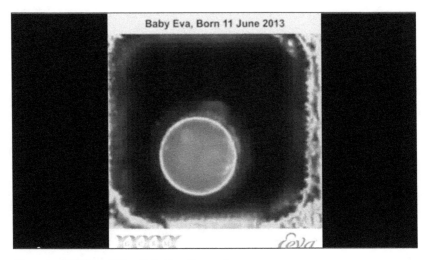

Figure 4.1. Still from Video *Baby Eva, Born 11 June 2013*.

an incubator for three to five days before they may be implanted in the womb. If more than one egg fertilizes and becomes an embryo, the embryologist will have to choose which embryo to implant. Conventional embryo selection requires embryologists to remove the embryos briefly from the incubator for a daily examination under the microscope. Time-lapse imaging technologies, by contrast, allow for continuous observation by taking photographs every 5 to 20 minutes while the embryos remain in the incubator. The resulting videos not only give increased insight into the embryos' appearance but also visualize a temporal dimension that remained invisible in the conventional method: the timing of cell divisions and the regularities of embryonic development. By matching the videos with growth patterns of embryos that developed into healthy fetuses, the time-lapse system suggests which embryos are most likely to grow into a baby.[5]

The efficacy of time-lapse embryo imaging remains contentious. Some studies suggest that this method may increase implantation, pregnancy, and live birth rates,[6] while others—including a Cochrane review—hold that the evidence of increased pregnancy or live birth rates is lacking or insufficient to justify the widespread clinical adoption of time-lapse embryo imaging.[7] And although the UK regulator likewise advises that "there's certainly not enough evidence to show that time-lapse imaging improves birth rates," it is currently on offer in the majority of UK clinics—often at an increased cost to the patient.[8] Meanwhile, some of the largest companies in the fertility sector have heavily invested in time-lapse imaging, including biotech company Vitrolife (EmbryoScope and Primo Vision) and pharmaceutical giant Merck (Geri and Eeva).[9]

With the clinical introduction of time-lapse imaging, embryo selection becomes a more visible step in the IVF process—one that requires new decisions and financial investments from patients, fertility clinics, and manufacturers. Forming a visual continuum with the egg's photograph discussed in the previous chapter, the first frames of these time-lapse videos depict the egg after fertilization and, as the cells divide, its subsequent transformation into an embryo. Emerging in the wake of influential visual reproductive technologies such as fetal ultrasound, time-lapse embryo imaging offers an even earlier encounter with prenatal life. And as the names of systems like EmbryoScope and Primo Vision suggest, the visualization of embryos is key to both the method and the marketing of time-lapse technology.

The observation of embryos is also instrumental in registering the *timing* of embryo development—or embryonic aging—as a key parameter for selecting which embryo(s) will be implanted in the womb.[10] The time-lapse systems film the developing embryos, quantify the visual information, and use this to predict their viability through algorithmic analysis. In doing so, time-lapse embryo imaging brings embryonic aging—e.g., the rhythmic regularity of cellular division—to the forefront of assisted reproduction. In other words, the precise timing of the embryonic aging process is central to this method of calculating embryo viability.

In keeping with this study's overall focus on aging and fertility, I here draw attention to the visualization, instrumentalization, and commercialization of embryonic aging in IVF. Drawing on the politicized history of imaging prenatal life, I analyze the rewriting of human origin stories with these prenatal images, in which embryos may be presented as individuals, collectives, or populations. What is at stake in the instrumentalization of embryonic aging in time-lapse embryo imaging is the creation of new risks, modes of value creation, and power relations in the fertility sector. The introduction of this technology must be situated in the context of consolidating fertility, biotech, and pharmaceutical

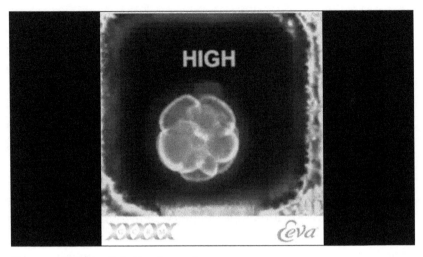

Figure 4.2. Still from *Baby Eva, Born 11 June 2013*.

companies, in which time-lapse embryo imaging may be employed to produce new kinds of biocapital. Whereas the earlier chapters addressed how embodied fertility became precarious in relation to the time of cryopreservation, here it is the time of embryonic aging that becomes a means of intensifying reproductive risk management and value generation in the IVF cycle. This method of embryo selection may then not just result in more or less "IVF success" but also affects the conceptualization and commercialization of aging at an embryonic level.[11]

Baby Embryo

The *Baby Eva* video shows a black-and-white image of a fertilized egg developing into an embryo. At the end of the video, the "HIGH" inscription above the embryo suggests a link between a HIGH prediction and a healthy baby.[12] This link between the prediction and the future child contributes to the framing of the embryo as an individual, an association that both has a politically charged history and aligns with the new treatment rationales of time-lapse embryo imaging.

This presentation of embryos as individuals fits into a wider trend of visualizing prenatal life at increasingly early stages of the reproductive process, in a visual continuum from gamete to baby—a trend that also emerged in the previous chapter. Following Eggfreezer's framing of the photographed egg as a "building block" of the potential future child, here the video portrays an origin story in which the embryo named "Baby Eva" is individualized as the coming into existence of an identifiable person.[13] In keeping with this individualized focus, the Eeva website presents its technology to intended parents by pointing out that "your embryo's journey is captured in video form during the critical first days of development." Thus positioning the video as a recording of a singular embryo, the website's use of direct address to consider "your" embryo emphasizes a parental responsibility towards this embryo and its journey—one that can be met by employing the technology at the "critical time" of the embryo's early existence.[14]

Described as "the ultimate home movie," the embryonic time-lapse videos read like the earliest recording of the future child's existence.[15] The recognition of these videos as "home videos," a genre associated with intimate family life, signals the kinship work implicit in individualizing the embryo as a potential family member to the intended parents. In these videos, the home video convention of filming significant events in children's lives to produce "future memories" meets an origin story that positions the incubated embryo as the beginning of children's lives.[16] In a similar way, the *Baby Eva* video firmly attaches the identity of the future child to these images and, by extension, suggests that the embryo's first cell divisions make up a significant, observable life event: a future memory for both the potential child and her parents.

The individuality of prenatal life, and its visualization in medical imagery, is center stage in scholarly discussions on ultrasound testing and fetal photography. Prenatal imagery has exceeded its medical function and plays a key role in patient experiences, reproductive politics, and the popular imagination of reproduction. Fetal images have been widely criticized for visually constructing an autonomous, individual fetus that appears to exist independently of its mother, thereby erasing the maternal body from view.[17] Anti-abortion campaigns have appealed to this medico-scientific imagery to extend personhood to the fetus and politicize the timing of its development, with the aim of reducing time limits on, and access to, abortion.[18] Fetal ultrasounds have also become widely recognized and circulated images of prenatal kinship. For many expectant parents, the encounter with the ultrasound image is an integral part of the pregnancy experience.[19] The presumed affect raised by these fetal images is moreover mobilized in anti-abortion US policies enforcing mandatory pre-abortion ultrasounds.[20] In these examples, the fetus's visual resemblance to the potential future child is capitalized upon to extend claims of individuality and personhood to it.

The image of the embryo, by contrast, has been used as an argument against its individuality. For instance, the embryo's image played a key role in ethical debates on the regulation of embryo research. In the United Kingdom, the visible development of the embryo's "primitive streak" 14 days after conception marks the moment until which embryos can legally be cultured *in vitro*. In the debates that led up to the establishment of this 14-day limit in UK law, proponents of embryo research used the embryo's image to argue against its individuality and pointed to its appearance as a cluster of cells that lacks recognizably human features. For example, one *Sunday Times* columnist explained that early embryos merely appear as "'stem cells' . . . stuck together like fluorescent frogspawn."[21] Here early embryos are disavowed as lacking distinguishable and observable human elements and resembling the less valuable reproductive tissue of another species.

While the embryo images functioned to dissociate the embryo from fetal imagery in these debates, the visual representations of embryos appear to work to the opposite effect in a clinical context. In Sheryl de Lacey's study of IVF patients viewing their embryos, the participants—all but one of whom became parents—described the experience of seeing embryos as an affirmation of them being "real":

> We've got a photo taken the day they [points to her twins] got implanted. So you look at it and you think "yeah, well there's Kylie and Jason sitting there." Martha points out the impact of the visual: "They're real [the embryos], they're very real and not many people see their children at eight and ten cells."[22]

The time-lapse embryo videos may similarly entail a significant visual encounter for patients, in which the embryos also present the active progression from fertilized egg to developing embryo.[23]

Compared to De Lacey's static embryo images, the time-lapse videos convey the embryos' liveliness even more vividly, not only because

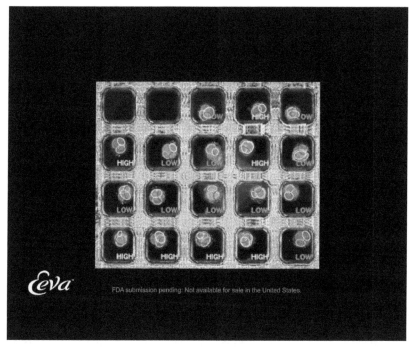

Figure 4.3. Still from *Eeva in Action (ASRM 2013)*.[24]

they are moving images but also because they create the illusion of time speeding up. In this they are reminiscent of early scientific films produced over a century ago that showed sped-up cell development. These videos of wriggling, dividing cells had the effect of both convincing audiences that "what they were seeing was really life" and making "the subject more real . . . than still images."[25] In the time-lapse videos, the speeding-up of playback time similarly makes the embryos appear more alive, as they wobble and divide in their microwells.[26] If the recording and playback speed had been the same, the cells would appear motionless, save for an occasional cell division. Yet as Baby Eva's embryonic development over the course of several days is compressed into a one-minute video, the increased speed dramatizes a much slower, less spectacular process and imbues the cells with a visible liveliness. The effect of recognizing the embryos' "realness" in the visual encounter that De Lacey's intended parents expressed may thus be intensified with embryo videos. This individualized liveliness of the embryo rendered real through accelerated motion has particular appeal in the ART context, where the association of embryos and future children is at the heart of the IVF practice.

Embryo Collectives: Grids of Potential

When the single embryo frame is zoomed out, a second set of images emerges that shows a grid of several embryos developing at the same time. A collective of embryos is growing side by side, each dividing its cells at different moments and wriggling independently within its square. The grid visually juxtaposes the differences between the embryos and thereby invites a comparison: some divide their cells steadily, while others lag behind. In doing so, the videos visualize the uneven development of the incubated embryos and the concomitant need for embryo selection. A valuation is attached to the active, inactive, or seemingly erratic behavior of the embryos in the last seconds of the video, when a red "LOW" or a green "HIGH" appears underneath each of them.

This grid image presents the group of embryos in a vastly different way from the single embryo that was celebrated as Baby Eva. In contrast with its individualized counterpart, the grid video depicts the potentiality of life that a set of embryos hold collectively—a potentiality that is not only dependent on the quality of the organic material, as is emphasized in discourses about age-related egg quality in OC, but can be actualized through an investment in the right technology for selection.

The time-lapse videos present the embryos as visibly fallible, as some cease to develop prematurely and others balloon to unusually large sizes. They thus visualize an alternative organization of the reproductive process in which not only sperm but also embryos function as a multitude that requires selection. Popular and scientific understandings of sperm selection typically present the female reproductive tract as the *in vivo* selection mechanism to prevent substandard sperm cells from interacting with the single egg released in ovulation.[27] In these embryo videos, it is the time-lapse system that similarly provides a selection mechanism to prevent substandard embryos from being implanted. The logic of embodied "natural" reproductive selection of sperm thus matches with a moment of *in vitro* technocultural selection of embryos.

By visualizing the need for selection in this way, time-lapse embryo imaging is part of a broader trend in which reproductive technologies are used as a means of improving the timing of reproductive processes. Whereas egg freezing is presented as a solution to female reproductive aging by *slowing* down cellular time, time-lapse imaging is discussed as a technology for *speeding* up the reproductive process. Embryologists sceptical of time-lapse imaging suggest that, even if the technology would improve selection over conventional morphological assessment, this would not improve pregnancy and birth rates because high-quality embryos could be frozen and implanted one by one.[28] Yet proponents suggest that time-lapse embryo selection is preferable to conventional selection to limit the number of implantations and shorten the time to a viable pregnancy. In keeping with this approach, large pharmaceutical companies such as Merck match their investment in the promotion and distribution of time-lapse technologies with a foregrounding of the concept of "time to live birth" (TTLB) as a measure of the effectiveness and efficiency of an intervention.[29] By showing the differential fallibility of an embryo collective, time-lapse embryo videos present a visual argument for embryo selection that may function more broadly as a technology to reconceptualize "IVF success" in temporal terms, as a speeding up of the reproductive process.

In the abovementioned *BBC News* item on the EmbryoScope, Dr. Fishel draws a link between *in vivo* and *in vitro* reproduction when he describes the time-lapse embryo-imaging apparatus as "almost like having the embryo in the womb with a camera on [it]."[30] Fishel's assertion suggests that the time-lapse embryo-imaging apparatus functions as an alternative, technocultural "womb" in which embryos can be observed through the integration of the camera.[31] The notion that the embryo videos show what we would see if we could put a camera in the womb not only naturalizes embryo selection as comparable to *in vivo* processes but also implies that the time-lapse apparatus in fact constitutes an improvement on the inconveniently opaque body as it allows embryologists and intended parents to observe, culture, and assess several embryos at once. Following Sarah Franklin's description of IVF as a model system that is "at once an imitation and a substitute for the *in vivo* process it models *in vitro*" and thereby "replicat[es] it in glass in a manner that both reveals how it works and changes this process into something else," time-lapse videos both reveal the embryonic aging process and visualize the embryos as a collective that requires selection.[32]

The framing of a single embryo representing Baby Eva and the grid image of embryos thus represent two very different origin stories. The former image, with its individualized embryo, appears to correspond to an origin story that has been upheld in pro-life debates that "life begins at conception," and indeed the image could be employed to visualize that standpoint.[33] However, the Eeva press release does not ascribe personhood to every embryo, but specifically frames this image with the text "Baby Eva, Born 11 June 2013." This particular embryo is therefore ascribed personhood *because* it was born; only after June 11, 2013, does it retrospectively gain individuality as an embryo.

By contrast, the grid image of the embryos, with its weak and strong elements, does not individualize the embryos but visualizes the need for their selection in anticipation of a potential pregnancy and birth. Auxogyn's Eeva website presents its embryo-selection method as the "difference you need for IVF success" and the test to "help reduce the risk of IVF failure."[34] This discourse of risk and success is matched in the grid image, which shows the embryo's observably arrested, erratic, or active development and overlays them with "high" and "low" inscriptions. With this visualization of the fallible nature of the embryos, the time-lapse grid image may be employed to reframe reproduction as technological achievement and the embryos as material that requires selection. While the textual framing of "Baby Eva" individualizes the embryo retrospectively, the "HIGH" and "LOW" inscriptions in the grid image show an anticipatory orientation towards the embryos, in which they figure as a collective with weak and strong elements that holds the potential for a future live birth.

What distinguishes these two framings of the embryo is less a matter of content—one is simply a zoomed-in version of one of the embryos in the grid—and more a matter of temporality. While the image of the embryo grid signifies an *anticipatory* potential throughout the process of selection and awaiting pregnancy, the single embryo *retrospectively* becomes meaningful as an individual once a birth, or even an ultrasound, has taken place that establishes individual personhood.

Datafied Embryo Populations

Alongside the embryo collective and the individualized embryo, there is a third type of embryo at the heart of time-lapse imaging: a historical population of datafied embryos that have previously been observed and selected in these systems. All major time-lapse systems are currently matched with proprietary algorithmic software packages, developed on the basis of data gathered from previously incubated embryos, which provide a data-driven tool for automatically selecting embryos for implantation. The time-lapse videos conclude with an assessment of each embryo—e.g., the "HIGH" or "LOW" displayed in the abovementioned images—which reflects the outcome of this algorithmic analysis.

Time-lapse embryo imaging systems thus do not only observe the small embryo cohorts depicted in the grid image but can also collect data over time and thereby translate a larger population of embryos into a body of visual and temporal information. When this data is used to create algorithms for selection, the *in silico* embryo populations provide an analytic frame for observing the incubated *in vitro* embryo collective. As a result, the embryo videos depict not only a synchronous comparison between the incubated embryos but also a diachronic one in relation to preceding populations. Through the lens of earlier observations caught in a database, the statistically rendered embryonic population frames the image of the developing embryo in the incubator's eye.

By matching the embryos' cellular growth patterns to previous embryonic populations' recorded developmental rhythms, time-lapse technology brings embryonic aging to the forefront in embryo selection.[35] With this shift, the timing of embryonic development becomes a key metric for determining which embryo can grow towards the fetal stage, which returns to the freezer, is discarded, or remains in the lab for further research. Giving new meaning to Franklin's "instrumental reframing of reproduction as technology," the time-lapse apparatus thus renders embryonic aging—its temporal regularities and its predictive value in anticipating future growth—into a technology.[36]

Paradoxically, in this process of making embryonic aging more visible in time-lapse technologies, human vision is displaced as the only lens employed for embryo selection. Not only are regularities of timing and textures that are not observable to the human eye detected through pattern-recognition operations, but the vast data sets that inform the assessment of the images become a component of what it means to "see" the embryo. Automated pattern recognition and algorithmic predictive analysis thus open up a new, data-driven way of seeing, an *in silico* vision, that integrates observation and calculation.[37] Reproductive decision making on the part of embryologists and intended parents becomes integrated with these new ways of seeing that increase the embryos' visibility to a greater number of people yet make the foundations of the decision-making process more opaque by relying on invisible data flows and algorithms. In other words, more people can see the embryos, yet what is seen—and what we should look at—shifts in datafied models of time-lapse embryo selection. What is at stake in viewing the embryo as if there were a camera in the womb is therefore not simply a question of making the embryos visible but of making this visibility legible as a tool for selection.

As the time-lapse embryo imaging apparatus incubates, observes, and assesses the embryo, the embryonic tissue is variably visualized as a prenatal individual, as a collective that requires selection, and as a datafied population that becomes integrated and instrumentalized in the time-lapse system. These approaches to visualizing the embryo follow from different temporal vantage points, in which the cellular tissue becomes meaningful retrospectively, anticipatorily, or, combining the two, as historical data for future selections. As the embryo videos become legible through the comparison with earlier populations, the visualization of the embryos' development is rendered into a tool for selection and embryonic aging becomes itself part of the time-lapse technology—and thereby holds significant commercial potential.

The Biovalue of Embryonic Aging

With the introduction of time-lapse technologies, embryonic aging has become instrumentalized as a highly marketable tool for selection. Embryonic aging is rendered valuable in the time-lapse system through its observation and transformation into cell cycle data, which may be used to derive parameters and algorithms that predict the viability of other embryos. In the translations from cell divisions to data to method, these technologies produce what Catherine Waldby calls "biovalue," which "refers to the yield of both vitality and profitability produced by the biotechnical reformulation of living processes."[38] In time-lapse selection, embryonic aging becomes the foundation for potentially increasing both vitality, by transforming the embryo selection procedure, and profitability, by both offering a new step in IVF that comes with an additional price tag and reframing embryonic aging as patentable property.

In the fertility clinic, time-lapse embryo imaging generates biovalue by bringing the embryo into the intended parents' view and presenting them with additional clinical and financial choices for their IVF cycle. In the embryo videos' grid of potential, the risk of implanting the wrong embryos becomes visible—and time-lapse technologies are presented as a way of reducing it. When time-lapse imaging is promoted as a visible way of relating to "your embryos," it suggests an individual and financial responsibility for managing the embryos' potential. Meanwhile, producers of the systems appeal to IVF clinics by making the business case for time-lapse embryo imaging both as a high-tech marketing tool and as a means to increase income per cycle, given that the estimated cost is significantly lower than the standard selling price per treatment.[39] Embryonic aging is thus at the heart of an expansion of the IVF cycle with time-lapse techniques, which may increase the biovalue of both a more profitable treatment cycle and, if only potentially, a more efficient use of the analyzed embryos themselves.

Time-lapse embryo imaging moreover provides the occasion for *patenting* embryonic aging as a tool for selection. As Waldby states, "The process of producing biovalue is also the process of technical innovation that enables the patenting of cell lines . . . as inventions, securing their status as intellectual property and possible sources of profit for their inventors."[40] Rather than generating new cellular life forms, time-lapse technology produces new forms of biovalue enabled by reframing the embryonic aging process itself—its visual registration and its function as a tool for predictive analysis—as patentable property.

Since 2011, the timings of cellular development have been patented as "predictive parameters" for embryo selection. Both US and European patent offices issued the first time-lapse patents to Stanford University, with exclusive licensing to Auxogyn (now Progyny), the company that produced the Eeva system. The patents describe the association of "good developmental competence" with temporal markers of cellular development, such as a "cytokinesis 1 that lasts about 0–30 minutes" and a "time interval . . . between the resolution of cytokinesis 1 and the onset of cytokinesis 2 [of] 8–15 hours."[41] Rather than describing only the method of time-lapse analysis, the patent also covers the time it takes for cells to divide and develop as part of Auxogyn's intellectual property.

With the issuing of these patents, the question arises to what extent the timing of embryonic aging is a natural phenomenon, and therefore unpatentable, or an essential part of a new, patentable invention. Jacques Cohen, chief editor of *Reproductive BioMedicine Online*, led a scholarly response to the Auxogyn patents and wrote a plea in this journal against "patenting time and other natural phenomena":

> Claiming cell cycle timing or duration as an invention that merits a patent would strike most students of developmental biology as an unlikely proposition but researchers at Stanford University have successfully done exactly that! The first three cell cycles in the human embryo developing *in vitro* are now owned by a corporation.[42]

Cohen argued that "the length of the cell cycle is not an invention and its key role in development is not a new observation; it is an indisputable and well-known fact of nature" that has been described since the late 19th century. A precedent of patenting temporal cellular phenomena, he claimed, will have long-term problematic effects.[43] In response, Stanford professor and inventor of the patent, Renee Reijo Pera, claimed that the patents cover the "assays intended to distinguish optimal [and suboptimal] embryos for transfer in IVF" and therefore entail a method rather than a natural phenomenon.[44]

In the ensuing riposte between Reijo Pera and Cohen, the former argued that the "diagnosis of embryo viability" does not address a "naturally occurring phenomenon" because there is "no need to distinguish quality amongst as many as 5–10 embryos (or even more) in natural conception; and in nature women simply do not conceive outside of the body."[45] Cohen responded that no studies have supported the premise that *in vivo* and *in vitro* cell cycles are fundamentally different processes; in fact, it is their close resemblance that has resulted in the birth of over five million children from IVF. "Arguing that those processes were somehow not natural (and therefore patentable)," he suggested, "may instigate an entirely different discussion, not unlike those that engaged the opponents of IVF in its early days."[46]

Yet what is at stake here is not so much the nature of the incubated embryos' naturalness but the reconceptualization of embryonic aging as part of the time-lapse technology and method. In time-lapse systems, every incubated embryo may not only produce a fetus but also generate a new data set that may be instrumentalized for future selections. The incubated embryos thus become nodes for data generation, which at once propel clinical and scientific knowledge production and steer embryological decision making for future selections. Once datafied as both tool and object of selection, the incubated developing embryo enters the realm of economic valuation not, in the first instance, as an exchangeable commodity but rather as a generative node in an ongoing automated process of data and algorithm production that anticipates and, potentially, enables future reproduction.[47] The key transformative aspect of time-lapse embryo imaging thus follows from the *data-generativity* of the embryo and the particular ways in which knowledge, reproductive value, and capital value become enmeshed in the datafication of embryo selection.

Algorithms for Embryo Selection

This datafication of embryo selection reconfigures the nature of reproductive decision making in IVF, as embryologists may now combine their visual assessment of the embryos with the algorithmic analysis of the machine. At a time when time-lapse distributors such as Merck are investing in a drive towards automation and standardization in IVF, decisions about embryo selection are becoming heavily reliant on large data sets and new interfaces through which the embryo, and its potential reproductivity, become legible. This shift relies on the emergence of specific algorithms developed on the basis of data taken from previous embryo populations, which have become products in their own right and are integral to the commercialization strategies of data-driven embryo selection.

When IVF cycles become data generating, the fertility clinic takes up a new role of gathering sizeable data sets on developing embryos and, in some cases, using these to develop in-house algorithms. Time-lapse system producers, likewise, are gaining access to uniquely large, privately held data sets about embryo development, which may be used to create new algorithmic products for embryo selection. For example, Vitrolife, producer of the popular EmbryoScope system, has access to embryo development profiles and implantation outcomes from over 30,000 embryos. Embryologists and IVF clinics worldwide have contributed to this data set since 2009, thus reportedly creating "the world's largest database of embryo development with known clinical outcome."[48]

Rather than being inherently valuable, these large-scale data sets extracted from developing embryos only acquire value when they are "reinstated into specific forms of labour and care—when data are collated, curated, interpreted and otherwise acted upon."[49] This work of rendering embryo data valuable in both reproductive and monetary terms is one of the new forms of labor emerging with datafication that becomes visible in the marketing of algorithmic software for embryo selection. CARE Fertility, for example, has developed its own proprietary algorithms for embryo selection using the Embryoscope. Beyond the potential for improving reproductive outcomes in their reproductive cycles, this process itself has become part of its communication to patients:

> Our scientists are world-leaders in time-lapse technology, and our CAREmaps technique is really highly developed; we've innovated models that can help us choose the best embryo more reliably, allowing us to see whether each has a low, medium, or high chance of success.[50]

Not only promoting time-lapse embryo imaging itself, the CARE website specifically markets its proprietary CAREmaps (morphokinetic algorithms to predict success) algorithmic model as the key to IVF success. The datafication of embryo selection thus creates novel algorithmic products, which are a testament to the introduction of new forms of bioinformatical labor in the fertility clinic. As CAREmaps shows, these algorithms may not only affect clinical outcomes but also aid the branding of both the clinic's innovative identity and an add-on technology that comes at an additional cost to intended parents.

The producers of time-lapse systems likewise use embryo data to develop new algorithmic products. Vitrolife's "largest database" of embryo data and known implantation data (KID) outcomes is translated into a valuable asset through its KIDScore tool. Clinics can purchase this software package along with the EmbryoScope, which consists of algorithms that measure the "implantation potential" of the embryos in the incubator and provide a "morphokinetic score" between one and five to embryologists, who can then "select the embryos ranked high with better chances of implanting and becoming a child."[51] The rival system Geri—distributed by pharmaceutical giant Merck—is similarly coupled with the Xtend Algorithm and Eeva software packages, which were developed on the basis of multicenter reference data on file at producer Progyny.[52] KIDScore, Xtend Algorithm, and Eeva software assign scores to the embryos to indicate which are more likely to survive. Given that these algorithmic tools rely on large sets of "known implantation data," this practice newly aligns the generation of biodata with the generation of biocapital. Social scientist Linda Hogle argues that a "tidal wave of efforts to extract value from health data has accompanied the big data phenomena, leading to considerable investments by pharmaceutical, medical device and health risk management companies"—and, in this case, leading to algorithmic products in their own right.[53]

The development of these algorithmic products relies on the presence of existing networks of data connectivities between pharmaceutical, biotechnological, and fertility companies, given that software such as KIDScore was developed on the basis of data sets sourced from IVF clinics across the world. The (contested) claim that such networked embryo data collection and comparison is feasible and reliable with these time-lapse systems is itself a key element in the marketization of these algorithmic products. After all, their selling point is not simply the promise of improved pregnancy rates but an improved workflow in the lab. Vitrolife emphasizes that KIDScore is easy to use and requires annotation of only a limited number of variables, which its predictive analytics method anticipates and preselects. This is presented as a beneficial effect because it can enable a "high level of consistency in embryo scoring in your clinic."[54] This discursive framing of the software points to "an overarching principle of interchangeability" underlying the promise of time-lapse embryo imaging, which applies not only to intra-clinic but also to inter-clinic variation.[55] It is this principle that motivates the claim that "KIDScore is universal to all clinics and can be used immediately without acquiring your own data first."[56] The upholding of a model of universality and interchangeable standardization is both a key driver and an effect of the datafication of embryo selection.

A next step in the development of this technology is to employ machine learning and integrate artificial intelligence into automated embryo selection. This approach is rapidly gaining traction in the IVF community; the two largest reproductive medicine conferences (ESHRE and ASRM) have recently seen a remarkable increase in the number of studies presented on these methods, while large companies such as Merck and Vitrolife used the events to showcase their investments in these approaches both through new products and at industry symposia.[57] In artificial intelligence approaches to embryo selection, large data sets with information about the incubated embryos and their viability can be used to automatically generate algorithms for selection. Based on pattern recognition methods, rather than preformulated hypotheses, artificial intelligence systems can use preexisting data of quantified embryo observations to self-learn and self-generate algorithms for embryo selection. If such algorithms can create higher success rates, the resultant selection methods are not necessarily based on biological understanding of the observed phenomena—but rather on algorithmic and statistical data analysis.[58]

At the time of writing, privately listed Australian fertility company Virtus Health is rolling out the first artificial intelligence (AI) product for embryo selection. Ivy, as it is called, has "taught itself how to select out the embryo with the highest potential to create a fetal heart." The data scientist who developed Ivy explains that

> it starts off with a completely blank canvas and it's not influenced by any previous human knowledge or bias. It has learned directly from thousands of embryos that have had a known fetal heart outcome and has slowly and stead[il]y improved itself to become better and better at selecting embryos.[59]

At the fertility clinics owned by Virtus Health, Ivy is touted as having "the potential to transform IVF medicine by shortening the timeframe to a successful pregnancy" because it provides a so-called "EmbryoScore predicting an embryo's potential to develop a fetal heart."[60] This approach is bound to have a wider reach as Vitrolife, which produces the Embryoscope, has partnered with Virtus Health to use AI for time-lapse embryo selection. Likewise, Merck, which distributes the Geri system, has launched new automated embryo analysis products that rely on AI technology.[61] The introduction of artificial intelligence in artificial reproduction is thus currently giving rise to new clinical and research practices, which directly affect which embryos are legible as viable and therefore implanted, preserved, or discarded.

The data-driven approach to embryo selection with time-lapse embryo imaging thus entails at once the clinical introduction of integrated apparatuses for reproductive data generation, the creation of connected networks of data sharing, and the production of biocapital out of biodata by means of algorithmization—all of which combine in a system that is marketed directly to patients and fertility clinics. The instrumentalization of embryo-aging data in the drive towards automating and standardizing embryo selection not only creates new forms of biovalue but also reorders institutional relationships between fertility, biotech, and pharmaceutical companies.

The Institutional Genealogy of Time-Lapse Embryo Imaging

The significant financial investments in time-lapse embryo imaging over the last decade are indicative of an infrastructural shift away from conventional to time-lapse embryo selection, thereby creating new power dynamics within the fertility sector. Swedish Vitrolife, the company that produces Primo Vision, saw a continuous increase in sales of the systems from 13 to 30 million SEK (Swedish krona) per quarter in the 2013–2014 period. In 2014, Vitrolife acquired Fertilitech and its EmbryoScope and more than doubled its sales.[62] By 2018, its time-lapse products were installed in over a thousand clinics worldwide, and Vitrolife reported almost 300 million SEK in global sales of time-lapse technologies.[63] After the company received regulatory approval for its Embryoscope system in China and the United States, two of the world's largest fertility markets, in 2018, sales were set to increase once again.[64] The distribution of significant numbers of machines to fertility clinics and laboratories—a majority of UK clinics have time-lapse systems—entails a shift both in the knowledge production about embryonic development and in clinical IVF practice.[65]

As fertility clinics invest in time-lapse imaging hardware and software, more patients are likely to come across this add-on technology and more embryo videos will come into circulation, both within the clinic and beyond. In the United Kingdom, for example, time-lapse embryo imaging has become more prevalent over the years. In the 2013–2016 period, 14% of all IVF patients used time-lapse selection; this went up to 22% in the 2016–2018 period.[66] Given that the time-lapse videos are also tools for patient communication, this increase means that more patients are likely to encounter these embryo videos. Clinics such as CARE Fertility have dedicated sections on their websites that use the embryo videos to market time-lapse embryo imaging to intended parents as a means to "predict success." Drawing on the aforementioned frame of the individualized embryo, the CARE website includes a video titled "Jaycie's Journey," which is presented as a "world first film" of a child filmed "from the moment of conception, from one cell, through to the one hundred trillion cells at birth using Embryoscope time-lapse imaging."[67] Instead of addressing the intended parents directly, Vitrolife's CEO Thomas Axelsson appeals to the clinics by stating that time-lapse imaging "improves clinics' profitability through the availability of additional services [and] marketing of improved treatment results."[68] CARE Fertility's inclusion of a "special download" of the time-lapse videos after embryo transfer as part of their IVF package is an example of such an additional service. The embryo videos thus fulfill multiple functions as diagnostic, patient communication, and marketing tools.

Significantly, these additional functions of the embryo videos are materialized in the EmbryoScope apparatus itself, which features a dedicated "EmbryoScope® Counseling App." This app, developed "to improve patient communication," can be used with a tablet to show intended parents the merits of time-lapse selection with the visual aid of embryo videos.[69] If they opt in, the treating doctor can show them their developing embryos on the app. In this way, the framing and distribution of embryo videos to the intended parents is built into the time-lapse system. Genea's time-lapse machine Geri takes this approach one step further with its "Grow" app, which allows intended parents to live stream videos of the developing embryos from the incubator to their smartphones. Such features could provide an extra selling point for future patients as they may provide reassurance and involvement during a time that is otherwise characterized by waiting for news from the fertility clinic.[70]

By bringing the embryos into view, time-lapse embryo imaging particularly lends itself to becoming a patient-driven technology that brings the embryo selection step in IVF procedures into the realm of intended parents' reproductive decision making. The move towards making time-lapse imaging more patient-driven presents a demand on fertility clinics' integrity to counterbalance the facts that, on the one hand, the intervention is not always suitable or required in all IVF cycles—especially given that evidence of its efficacy is currently limited—and that, on the other, there are significant financial stakes involved, given the investments made in this technology by clinics and producers alike.[71]

More than simply an add-on to the IVF cycle, time-lapse embryo imaging is at the center of a broader shift in the production of value through the consolidation of previously separate fertility services. This trend of consolidation is played out in major fertility companies, such as Merck, Cooper Surgical, Vitrolife, and Progyny, which all share the mission of creating a portfolio that covers each step of the IVF cycle. After their initial production in smaller biotech start-ups (Fertilitech, Auxogyn), as of 2015 all four major time-lapse machines are currently owned or distributed by two companies that sell not only time-lapse machines but also other products required for treatment. Vitrolife, the time-lapse market leader that owns both the Embryoscope and Primo Vision, presents itself as providing "an unbroken chain" of products for "every step during the fertility treatment," including culture media, culture dishes, pipettes, and needles.[72] Here time-lapse embryo imaging has become a link in the unbroken chain of IVF treatment.

Pharmaceutical giant Merck, with a revenue of over $40 billion in 2018, aims to be a "holistic fertility provider" by distributing the Geri and Eeva time-lapse embryo systems alongside its fertility drug portfolio as part of a mission to cover "every stage of the reproductive cycle."[73] Offering, in business terms, "turnkey" or "end-to-end" solutions in fertility care, these consolidated companies have a stake in an increasing number of steps and aspects of fertility treatment. As the market leader in fertility pharmaceuticals, Merck previously focused primarily on selling hormonal drugs used in IVF cycles. In 2014, Merck began to expand its drug portfolio with lab-based fertility biotechnologies, stating that it recognized the importance of these technologies in improving IVF outcomes. This portfolio expansion occurred around the same time as the introduction of biosimilars of Merck's major fertility drugs—including those for follicle stimulation and the triggering shot for inducing ovulation before egg extraction.[74]

After commercializing and distributing Progyny's Eeva and Genea's Geri systems alongside one another, Merck integrated the two systems in 2017. Bringing together Eeva's software and dark-field microscope with Geri's incubator and bright-field microscope, the merging of the two machines materialized another consolidating move in the genealogy of time-lapse embryo imaging. Merck, in turn, continued this consolidating trend by partnering with fertility- and genetics-focused biotechnology companies Genea and Illumina to create the Global Fertility Alliance, which was aimed at "raising awareness of the need for standardization and automation in In Vitro Fertilization (IVF)."[75]

Amid these consolidating institutional contexts, there is at once scientific, clinical, and corporate interest in increasing automation and standardization in embryo selection with time-lapse embryo imaging. This technology provides the conditions of emergence for the creation of novel data infrastructures and large data sets on embryonic aging. This accumulation of data becomes a locus of value creation in its own right as producers market not only machines but also proprietary algorithms for selection, which have been developed on the basis of embryonic aging data gathered from globally dispersed time-lapse apparatuses. What is of interest in the coming years is, then, how technological developments and consolidating companies affect the accumulations and flows of datafied embryo populations, whose incubated imagery becomes valuable in its aggregation across time and space. As the basis of these data flows, the embryo videos become instrumental in the redistribution of the value of and responsibility for embryonic aging between patients, clinics, and corporations.

Conclusion

By following the journey of the egg, the preceding chapters have made it clear that egg freezing introduces new technologized modes of managing female reproductive aging for a growing group of fertile women. The time of cryopreservation, of preventable loss and extendable potential, can shift the temporal organization of fertility across the life course, as it gains a more distributed and precarious character in the context of OC. This chapter highlights how the time of embryonic development likewise becomes a locus for intervention and investment through the introduction of time-lapse embryo imaging. Whereas egg freezing expands the target group for IVF treatment, time-lapse embryo imaging expands the number of steps and treatment choices within each IVF cycle. In doing so, time-lapse embryo imaging entails a shift in clinical practice that foregrounds embryonic aging in human origin stories, instrumentalizes this developmental time in increasingly standardized and quantified IVF practices, and commercializes it amid trends of widespread consolidation in the global fertility sector.

The newly visible accounts of embryonic aging tell stories about both individualized beginnings of life and the need for their technologized, data-driven management in the IVF cycle. Time-lapse technology makes embryo development visible to intended parents as the earliest moments of their (potential) future children's lives, and its marketing relies on the association of viable embryos with born individuals. Yet the embryo videos simultaneously complement these individualized understandings with one in which groups of embryos collectively hold a potential for "IVF success" that is contingent on technocultural—as a variation on natural—selection.

Time-lapse technologies foreground embryonic aging as a key element both in conceptualizing the embryos' viability and in mitigating their fallibility. They compare the development of embryos in the incubator to the temporal growth patterns of earlier embryonic populations, which provide a predictive prism for embryo selection. More specifically, embryonic aging becomes an instrument for selection through its translation into data sets and an algorithmics of viability prediction. Bearing names like KIDScore and EmbryoScore, such algorithms become products in their own right, which complement the new reproductive data infrastructures established through the growing sales of time-lapse systems. The clinical instrumentalization of embryonic aging in time-lapse imaging thus generates biovalue by increasing profitability and, potentially, vitality in embryo selection.

What is remarkable about the commercialization of time-lapse technologies is the way in which strategies of patenting, direct-to-consumer branding, algorithmizing selection, and acquiring the whole IVF supply chain are combined into a total system for data-driven embryo selection. This multipronged move towards datafication, and the concomitant promise of automation, standardization, and data/capital accumulation in a more networked mode of embryo selection both reflects and reinforces a consolidating trend in the fertility sector—characterized by mergers resulting in larger fertility chains, online platforms adopting a key role in the organization of fertility care, and the portfolio expansion of pharmaceutical and biotechnological companies to cover each step of the IVF cycle.

Time-lapse embryo imaging thus couples the production of biovalue to a conceptualization of embryonic aging as at once a visible, culturally significant process in an individual's origin story, an added financial and clinical treatment option for IVF patients, and a phenomenon that companies may commercialize as patentable property and tool for selection. The resultant clinical operationalization of visible embryonic aging as a technology for selection positions cellular temporality at the basis of what is seen to count as a viable life that may be implanted in a woman's body. While time-lapse embryo imaging visualizes, instrumentalizes, and commercializes the aging of the embryo, in the next chapter I discuss how its subsequent implantation politicizes the age of the intended mother.

5

Postfertile Conceptions

Egg Freezing and the Reinvention of Older Motherhood

The journey of the frozen egg may follow all the stages I have addressed in the previous chapters: anticipation, extraction, cryopreservation, fertilization, incubation, and embryo selection. However, the act of choosing motherhood—whether or not a birth will follow—only presents itself at the next step, in which the embryo enters the intended mother's womb and a pregnancy may ensue. It is at this stage that the question of aging emerges perhaps most pertinently. Here the different elements of distributed reproductive aging—from the cryo-eggs' frozen time to women's age-specific reproductive embodiment and the aging of incubated embryos—come together, potentially resulting in the familiar temporal hybrid of embryonic and adult aging in pregnancy. And because frozen eggs offer a chance of establishing such a pregnancy in spite of age-related infertility, egg freezing raises new—and old—questions about having children later in life.

Condemnations, celebrations, and regulations of the "older mother" abound in the history of IVF—and egg freezing emerges in the wake of these earlier cultural negotiations of aging and motherhood. For those women with the wealth and health to access it, IVF has created the possibility of having children later in life, in spite of age-related subfertility. Albeit with limited success rates, IVF has improved chances of later conception with one's own eggs. But the more dramatic age-related shift followed from the possibility of using younger women's donor eggs to establish pregnancies in older women. Donor-egg IVF enabled women who experienced age-related infertility to carry and give birth to children, even if their own eggs were no longer viable.[1] The reconfigured meanings and materialities of later reproduction after IVF led to institutional regulations and public discussions that revolved around the question of "How old is too old?"[2]

With respect to this question, the Netherlands adopted the 2003 Model Embryo Act, which established 45 years as the maximum age at which women may undergo IVF.[3] This act followed earlier legislation— the 1997 IVF Planning Decree—which motivated the age cap with reference to concerns about the health risks associated with older motherhood, the welfare of the child, and the limited available research on later pregnancy with donor eggs.[4] Since then, Dutch gynecologists have argued that, while international experience suggests that there are indeed higher complication rates, the maximum age cap could nevertheless reasonably be raised to 50 years.[5] Thus in 2009, when the Amsterdam Medical Centre (AMC) proposed to start elective egg freezing, it also suggested increasing the age cap for using frozen eggs to 50.[6] Two years later the minister of health approved elective OC but maintained the 45-year age limit.[7] While the use of OC was thus eventually deemed acceptable, the maximum age cap remained unchanged.[8]

In contrast to the Dutch model, the United Kingdom and the United States do not set a fixed maximum age for fertility treatment, instead leaving the decision to the treating consultant and clinic. Rather than regulating access by chronological age, clinics may do extensive testing at later ages to determine women's suitability for treatment. Some centers, like the Bridge Clinic in London, specifically market to women over 40. While UK and US clinics routinely offer treatments beyond the Dutch 45-year limit, the National Health Service (NHS) shares the Dutch Health Care Insurance Board's policy of only covering IVF costs for women up to 42.[9]

The question of age-specific access to reproductive healthcare, as well as the popularity of egg freezing, relates to wider demographic trends of people having children later in life. Average childbearing ages have been increasing, although current trends are often presented in relation to the 1970s and 1980s, when averages were unusually low compared to earlier decades:

TABLE 5.1. Average Age of Women Having Children			
	The Netherlands	UK	US
1950	30.6	28.8	26.7
1980	27.5	26.9	25.6
2015	31.1	30.3	29.1

Sources: ONS 2016; Van de Pas 2019; HFC 2019.

Since the 1980s, paternal ages have also gone up; men are consistently on average three years older than women when they have a child.[10] Along with these developments, there has been an increase in unwanted childlessness.[11] In keeping with the later age of reproduction in the general population, women seek fertility treatments at increasingly older ages. For example, British women were on average 33 years old when they underwent fertility treatment in 1992 and, by 2016, this had risen to 35.5.[12] During this period, fertility treatments also became more popular: annual cycles more than tripled, from 18,300 to 68,000.[13]

As IVF expanded the possibilities of later childbearing amid these demographic trends, "older motherhood" became a politicized social construct. This is a relatively recent development in Western European societies; throughout the 20th century, so-called older motherhood was a common phenomenon. Although Dutch women had their first child earlier, the average age at childbirth in 1950 (30.6) approximates that observed in 2015 (31.1).[14] In spite of the absence of IVF in 1945, an equal number of children were born to women over 45 in 1945 and 2015 in the United Kingdom, as women had less access to birth control and more children throughout their lives.[15] In the 1920s, 42 was the average age for a British woman to have her last child. Yet over the course of the 20th century, ages that had once been unremarkable became considered "too old," and the women who pursued motherhood at this age, a social problem.[16] What was new, in fact, was not so much older motherhood but so-called delayed motherhood, as reflected by the increase in the maternal age at the birth of the first child.[17] Although objections to late reproduction may be presented as health or welfare concerns, the historical specificity of the unease with older motherhood suggests that they may equally be motivated by other factors, such as norms governing the appropriate timing of reproduction and popular attitudes to technologized extensions of the reproductive life span.

This chapter addresses the new ways of attaining fertility and motherhood with frozen eggs after the end of the reproductive life span, which both reflect and transform existing notions of "older motherhood." I distinguish three new forms of technologically mediated older motherhood that co-emerge with egg freezing. First, as a counterpart to the anticipatory logic of OC, the older motherhood enabled by cryo-eggs gains a more premeditated, potentially "willful" character.[18] When postfertile conceptions are the result of a reproductive intervention much earlier in life, younger women become newly implicated in the politicization of older motherhood. Second, as an alternative to donor eggs, frozen eggs allow women to conceive biogenetically related children at later ages. The concomitant reconfiguration of aging and kinship in this new form of genetically related older motherhood is the focus of the second section, which analyzes online accounts of women who have thawed their frozen eggs. The third form of older motherhood occurs at a later stage, after the intended mother's death. With OC, for the first time in history, posthumous conception and motherhood become technical possibilities. This admittedly rare new form of motherhood nevertheless widely affects women who freeze their eggs through informed-consent forms, which confront all patients with the question of their death and reproductive legacy. This chapter addresses these three new configurations of fertility and motherhood by focusing on how egg freezing reaffirms and transforms the intersections between reproductive aging and willfulness, kinship, and mortality.

Willful Conceptions

As a reproductive technology aimed at having children at a later age, egg freezing provides the occasion for revisiting the controversies surrounding "older motherhood" that emerged with egg donation in the late 20th century. After the first postmenopausal women gave birth using younger women's eggs in the 1980s, donor-egg IVF became increasingly popular, accessible, and controversial over the following decade. Older mothers received intense media scrutiny, and new legal limits restricted the extent to which donor eggs could expand the age range for women's reproduction. As the Dutch government established national age limits to donor-egg IVF in the 1990s, the United States and United Kingdom were likewise hesitant about older motherhood, even if they did not set maximum maternal ages.[19] Given that both donor eggs and frozen eggs can push physical and cultural age-related limits to childbearing, the history of controversy surrounding older motherhood provides some origin stories for the more recent responses to egg freezing and the new stretching of maternal age limits that it enables.

The 1998 documentary *Granny's Having a Baby* gives insight into this recent history of politicized constructions of older motherhood by telling the story of Liz Buttle, who became a mother at 60. As the film demonstrates, the main concerns raised about older motherhood in popular and medical discussions were associated with health risks and children's welfare.[20] Yet a critical reading of the documentary shows that another key dimension of the public controversies on late reproduction pertain to a wider cultural logics of aging through which older motherhood becomes legible and regulated. I approach Buttle's story not so much as an exceptional instance of late, technologized reproduction that invites ethical judgment but rather as a limit case that provokes the articulation of an often implicit, gendered politics of reproductive aging that affects all women—whether they become mothers or not.

A Channel 4 documentary aimed at a general audience, *Granny's Having a Baby* magnifies some of the popular attitudes towards older motherhood at the turn of the millennium.[21] Throughout, the documentary positions older mothers—and Liz Buttle in particular—as subjects of public concern that invite moral judgment. This framing of older motherhood as a problematic social phenomenon is evident from the start, as the documentary opens with a portrait of Buttle's face and the voiceover announces, "This is Britain's first pensioner mother." More portraits follow hers: "This is the professor whose clinic she duped to get fertility treatment" and "This is the miracle baby whose birth sparked a huge row about older motherhood." Much as crime television shows "present us with fables about the nature of our society and the punishments we can expect if we deviate from its rules,"[22] *Granny's Having a Baby* gives insight into the intersection of different cultural systems of aging that inform reproductive age norms and the "huge row" that may ensue when people deviate from them.

With an establishing shot of the Welsh countryside, the documentary introduces Buttle as she wakes up in bed and breastfeeds baby Joe. "Oh dear," Liz responds to him, "you want to come up and have your breakfast." She lifts her shirt and the baby latches onto her breast. As the camera zooms in on the child and Buttle's breast, the voiceover says, "Liz Buttle is Britain's oldest mother. Joe was born when she was 60." By introducing Buttle while she is feeding, the documentary visually establishes her as the baby's mother, thereby distinguishing her from the many women her age who care for infants.

Bringing together aging and maternity, the image of Buttle's breast becomes a symbol of older motherhood and the social provocation associated with it. Given the breast's dual cultural association with both sexuality and maternal nourishment in contemporary Western societies, breastfeeding is bound by strong privacy conventions. This is most obvious in the relative absence of—and controversy surrounding—public breastfeeding. Britain's comparatively low breastfeeding rates—only 25% of new mothers breastfeed for six months—have been linked to a politics of public space that constrains breastfeeding.[23] Pressure on women to be "discreet" in public spaces suggests that the maternal nourishing breast cannot be decoupled from its "cultural coding . . . as primarily sexual," and must therefore remain covered.[24] Within this cultural context, introducing Buttle with a scene of breastfeeding frames her maternity with visual codes that signal transgression.

This rhetorical effect is intensified because the scene's transformation of private into public breastfeeding exposes the body of a mother of advanced age. The image of Buttle's breast is situated within television and film conventions that produce a "lopsided mirror to life," in which "only older men are allowed to grow old on screen."[25] Large-scale studies of Hollywood cinema affirm this ageist and sexist double standard: there are more roles for middle-aged and older men, male actors are on average 6–10 years older, and their average earnings per film reaches a peak at 51 years—compared to 34 years for their female counterparts.[26] Susan Pickard moreover notes that, when there are roles for older women, they are often played by younger ones; thus Angelina Jolie plays Colin Farrell's mother despite only being one year his senior, and 37-year-old Maggie Gyllenhaal was rejected in casting for being "too old" to play the lover of a 55-year-old man.[27] Not only do women disappear from the screen with age but the cultural policing of body revelation intensifies with age, particularly during the time after the presumed loss of fertility. Julia Twigg observes this phenomenon in the tendency for older women's clothes to be less revealing and more muted in color—noting the distinctive, moralistic ways in which condemnations of "overly sexual display" fall particularly heavily on older women.[28] In the context of Buttle's ironically asexual reproduction and her bodily revelation in the documentary, this raises the question of how reproductive aging norms are linked to the age-specific sexualization and desexualization of women's bodies throughout the life course.

Buttle's characterization as "pensioner mother" also references the intersection of age norms and labor relations. The notion of a "pensioner mother" is a conjunction of two life courses that would normally follow one another but now occur at the same time. Although eligible for state pension, Buttle emphasizes her active working life as a farmer throughout the documentary. While breastfeeding Joe, she tells him, "Mommy's got to get to work," and later explains to the interviewer, "I do all the things I used to do. I still do the same work, chopping wood, putting the horse on a rope. Compared to farming, looking after a baby is not any work at all." Buttle thus rejects the pensioner identity by presenting herself as a capable farmer whose physically demanding work is a testimony to her continued fitness and ability to raise a child. Rather than a threat to motherhood, as associated with the trope of wanting to "have it all," Buttle presents her work as a qualification for motherhood. Here labor acquires an almost symbolic function as an expression of "successful aging" and continued functionality—challenging a notion of pensioner identity as a disqualification for productive and reproductive labor alike.[29]

Implicitly responding to criticisms that a pensioner is too old to become a mother, Buttle's claim to continued (re)productivity expresses a "type of late modernity notion of citizenship for aging individuals based on principles of agelessness, health, [and] independence." This "successful aging" approach contrasts with Buttle's critics' views, which "reduce ageing people to their bodies and the risks of bodily decline, illness and disability."[30] The documentary features these critics through a compilation of street interviews in the nearby town of Lampeter. "I think it's disgusting really," says one of two young women, giggling nervously. "She'll be dead when he's 15." Her friend nods in agreement. An adult man remarks, emphatically disapprovingly, "It's a health risk at any age. At 60, it's not going to do her any good. I'd be surprised if she lives to be 80." With a cut to Buttle coughing as she drives her car, the documentary invites the viewer to share their concern about her mortality.

These strong condemnations cannot simply be explained as concern for the welfare of the child or even the health of the mother, but point to the specificity of older motherhood as an ethical category. The disapproval does not only follow from the risk of Joe becoming an orphan or a carer early in his life, as such unease is unlikely to be voiced in similarly strong terms about a child born to parents of average child-bearing age who suffer from life-threatening diseases.[31] It is also not a concern with older parents in general, as older fathers do not challenge normative expectations about reproductive timing as much as older mothers do.[32] Indeed, Peter Rawstron, Buttle's then partner and only three years her junior, did not receive similar criticism about his age or his continued commitment to Joe's upbringing. In fact, Rawstron left Buttle and baby Joe weeks after the documentary was shot. Children are commonly raised by grandparents or older carers without provoking disgust. Rather, it is the particular transgression of older motherhood—combining the particularities of health risks, gender, and age—that Buttle epitomizes through the perceived willfulness of her decision to disregard medical, physical, and cultural standards and have a child.

Willful Older Motherhood

Sara Ahmed theorizes willfulness as a conflict between the "individual will" and the "general will": "The willful character is the one who poses a problem for a community of characters."[33] More specifically, Ahmed describes a historically pervasive "reproductive will" that follows from an understanding of the womb as embodying an impetus to reproduction: "If women exist as wombs, as child makers, then they inherit the reproductive will, as that which if thwarted or blocked, causes illness and damage. Nonreproductivity can thus be treated as a willful object."[34]

Buttle's story draws attention to the age-specificity of the reproductive will. Ahmed suggests that because adulthood "is imagined as leaving playfulness behind" and becoming (re)productive, "nonreproductive adult bodies can appear as willful children, or perhaps willfully childlike, as selfish, . . . as refusing the demand to grow up."[35] In Buttle's case, there is a reversal of this logic; precisely her reproductivity is criticized as a "selfish" refusal to transition into a life course no longer associated with childbearing. Buttle's perceived willfulness follows from her reproductive act against a general nonreproductive will that is expressed in the documentary as a public disapproval of her older motherhood. A young woman, for example, says, "If it's naturally done, it's naturally done," but thinks Buttle's use of reproductive technologies is "a bit of a farce." Whereas Ahmed speaks of a historical tradition in which the womb is conceptualized as having "a will of its own: . . . *the will-to-reproduce*," the response to Buttle appears to suggest the temporal conditionality of this will through its reversal into a *will-not-to-reproduce* after a certain age.[36]

Rather than the womb as such, here it is the onset of age-related infertility that is associated with the will-not-to-reproduce; the use of reproductive technologies signifies the willfulness of Buttle's decision to reproduce in spite of it. Possibly anticipating objections against her use of donor-egg IVF, Buttle initially claimed that Joe had been conceived accidentally in "the back of [Rawstron's] blue Maestro van," after she had supposedly "given up thoughts of babies" because of her age.[37] But the news that her conception was not "naturally done" emerged soon after Joe's birth and contributed to the controversy. In Buttle's case, it is thus not only the occurrence of older motherhood outside "normal reproductive years" but an intended mother's deliberate choice to pursue it with reproductive technologies that is seen as a willful transgression of the chrononormative limits to reproductivity.

In their analysis of Dolly, the cloned sheep, Franklin and Roberts argue that the sheep's significance followed not only from the embodiment of a new means of biological manipulation but from its breach of "some of the biological limits formerly assumed to act as a natural boundary." Dolly represented the loss of the idea that "there is anything like a biological barrier or limit beyond which humans cannot go."[38] In a similar sense, Buttle's exceptional late reproduction not only aligns with social constructions of the "unnaturalness" of older motherhood but also highlights a more general loss of a temporal biological limit to fertility. The possibility of donor-egg IVF displaces the onset of age-related infertility as an absolute barrier to pregnancy and replaces it with a sociality of reproductive wills. Appeals to medical risks have been upheld as apolitical motivations for regulating the temporal transgressions afforded by donated eggs. However, only if we pay attention to how notions of reproductive aging entangle—as they did in Buttle's case—with gendered labor relations, regulations of sexuality, the gendering of nature, and histories of women's agency over reproductive decision making do we get a fuller sense of the uneven distributions of wills and willfulness through which chrononormativities of female fertility are reestablished and resisted.

OC and Premeditated Older Motherhood

Following the history of public ambivalence towards older motherhood that is so overtly expressed in Buttle's case, egg freezing enables a new form of willful older motherhood characterized by premeditation. As noted, the willfulness of older motherhood is reinforced by the use of reproductive technologies, which suggest a more agentic choice rather than an accidental conception in the back of a van. OC takes this one step further by positioning the agentic choice for having children later in life in the fertile life phase. If the first phase of egg freezing simultaneously represents an active choice not to have children at present and a willingness to conceive after the onset of age-related infertility, the second, egg-thawing phase enables a form of premeditated older motherhood that follows from the earlier anticipatory act. Both nonreproductivity in the fertile life phase and reproductivity after "normal childbearing years" are widely criticized;[39] OC's specific willfullness follows from their combination in its potential violation of both the "reproductive will" earlier in life and the will-not-to-reproduce after age-related infertility.

By bringing reproductive decision making about childbearing after age-related infertility into the purview of younger women, concerns about older motherhood, and its attendant reproductive aging norms, are transposed earlier into the life course. Although women opting for OC may not embody the identity of the older mother at the time of egg extraction, the act of freezing itself signals a willingness to harness reproductive technologies to have children beyond the onset of age-related infertility. The willfulness of doing so is a central axis in the public discussions of egg freezing. As we have seen in the earlier chapters, many of the objections to older motherhood and its relation to notions of labor, nature, technology, and risk were revisited in the initial responses to women freezing their eggs, whether in representations of egg freezing as yet another means for career women wanting to "have it all" or in the rejection of technologically enabled transgressions of natural limits to fertility. Critics pointed to women deliberately "postponing" motherhood and deprioritizing it in favor of careers or fun. More empathetic accounts highlighted the lack of willfulness and deliberate delay, instead presenting egg freezing as a response to relational concerns about absent or unsuitable partners, which were understood to be less within one's own control.[40]

Much as donor eggs shifted the temporal limits to age-related infertility and provoked the adoption of legal age limits against a specter of a potentially limitless extension of fertility, so the introduction of egg freezing is reconfiguring the relationship between physical, technologically assisted, and regulatory temporal limits to fertility. This is evident in the 2011 Dutch legislation on egg freezing, which reinstated the 1997 age limit of 45 years. Although an increase to 50 years was suggested when the egg freezing discussion started two years earlier, the Dutch Association of Gynecologists' (NVOG) statement on egg freezing reaffirmed 45 years as the profession's accepted age limit, and Health Minister Schippers reiterated that medical risks preclude raising the age limit for using frozen eggs.[41] Yet only three years after the 45-year limit was upheld, "recent medical developments"—presumably including egg freezing—motivated the minister to request the NVOG's reconsideration of the age limit, which resulted in the 2016 adoption of a 50-year limit to donor-egg and cryo-egg IVF.[42] The gynecologists argued that international experience, the societal need for medical possibilities that would allow later motherhood, and the limited increase in medical risk warranted raising the maximum age limit.[43]

This shift points to a tension within egg freezing. On the one hand, the destabilization of age limits to fertility emerging with egg freezing has been counterbalanced with public articulations of the "normal reproductive years" appropriate for the timing of women's childbearing. In the face of their potential transgression with egg freezing, these age limits have become newly politicized not only at the time of egg thawing but at much earlier ages when women can consider freezing their eggs in anticipation of motherhood later in life. On the other hand, as will become clear in the next section, egg freezing renders these age-related fertility limits newly flexible in ways that allow for the creation of new reproductive age norms that instead encourage fertility extensions and reflect a broader, gendered "will to youth."[44]

Postfertile Extensions: Conceiving Motherhood with Frozen Eggs

With OC emerges the possibility of not only carrying but *conceiving* children at later ages with frozen eggs. The suggestion that female fertility can be extended through this procedure raises questions about the centrality of conception in contemporary understandings of fertility. How does the introduction of egg freezing shift notions of older motherhood, and the interrelation between fertility and aging, in ways that point not only to the age-related transgressions that were central in Buttle's case but also to new modes of achieving "reproductive success" later in life? And what exactly is extended when people freeze their eggs?

In order to better understand the notion of fertility extension, I attended an open evening titled "Fertility over 40" at the Bridge Centre, a London fertility clinic. Michael Summers, a consultant in reproductive medicine, gave a PowerPoint presentation that included slides with the familiar selection of downward graphs detailing female age-related fertility decline and dwindling IVF success rates. These graphs were contrasted with those presenting the results of donor-egg IVF, which showed much more favorable live birth rates that remained stable as the x-axis of women's age progressed from late thirties to late forties. Up next was a collage of photos of Hollywood actors who had been pregnant in their forties. Summers told the audience that the celebrities in his PowerPoint had probably all conceived through egg donation, even though they may not have affirmed publicly that this was the case.

These two elements of Summers's presentation are not exceptional or unusual. Celebrity pregnancies in women over 40 are a popular topic in entertainment media and—as became clear in chapter 1—fertility statistics are an integral part of popular discourses on reproductive technologies.[45] While the celebrity images have been criticized for "weaving into our cultural fabric that age is no longer a barrier to having a baby," gloomy fertility statistics of reproductive decline have been used to popularize the opposite message.[46] In Summers's presentation, the donor egg provides a resolution for these opposing messages: although fertility declines with age, with donor-egg IVF women can continue to have babies. The actors' portraits thus do not support the promise of unproblematic continued fertility but rather an age-specific need for fertility treatment. Because the eggs' age, rather than the woman's, is presented as the limiting factor, donor-egg IVF introduces an additional age bracket in the progression from age-related fertility to infertility within which gestational motherhood may be attainable, but genetic relatedness is not.

Summers's presentation of egg donation as a widely practiced treatment—especially among celebrity women—suggests that the likelihood of genetic relatedness becomes contingent on maternal age and, accordingly, age becomes a factor in questioning maternal genetic kinship. In other words, in Summers's presentation, the expected use of donor eggs, and the concomitant question of relatedness, emerge as a function of the actors' chronological age. In this way, through the recognizable incongruities between a woman's age and her reproductivity, invisible interventions like IVF and egg donation become visible in pregnancies that would otherwise be impossible, such as those by women who are recognized to be past childbearing age. By rendering the use of reproductive technologies visible, older motherhood thus becomes *a marker of a technologically interventionist motherhood.*

Egg freezing, however, presents a different logic in the relation between biotechnological intervention, kinship, and aging. As in effect a form of egg donation to a future self, egg freezing removes the kinship compromise associated with egg donation. It offers the promise of an alternative form of older motherhood that extends beyond age-related limitations of egg viability, but nevertheless maintains a maternal genetic bond.[47] In this way, OC may stretch the lines of maternal genetic descent beyond the temporal distance that normally divides one generation from the next—a *genealogical stretch* as it were. As a result of cryopreservation, it may no longer be possible to infer maternal genetic relatedness—as a function of egg donor use—from a woman's age alone.

The Will to Fertility: Extending Successful Reproductive Aging

Yet the aim of Summers's inclusion of the celebrity mothers was not to question relatedness but to introduce positive imagery of older motherhood and thereby normalize donor-egg IVF. In contrast with Buttle's case, Summers's PowerPoint presents donor-egg IVF over 40 not as a transgression of age or kinship norms but as a sign of successful aging. The celebrities' continued reproductivity fulfills what Michelle Smirnova calls the "will to youth," or "the imperative of the aging woman to promote her youthful appearance by any and all available means." Susan Bordo similarly argues that celebrities "have established a new norm achievable only through continual cosmetic surgery in which the surface of the female body ceases to age as the body grows chronologically older."[48] The birthing of their "miracle babies" may be another variation of this type of medically mediated female successful aging project, in which the "will to youth" is transposed to uterine interiority in alignment with the body's surface appearance. The fact that almost half of all UK media articles on older motherhood focus on celebrity stories suggests that Summers's inclusion of celebrity images is indicative of a broader "new norm" pertaining to fertility, in which having children later in life is a form of elite, aspirational reproduction that affirms continued youthfulness and reproductive functionality.[49] In other words, the "will to youth" is expanded to include a "will to fertility."[50]

Egg freezing epitomizes this will to fertility when it is presented as a technology for successful reproductive life course management. Media tropes that position egg freezing as a means of "taking control" of the biological clock, and marketing slogans such as Eggbanxx's "Smart Women Freeze," position extended fertility and future motherhood later in life as a sign of success, aspiration, and control. The egg freezing network Extend Fertility, for example, writes,

> Bottom line: women in the US are increasingly having their first child later, and studies show this could be extremely beneficial for them and their babies. Think you might be in this camp? Consider planning ahead by freezing your eggs now.[51]

Rather than a threat to "normal limits" to reproduction, older motherhood is here presented as "extremely beneficial" for both mothers and children. Now rendered into a beneficial approach to reproduction, older motherhood becomes a sign of successful reproductive aging that is the outcome of planning earlier in life. If you plan ahead, Extend Fertility suggests, your eggs will be "preserved until you're ready for them."[52]

The implication that you will be "ready for them" later in life, when you are no longer fertile, is consistent with contemporary media portrayals of older motherhood. In their analysis of 719 UK media articles about older motherhood, Mills and colleagues describe how later childbearing was presented as an acceptable reconciliation of competing social expectations, including career achievement, financial security, and social and relationship fulfillment. Rather than "hav[ing] it all at once," they argue, a temporal separation between career advancement, personal gratification, and motherhood was represented as desirable, and even necessary to ensure a high standard of "intensive mothering."[53] In keeping with this media analysis, Lauren Jade Martin's study of women's experiences of the "biological clock" confirms that, alongside intensive mothering, her participants also favored later childbearing in order to meet a host of conditions for optimal childbearing, including financial stability, a supportive relationship, and career achievements.[54] Yet as relationship patterns shift, higher education lengthens, and tuition fees and student debts rise while employment and housing becomes more precarious, the ideal of having children only once a set of conditions are met becomes increasingly unattainable during the years when most women are fertile.[55]

As major OC companies promote egg freezing as a means of extending fertility, they suggest a model for successful reproductive aging in which the timing of childbearing is less constrained by age-related fertility decline, and instead determined by "when you are ready." However, beyond a personal consideration, this notion of "being ready" is situated in socioeconomic systems in which readiness is increasingly poised to arrive at a time when medical interventions are required to conceive. In other words, the popularity of egg freezing, and the fertility extensions associated with it, emerge at time when the conditions for readiness are potentially only met after the onset of age-related infertility, at a point in time when having children is beyond the physical ability of many women.

Extending Families: Kinning with Eggs

As a method for conceiving later, "when you are ready," egg freezing can also function as a kinship technology for establishing a type of motherhood that—unlike third-party egg donation—maintains a biogenetic relatedness to the child. Importantly, later conception with frozen eggs also maintains the possibility of conceiving with a male partner or sperm donor and establishing a particular chosen family form. Implicit in this fertility extension is, then, also a *kinning extension*. And in order to understand the complexities of the kinship and fertility extensions that the frozen eggs afford, I turn to the stories of women who have tried to conceive with their frozen eggs.

The second phase of egg freezing appears straightforward: when you are ready to have a child, you can come back and attempt to get pregnant with your frozen eggs. Yet the accounts of women who decide to do so show that a host of reproductive decisions surround thawing one's eggs. It requires deciding whether and when to attempt to become a parent, anticipating to what extent one is still fertile, navigating who will provide the sperm, deciding whether to try fresh or frozen eggs first, and coming to terms with the non/reproductive outcomes. Although this second half of the egg freezing procedure remains largely unrepresented in media discourses, detailed blog accounts by women who attempted to have children with frozen eggs—including *Egged On* (UK), *Eggsurance* (US), *Egg Freezing Diary* (UK), and last chapter's *Eggfreezer* (US)—give insight into the numerous reproductive pathways that follow egg freezing.

These blogs are among the first public accounts of the later stages of egg freezing.[56] The most prominent is Brigitte Adams's blog. As one of the first high-profile patient-run egg freezing websites, Adams's *Eggsurance* has received widespread popular and media interest, which turned her into "the face of egg freezing." Her story is that she froze 11 eggs in 2012, when she was 39. Egg freezing, she told the *New York Times*, gave her "this incredible calmness." No longer was she under "such pressure that the next guy [she] dated would be daddy material."[57]

Five years later, she decided to use her frozen eggs to become a single mother by choice. The 11 frozen eggs produced only one potentially viable embryo to implant, and she was "over the moon" with her initial positive pregnancy test. When, 48 hours later, the second test was negative, she wrote to a friend, "I am disgusted by the egg freezing process and the hopes I pinned on it." After the initial shock, she reflected on her blog,

> The girl who starts the first egg freezing website and becomes egg freezing's poster child fails with her frozen eggs. It was a cruel irony. I felt like a fraud. How could I champion something that didn't even work [for me]? . . . I was ready to close [up] shop and abandon the site and telling the rest of my story.
>
> I realized that bottling up my egg freezing experience would not help. As more and more women come back to use their frozen eggs, not everyone, like myself, will be successful. We will hear more stories like mine that will, hopefully, help women set realistic expectations.[58]

One such story is Alice Mann's (pseudonym) detailed account of egg freezing. In 2014, Mann was 36 and started her blog, *Egged On*. She went through three rounds of OC and invested a total of £13,755 to freeze 14 eggs. In her words, "The idea was that I'd freeze my eggs, find the man of my dreams, and have kids with him, using my frozen eggs if necessary."[59] Three years later, however, she decided to become a single mother with the frozen eggs. The eggs did not produce a pregnancy, and she continues to undergo IVF with her "fresh" eggs.

A woman writing under the pseudonym Kopaylopa likewise underwent three cycles and froze 13 eggs in 2013, when she was 38. Three years later she decided to thaw the eggs and attempt single motherhood. She subsequently gave birth to a healthy daughter who was conceived from one of the frozen eggs. These women's public accounts of egg thawing highlight how extending fertility intersects with new modes of extending kinship and the political-economic histories of the family form that underlie them.

The stories of these women confirm the importance of the potential future male partner that most studies of OC report. Perhaps more so than a kinship technology for establishing a maternal genetic bond, the frozen eggs materialize a continued possibility for a nuclear family in which the patrilineal connection remains uncompromised. Mann's embryologist articulated this rather straightforwardly when she considered fertilizing some of her eggs at the time of freezing:

> He said to me, "If you can get ten eggs, I'd freeze ten eggs. The techniques around eggs are improving all the time, so our success rates with eggs are getting better all the time. The thing is that if you freeze embryos, and then you meet somebody, those embryos aren't really any use to you." Obviously, he's working on the—fairly reasonable—assumption that a future partner is going to be less likely to want to raise a child who isn't genetically his.[60]

Egg freezing here functions as a kind of anticipatory "kinship work."[61] Both Mann and the embryologist position egg freezing as a means to enable a genetically unified family in which kinship affirmation through biological substances contributes to continued parental commitment. Even though freezing embryos would result in higher success rates, the eggs are frozen unfertilized to preserve future kinning possibilities. In this case, the fertility extension afforded by the cryo-eggs is, then, also an extension to another: a means of meeting the presumably continued fertility of a future male partner.

Reflecting the importance of the future partner in egg freezing, the bloggers frame the perceived period of fertility extension specifically as a time to meet someone:

> Your body and your eggs just keep getting older, which is why freezing them is actually a pretty smart idea, because it gives you a little more time so that you can try to find that one diamond in the crap heap of American men.[62]

Egg freezing thus initiates an extended period of waiting and dating, during which a future family can be imagined in spite of fertility decline. Mann describes this tension between fertility anxieties and family aspirations:

> If you're single and want the possibility of children, your mid-30s robs you of that, however hard you rail against it, however much you wish it weren't the case. And even though I thought freezing my eggs would give me breathing space—and to some extent it did—that shadow never goes away entirely. And it's exhausting.[63]

Mann's experience affirms the widespread finding that most women cite an absent partner as the main reason to freeze their eggs.[64] For them, egg freezing functions as a means to "temporarily disentangle" parental and partnership projects by bracketing childbearing and gaining more time to find the right person to start a family with.[65] Egg freezing, then, offers a means to "anticipate coupledom" and "reinforce the genetic relatedness of offspring."[66]

Marcia Inhorn argues that it is not coincidental that specifically highly educated, professional, single women are freezing their eggs. Apart from the fact that the high costs of egg freezing exclude large sections of the population, she points out that the so-called fertility penalty for meeting educational and employment aspirations is significant. As women aim to be established in unforgiving labor and housing markets and reach financial and relationship security before they have children, many find themselves—or expect themselves to be—unable to conceive once these conditions are met—if, indeed, they ever are. This fertility penalty is coupled with a situation in which there are only three college-educated men for every four college-educated women in the United States. Inhorn argues that the combination of a "massive undersupply of college-educated men" and the low rates of educational "intermarriage" create a situation in which specifically highly educated heterosexual women are interested in egg freezing as a "stop-gap" measure while they look for a male partner.[67]

Alongside the demographic constraints, the privileging of relationships over singlehood itself is characteristic of a contemporary predicament that egg freezing brings to the limelight. In her work on the sociotemporal dimensions of singlehood, Kinneret Lahad argues that being single is, to a large extent, discursively framed as a liminal, transitory stage on the way to couplehood and family life.[68] She describes the prevalent conceptualizations of coupledom as essential to self-fulfillment while singlehood represents "a waiting period, during which one must do all in one's power to exit the waiting mode."[69] This emphasis on choice and agency in achieving partnerships itself reflects a neoliberal ethos of self-managing singlehood, in which there is little consideration of the sociocultural structures from which these very choices emerge.[70] In the face of both a neoliberal emphasis on individual accountability for making romantic arrangements and the continued hegemony of traditional relationship and family norms, the absence of a partner can be experienced as not merely an inconvenience but a social failure. To a large extent, Lahad argues, this sense of failure is contingent on aging; "waiting for Mr. Right" shifts from representing a romantic longing earlier in life to an increasing inability to attain hegemonic hetero-nuclear family forms later in life.[71]

This dynamic between agency and failure in relation to singlehood is a recurring theme in the bloggers' accounts of the waiting and dating period enabled by frozen eggs:

> I felt like a failure before I froze my eggs. *What was wrong with me? Why was I still single and childless at 39?* . . . Once I froze my eggs those ugly feelings of self-pity started to dissipate.[72]

Mann likewise related her experience of singlehood as failure, to which egg freezing provided a resolution:

> I once thought that freezing my eggs was an admission of failure, that it was me putting my hands up and saying "I haven't been able to do what everyone else has." I don't see it like that now. I see it as a sensible, self-preserving, pragmatic decision.[73]

In the context of the perceived social failure associated with singlehood, egg freezing provides a means of realizing the agentic self-empowerment that Lahad describes. Yet rather than a relationship as such, it can be the cryo-eggs—and the potential for family and partnership they represent—that provide a resolution to unwanted singlehood.

The use of frozen eggs as a means to extend the period of waiting and dating, thereby prolonging the time frame within which the future partner may arrive, is situated within a particular political-economic history of the family form. The family form that these egg freezing accounts reference is both a dominant cultural norm and at the heart of a neoconservative and neoliberal political project that Melinda Cooper describes in *Family Values* (2017). Cooper offers an alternative to a reading of neoliberalism that emphasizes the exaltation of the atomized individual. She makes the case that the political history of neoliberalism relies on and reproduces the family form through the installation of the family—rather than the state—as the "privileged site of debt, wealth transfer and care."[74]

Egg freezing has been framed as an expression of a neoliberal logic of self-investment in future fertility. Rather than shifting social structures to facilitate reproductive decision making throughout the life course, egg freezing is a quintessentially individualist technology that self-responsibilizes women to achieve continued fertility. Yet the fertility created through this procedure is not only individual in nature but often becomes meaningful in its extension to the other, to the potential future partner with whom an imagined family form may be attained. Cooper alerts us to the interlinking of the politics of economic redistribution and cultural recognition in this family form. These two aspects are intertwined both in the earlier construction of the Fordist family, which positioned "white, married masculinity as a point of access to full social protection," and in today's politics of distribution, in which the legally and culturally legitimized family functions as a primary wealth-transmitting mechanism of inheritance, social security, and gendered provision of care.[75] This coincides with a move from the Fordist family wage to the ideal of the two-earner family, which, in turn, coincides with the rise in paid working hours required to support a family under financialized capitalism.[76]

So when egg freezers emphasize the importance of the absent male partner, this need not simply reflect a romantic or individual preference, or even solely a cultural norm. It may also be rooted in the political divestment of social welfare from the state to the private family and the concomitant redistributive logic that foregrounds the family as the key social unit through which citizenship rights and obligations—including care and financial security—may be obtained. And it is the neoliberal logic of private investment and indebtedness, rather than public welfare, that is matched in the egg freezing practices. This happens not only through the self-responsibilization of women for their future fertility but also through the positioning of the family as itself a redistributive unit that requires investment—of eggs and capital alike.

* * *

While egg freezing is described as a means to establish a desired family form in the future, the trajectory after OC can equally be a time to come to terms with single motherhood. For example, while she was ready to have a child with a partner, Alice Mann needed three years to adjust to an alternative imagined family model and attempt to become a single mother:

> I felt like I had—albeit in my own time, which let's be honest was about three years—come to a decision about something that I felt financially, emotionally and practically capable of taking on all by myself. I felt a bit like Superwoman.[77]

And Adams describes that the key step in being ready to use her frozen eggs was "being OK with being single."[78] So while egg freezing clearly functions as a kinship technology that holds the promise of a future conception with a chosen partner, these stories highlight how it equally enables a move towards having children without a partner. In other words, although freezing eggs is typically framed as a possibility of inhabiting nuclear family forms, thawing these eggs may in fact require the opposite: coming to terms with single motherhood.

Extending Reproductive Loss

Although egg freezing is often presented as a means to extend fertility beyond its age-related loss, the women's stories show that OC's second phase can be contingent on different kinds of fertility loss. Indeed, women can use their frozen eggs if the eggs in their body are no longer viable. But frozen eggs can also function as a back-up option in IVF, only to be used if fresh eggs fail. Alternatively, frozen eggs can be a preferred option for presumably fertile women in order to benefit from the cryo-eggs' relative youth. Reflecting these different "frozen-only," "fresh-first," and "frozen-first" treatment rationales, the egg freezers' stories elucidate the nature of the fertility losses that precede, and accompany, egg thawing.

Exemplifying the fresh-first approach, Kopaylopa decided to try to have a child on her own two years after freezing her eggs. She visited the fertility clinic and received the following advice: "It's likely to be fresh IVF cycles until I'm either pregnant or running low on resources . . . , and then (and only then) will we move on to the frozen eggs."[79] Rather than egg freezing extending her fertility, it functions instead as a back-up option. In other words, in Kopaylopa's case, the frozen eggs are not a preferred source of ongoing reproductive potentiality to be used when she is ready for motherhood, but their use is contingent on failed IVF cycles.

Mann's experience, by contrast, reflects a frozen-first approach. A couple of years after egg freezing, she returned to the clinic for fertility tests to check whether she could wait a little longer to start trying to conceive. In contrast with Summers's emphasis on the egg's age—not the woman's—as the crucial factor in reproduction, and notwithstanding the fertility extension associated with her frozen eggs, tests of her embodied fertility became the instigating factor in Mann's decision to start trying. Although the test outcomes were positive and gave her "permission to procrastinate," Mann soon decided that "I want to try, of course I want to try."[80] Although she was presumed fertile, her eggs were thawed at the first attempt at conception, as her doctor explained:

"Even though your ovarian reserve is good, we're going to use the frozen eggs," she said. "The older you are, the more likely your eggs are to be chromosomally abnormal."[81]

Although Mann's ovarian reserve was deemed sufficient, the age difference between the eggs in her ovaries and those in the freezer became an indication to use the latter. Ironically, the fertility tests that Mann used to determine her reproductive timing decisions were not the determining factors in her treatment plan. The fertility loss that became an indication for OC was, rather, the difference in the passage of time between Mann's cryo-eggs and her embodied eggs.

In addition to these fresh-first and frozen-first options, there is the frozen-only approach, which is reflected in Brigitte Adams's story. Adams returned to the IVF clinic at age 44 and approached the frozen eggs as her only option for having her "own" child. When she froze her eggs, she was adamant about two things:

1) I would NOT be a single mom
2) I would NOT try to get pregnant after age 42

Fast forward five years: I am still single, a few days shy of my 44th birthday and finally ready to use my frozen eggs. What changed? I chalk it up to three things: accepting my path, being OK with being single and having a kick ass family.[82]

Although she had strong ideas about age-related limits to conception, in retrospect Adams adjusted her reproductive timing decisions primarily with reference to relationships and readiness rather than an imagined biological clock. It was precisely egg freezing that allowed her to "move on" and organize her reproductive decision making according to these other time lines:

By taking my fertility into my own hands, I was finally able to accept that, thought [sic] my life had not followed the perfectly linear path I had expected, I had done everything I could and was finally able to move on.[83]

As part of moving on, she was no longer concerned about reproductive aging in the same way she had once been—not only because a sense of reproductive possibility had been displaced to the eggs but also because she had done everything she could. The decision to use the frozen eggs was contingent on the loss of the expectation both of finding a partner and of being able to conceive: "I made this decision once I finally acknowledged to myself that the chances of Mr. Right galloping up on a white horse and whisking me off to coupledom were about as likely as me getting pregnant naturally (about less than 1% at age 44)."[84]

If the decision to thaw eggs is contingent on different forms of fertility loss, the clinical process of the second phase of egg freezing itself involves a cascade of fertility gains and losses—rather than a straightforward extension. When frozen eggs represent the final option for conceiving without donor eggs, as Adams describes, the failure of the frozen eggs represents a particular kind of fertility loss that did not exist before. More so than if she had not frozen her eggs in the first place, the loss of fertility occurs again and again. Adams's fertility loss first emerges as the experiences of reproductive aging that drive the egg freezing decision, then as a motivating factor for thawing them, subsequently in the appearance of the fibroid, in the disappointing results in the transition from eggs to only a single embryo, and finally in a chemical pregnancy that is lost after 48 hours:

> I can barely see straight and not sure I should even post this . . . I was told on Saturday that I was pregnant. I was told on Tuesday the embryo had died. I have no more eggs to try. I have no more eggs to retrieve. I have no energy to try again. I am mourning the loss of a baby and the loss of ever having a biological child.[85]

Egg freezing thus offers a multiplication of fertilities—in the body and in the freezer—which may be lost at different points in time. In this way, the fertility extension associated with egg freezing creates a situation in which fertility can be lost later in life, at the time of egg thawing.

This belated fertility loss, moreover, has a different character when it is tainted by the logic of retrospective regret:

> No one talks about part 2 of egg freezing. We need to start. If I could do it all again I would:

- Freeze multiple rounds
- Freeze embryos
- Really understand my AMH and FSH levels
- Stop working so many hours at shitty jobs
- Not count on my frozen eggs to work.[86]

While Adams had earlier assured herself that she could move on if the eggs would not be successful because she had done "everything she could," her response to losing the frozen eggs is retrospective regret at not having frozen more eggs. In the post reflecting on her lost eggs, the first recommendation she gives to her former self is to freeze more eggs. In this sense, the grief associated with fertility and pregnancy loss is compounded with a self-responsibilized retrospective regret associated with the agentic possibility of freezing ever more eggs for later.

Grief is also the affect described by Eggfreezer, whose story we followed in chapter 3. Four years after her blog went dormant, Eggfreezer returned to Blogspot to share the following message:

> 7 years later, I went to use the frozen eggs, and 100% died immediately on thaw. They were supposed to survive thaw with over a 90% success rate. Instead, every single one died. . . . These eggs were so good, Dr. B told me at the time that he wouldn't let me do another freeze cycle because I had so many perfect 32 year old eggs. This is unfathomable. I cannot begin to explain the grief I am feeling.[87]

After describing the eggs as "starting building block[s] of a future human being" and "fully sufficient and necessary to make that human my biological child," Eggfreezer here links the loss of those eggs to the loss of the imagined future child and the kinship bond that binds them.[88] The disconnect between the outcome of the thaw and her expectations for the eggs' reproductive potential, rationalized on the basis of their quantity and age-related quality, results in epistemic dismay: this is unfathomable.

More so than reproductive failure after unsuccessful incubation, fertilization, or egg collection in IVF, Eggfreezer's case shows a new, OC-specific form of fertility loss that occurs after a successful egg collection. This extended fertility loss is characterized by the combination of a calculus of fertility that suggests a distributed form of ongoing fertility associated with the 32 cryo-eggs (see chapter 3)—in this case over the course of seven years—and a particular reproductive loss occurring between egg collection and fertilization when the eggs don't thaw correctly. What is lost with Eggfreezer's eggs is not only the potential future "own" child but the personal investment in the eggs as symbols of fertility that bore the expectation of a longer trajectory of fertility gains and losses through future IVF procedures. Adams's and Eggfreezer's stories illustrate how age-related fertility loss after egg freezing is intensified both through a course of "little victories [and] little disappointments" and by being charged with earlier affective, financial, and bodily investments.[89]

So alongside the promise of continued fertility and genetically related motherhood, egg freezing also extends a cascade of fertility gains and losses. The possibility of kinning with a future partner through frozen eggs enacts the link between relationships and reproductivity; it shows how ideas about relatedness, singlehood, and family ideologies are materialized and articulated through frozen eggs. The online stories discussed in this section revealed the new and later kinning possibilities that frozen eggs hold, which may resolve a sense of failure associated with singlehood and fertility decline. Yet in doing so, egg freezing also sets women up for an alternative course of fertility losses—of embodied, frozen, and partnered reproductivity. These losses are intensified both through constructions of agentic retrospective regret and as the counterpart of the affective and effective investment in the frozen eggs over the course of the cryopreservation period. Egg freezing, then, extends not only fertility but also its loss.

Posthumous Conceptions

Cryopreserved eggs create the possibility of circumventing not only the end of fertility but also the end of life itself. Once frozen, eggs can retain their reproductive potential irrespective of the aging and eventual death of the body from which they originated. In other words, the eggs may outlive the woman who froze them. The eggs' continued viability thus opens up the possibility of a third new, and unusual, form of reproductivity emerging with OC that is altogether decoupled from the vitality of the living body: posthumous fertility.

This type of fertility can lead to posthumous motherhood through the fertilization and surrogate gestation of frozen eggs. This approach has not yet resulted in the birth of any children; even to living women, the number of children born from frozen eggs is relatively small.[90] However, as is the case with OC more broadly, the *possibility* of this new way of becoming a parent in itself affects both the practice of egg freezing and the cultural imagination of fertility. Particularly the informed-consent procedures stage a structural encounter with this possibility of posthumous fertility, as every woman who freezes her eggs must decide on the destination of her eggs in the future, including the future beyond her own death. Through these informed-consent procedures, the willfulness of egg freezing thus also stages an encounter with what is in effect a will.

Technically, posthumous motherhood is already possible through the gestation of frozen embryos. IVF procedures frequently produce more embryos than can be implanted in the womb, which are routinely frozen for future use. If the intended mother dies, these frozen embryos can still be implanted into another woman's womb. This happened in the case of the Chinese baby Tiantian, who was born four years after his parents died in a car crash. Tiantian's grandparents won the right to the frozen embryos after a lengthy legal battle and, because surrogacy is illegal in China, commissioned a surrogate in Laos to carry the pregnancy.[91] Frozen eggs likewise offer possibilities for reproduction after death, including posthumous conception.

As Tiantian's case illustrates, the posthumous possibilities of frozen eggs and embryos raise a range of ethical issues. The ethical bodies of the European and US professional societies in reproductive medicine (ESHRE and ASRM) both emphasize the importance of informed consent in posthumous reproduction. Making no distinction between gametes and embryos, ESHRE's discussion of this practice revolves around the notion of a couple's shared "parental project" and asks whether the frozen cells materialize continued reproductive intent.[92] As previously discussed, women often freeze their eggs when they are single, which implies a "parental project" of a different kind—one that has an anticipatory orientation and is limited to the gametes of a single individual. Unlike the embryo, the egg leaves the choice open for a male partner or sperm donor. This openness presents a unique situation, both in the posthumous use of eggs—and in the anticipation thereof through informed consent.

One such posthumous parental project emerged in the British case of Mr. and Mrs. M. and their daughter A., a young woman who was diagnosed with cancer at 21 years old. Soon after her diagnosis, A. wanted to have IVF treatment, but was too ill. When she experienced a period of remission from the cancer a couple of years later, she underwent, "in considerable pain," an egg freezing cycle that retrieved three eggs. Prior to treatment, A. signed a consent form stating that she wanted the eggs to be stored for later use in the event of her death. However, according to her mother, she was not given a second consent form to specify how, and by whom, the eggs might be used posthumously. A.'s mother, Mrs. M., later recalled that her daughter had been under the impression that she had signed all the necessary forms and that A. wanted a child "more than anything else in the world." Indeed, when visited by a newly pregnant cousin, A. had told her mother that she already had her babies: "They are just on ice, aren't they, Mum?"[93]

In January 2010, when it became clear to A. that she would not recover from her illness, she told her mother,

> They are never going to let me leave this hospital, Mum; the only way I will get out of here will be in a body bag. I want you to carry my babies. I didn't go through the IVF to save my eggs for nothing. I want you and Dad to bring them up. They will be safe with you. I couldn't have wanted for better parents, I couldn't have done without you.[94]

A. also spoke with one of her friends about her mother carrying her child in case she could not do so herself. In the last stages of her illness, according to her mother, A. repeatedly said she wanted her babies. Shortly after, in 2011, she died from an infection. Her mother was very clear about A.'s intentions with her cryo-eggs:

> I have absolutely no doubt in my mind that, as far as A was concerned, her eggs held a life force and were living entities in limbo waiting to be born. She was clear that she wanted her genes to be carried forward after her death.[95]

After A.'s death, her parents requested permission from the HFEA for the eggs to be exported to the United States, where a clinic had agreed to fertilize them with anonymous donor sperm and implant them in Mrs M.'s womb. However, the HFEA declined permission because, although A. had signed a consent form giving permission for her frozen eggs to be used after her death, other forms were missing that recorded her consent for the "export of the gametes, their admixture with donor sperm, the use of a surrogate and the use of the gametes in treating A.'s mother, rather than A."[96] The disagreement between A.'s parents and the HFEA led to several high-profile court cases. These were initially decided in favor of the HFEA, but A.'s parents later won on appeal. It has not been made public whether Mr. and Mrs. M. have been able to have a grandchild with A.'s eggs.

A.'s intergenerational, familial, parental project is thus one example of the new modes of family building enabled by egg freezing. A.'s case shows how relevant the possibility of posthumous fertility can be in the lived experience of finitude, even if the outcome of the future IVF treatment will never be known by the woman who froze her eggs. For A., her eggs signified her babies "on ice" that were waiting to be born, even if she would not live to meet them.[97] The eggs also consolidated the kinship bonds with her parents by coupling parental and grandparental roles, holding the potential of future children in the face of their daughter's death. In this way, the eggs reconfigure the relationship between fertility and mortality by balancing imminent death with the promise of latent life. Particularly when she was facing the end of her life, the fact that, according to her mother's testimony, A. understood the eggs as "living entities" suggests that they played an important role in her coming to terms with her mortality, as a "life force" that would outlive her own.

Although A.'s is an extraordinary case, indeed the first of its kind, the practice of egg freezing at large stages a structural encounter with finitude and the possibility of posthumous reproductivity and motherhood. As A.'s story shows, this is particularly pertinent for women who freeze their eggs prior to cancer treatment, an experience that demands a confrontation with mortality in its own right.[98] Yet also for women who freeze their eggs in anticipation of age-related infertility, the informed-consent procedure invites a consideration of the eggs' posthumous destination.

This is particularly the case in the United Kingdom, where informed consent is the cornerstone of the HFEA's regulation of reproductive technologies. The HFEA provides fertility clinics with standardized consent forms, which their patients must sign prior to treatment. The consent form for the storage of eggs states that the Human Fertilisation and Embryology Act 1990 requires patients to choose "what you want to happen to your eggs or sperm if you die or lose the ability to decide for yourself."[99] This section is a substantial part of the consent form and states that the gametes will "be allowed to perish" in case no consent is given. Forms for consent to treatment and egg storage ask whether women want the eggs to be used posthumously for the treatment of a partner, the treatment of others, or training purposes.[100] The options of reproductive donation require corresponding forms for egg donation and surrogacy arrangements, which address the eggs' fertilization and gestation in the event of death.[101] It was one of these latter forms that was missing in A.'s case; only in the appeal case were her reported statements that she wished for her mother to be the surrogate recognized as providing the consent that these forms were designed to record. The HFEA's informed-consent forms thus address posthumous reproductive use of gametes explicitly, thereby positioning it as an institutionally acceptable choice rather than an exception, as is the case in the Dutch context.

In the Netherlands, there is no uniform consent form analogous to that of the HFEA. Rather, each clinic has formulated its own statements of consent. Considering the forms of the University Medical Centre Utrecht (UMCU) and of the clinic MCK Fertility Centre (MCK), it is clear that the standard procedure is to let a woman's eggs perish after her death. If a woman freezing her eggs at the UMCU or MCK chooses to bequeath her eggs to another party after her death, she will need to make, respectively, an official request or a notary statement that explicates who may inherit and use the eggs.[102] The informed-consent forms both point to the possibility of posthumous motherhood and complicate the pursuit thereof, whether by administrative procedures or by stating—as MCK does—the clinic's policy of not working with gametes of deceased people. The forms' acknowledgment that the eggs can nevertheless be transferred to another clinic point to the fact that the frozen eggs' mobility opens up a regulatory flexibility in which patients can move their cells to institutional and national contexts that align with the intended parental project—just as A.'s parents attempted to do by exporting her eggs from the United Kingdom to the United States.[103]

Although the British and Dutch medical authorities differ in their approaches, both adhere to the ESHRE's standpoint that informed consent is crucial in "enabl[ing]" patients, and should be in place even if clinics do not themselves carry out posthumous treatments.[104] By calling it "enabling," the ESHRE positions informed consent as a means for patients to exert agency over the extracted eggs. Yet, as has become clear above, the forms also represent an institutional agency through the particular presentation of the available choices. The acknowledgment of the possibility of posthumous motherhood by an "institution of expertise" is situated in medical systems that enjoy a degree of preexisting trust from their patients.[105] The inclusion of certain choices as standard options for which consent can be given through formalized procedures, or by a tick of the box, normalizes these forms of posthumous reproduction as acceptable decisions that patients may consider in the egg freezing process. Their exclusion from the informed-consent procedure, or the requirement for a separate declaration, suggests the opposite and functions as a discouraging measure.

The informed-consent forms thus represent a meeting of individual and institutional speech acts. Through their ongoing power in directing the future pathways of frozen eggs, these speech acts of informed consent exemplify Judith Butler's understanding of performative utterances as "forms of authoritative speech . . . that, in the uttering, also perform a certain action and exercise a binding power."[106] In the contract of informed consent, ticking the box functions, quite explicitly, as a citation of authoritative speech that has binding power in determining the egg's destination. In other words, it is individual consent by institutional citation. Butler notes that "performativity must be understood not as a singular or deliberate 'act' but, rather, as the reiterative and citational practice by which discourse produces the effects that it names."[107] Informed consent can be understood as a citational practice of clinics and patients alike, in which posthumous motherhood is produced through its linguistic recognition. The continuity of consent stretching into the future, long after the ticking and signing, suggests that the "sphere of operation" of these speech acts is not limited to the present time of utterance—particularly given that the conditionality of "when you die" pertains to a time to come that is not yet manifest. In *Excitable Speech*, Butler addresses the "open temporality of the speech act" by qualifying the "moment of utterance" as a "condensed historicity: it exceeds itself in past and future directions."[108] In keeping with this understanding of the speech act's temporality, the informed consent to the posthumous use of cryopreserved eggs can be read as a future performative: a speech act that harks back in time through its citation of authoritative speech, yet takes effect not only during, but also long after, its utterance.

Because these declarations of the eggs' posthumous destination concern the time after death, the informed-consent practices function as a kind of will writing.[109] In "The Pleasures and Perils of Inheritance," Daniel Monk reflects on the writing of wills as a practice of "facing death [and] reflecting on one's legacies" that "bring[s] to the fore constructions of memory and identity, intergenerational relations, and the complexities of doing and undoing family and kinship."[110] Wills, he argues, are the means of the living to organize their legacy and pass on what is important in people's lives to the time after death. Egg freezing in anticipation of age-related infertility is oriented towards the biomedical passing on of bodily material to a future self. However, as we have seen in A.'s case, the practice may also entail passing on eggs to others after death, to continue an existing parental project—or start a new one. In this way, the speech act of informed consent not only has future world-making effects but also effectuates the "doing and undoing" of the kinship relations ascribed to the egg before and after death.

Egg freezing, then, presents people with a hitherto nonexisting possibility of leaving eggs-as-legacy. The emergence of this novel cellular legacy follows a history in which practices of reproduction and inheritance have been intimately entwined. In *Willful Subjects*, Ahmed writes, "The child is the one who *promises to extend the family line*, which requires the externalization of will as inheritance."[111] Monk similarly references a history in which inheritance "has long been . . . almost the raison d'être of conventional, albeit subtly shifting familial practices," particularly for women, who "hav[e] served as passive vehicles for the transmission of names, wealth and continuity across generations."[112] Egg freezing provides new ways for extending the family line beyond one's own lifetime, as frozen eggs can both comprise and redirect inheritance.

The use of egg freezing to ensure familial continuity after death may be observed in the case of 17-year-old Chen Aida Ayah. This Israeli young woman was hit by a car in 2011 and was declared brain dead a week after the accident. In the first case of its kind, the family received permission of the local court of Kfar Saba to extract and freeze Ayah's eggs for future reproductive use by a family member.[113] This case illustrates how OC provides the conditions of possibility for imagining and legally arranging the prolongation of the child's promise to "extend the family line" to the time after death.[114] Within a framework in which inheritance is intimately bound up with reproduction, the cryopreserved egg may attain a double function as both the reproductive means for maintaining familial continuity and the inheritable object itself.[115]

In the speech act of giving consent to posthumous reproduction— lacking in Ayah's case of posthumous extraction—the egg's double function provides the occasion for establishing *intended kinship* bonds prior to conception. Frozen eggs leave options open to determine the intended kinship bonds with a genetic father or donor as well as a gestational mother or surrogate in the context of a "parental project" after death. Women in relationships may leave their frozen gametes to their partners, much as men have done in a growing number of cases of posthumous conception with frozen sperm.[116] A woman's male partner could fertilize the frozen eggs posthumously, while a female partner could carry the embryo made with the frozen egg. Alternatively, as A.'s case shows, women may decide to leave their cryopreserved oocytes to friends or family members for an alternative parental project. In each case, the posthumous reproductive intention, and particularly the specification of "named recipients" in informed consent, may generate a "doing and undoing" of intended kinship bonds prior to conception through the figure of the egg.[117]

The expression of informed consent to the posthumous (dis)use of the oocytes entails the discursive production of the eggs as socially significant entities that may become differently recognized as the patient's legacy at the time of death. The classification of eggs as valuable or surplus material—and the concomitant willingness to donate them to other couples or research labs—has been studied widely.[118] An important aspect of this informed-consent process is its temporal dimension, and specifically the way in which the meanings ascribed to the cells are contingent on the passage of time, whether organized by the age or the vitality of the woman who froze her eggs.

The informed-consent forms organize the shifting symbolic significance of these eggs at the time of death as, for example, familial legacy, research material, or an extension of physical embodiment. As A.'s case illustrated, in posthumous fertility treatment, the eggs' legacy may take the form of *potential progeny*. Alternatively, when the eggs are used for research posthumously, the woman's death provides the occasion for a redirection of the eggs' significance from serving a "personal goal" of having a genetically related child to serving a "public goal" of improved medical science and public health.[119] In being passed on to research, the legacy of these eggs may be conceived as a contribution or "giving back" to biomedical science. The posthumous destruction of the eggs, in turn, reenacts the death of the woman's body at the cellular level.

In the informed-consent procedure, the consideration of these future destinations of the eggs entails a confrontation with one's own finitude. With modernity, anthropologist Margaret Lock argues, death and "associated beliefs about transcendence were disentangled from the realm of the sacred" and remade into a "medical matter." From the mid-19th century onwards, the physician's pronouncement of death has come to signal "the end" of the body and person. With the loss of the cultural currency of "imagined futures after death," time becomes "compressed into the individual life cycle."[120] As the afterlife was displaced by the finitude of the medically conceived body, so the continued viability of cryopreserved bodily material may provide alternative "imagined futures after death" that are based on the temporal plasticity of the cell. When frozen cells are understood as "part of me," as in the case of Eggfreezer (see chapter 3), or as "my babies," in A.'s words, it is medicine that facilitates a futurity beyond death through the continued viability of frozen bodily material. The informed-consent forms, accordingly, present both a confrontation with finitude and a possibility of cellular reproductive continuity "if you die," thereby shifting the finality of mortality: a life extension of a different kind.[121] The possibility of posthumous motherhood thus opens up a reconsideration of the relation between reproductivity and death, in which the end of reproductivity becomes a matter of consent and an agentic choice rather than a biological necessity.

Conclusion

Egg freezing introduces new ways of conceiving children, being fertile, and becoming a mother later in life—and even after death. As a means of circumventing age-related infertility, egg freezing practices reveal what is at stake in shifting the temporal parameters of female reproductivity. Long-standing public preoccupations with so-called older motherhood, which became particularly controversial and newsworthy after donor-egg IVF, are revisited in the context of egg freezing. Yet today the possibilities of later motherhood and extended fertility are also framed in light of gendered "successful aging" and promoted as signs of a form of elite, aspirational reproduction. The frozen eggs that enable reproductivity later in life, however, can not only extend fertility but also bring about its loss in new ways. This chapter discussed three novel reproductive pathways emerging with frozen eggs, which both challenged and reinforced the contentious relations between reproductive aging, fertility, and motherhood.

First, the possibility of a type of premeditated, willful older motherhood emerges with egg freezing. The association of older motherhood with willfulness became apparent in Liz Buttle's story, which, as a limit case, revealed how norms regarding the appropriate timing of reproduction may be expressed as health and welfare concerns, but are nevertheless informed by historically specific cultural systems of aging pertaining to gender, sexuality, and labor relations. Both the criticism of Buttle and the public objections to egg freezing for its transgression of "normal reproductive years" reaffirm existing chrononormativities that are threatened by the introduction of new technologies that enable later reproduction. By eliciting the articulation of these chrononormativities, Buttle's case reveals the temporal conditionality of Ahmed's "reproductive will." By extension, the willfulness of OC's older motherhood follows from the transgression both of the will-to-reproduce earlier in life and of the will-not-to-reproduce after age-related infertility.

Whereas Buttle's case draws attention to the transgressive framing of older motherhood, narratives about celebrity older motherhood conversely reference it as an achievement of successful aging and a sign of continued functionality. The prevalent and highly gendered "will to youth" thus finds its counterpart in an ongoing *will to fertility*. Given the growing popularity of egg donation later in life, new mothers' ages may begin to function as a marker of a decreasing probability of genetic relatedness and an increasing likelihood of a technologically interventionist motherhood, rendering the otherwise invisible use of ARTs recognizable. However, frozen eggs can shift the logic of this age-related recognizability of genetic relatedness. The ability to conceive after age-related infertility with cryo-eggs points to the second form of older motherhood of interest: genetically related motherhood later in life.

While egg freezing opens up the possibility of a fertility extension resulting in genetically related older motherhood, it also extends the potential of establishing genetic ties within a family unit. It thus not only enables an extension in time but is frequently motivated as *an extension to another*. Frozen eggs represent a kinning extension not only to the child but also to the imagined future male partner. This need not only reflect a romantic preference but also a neoliberal diminution of social welfare in favor of a repositioning of the family as the key redistributive social unit—which requires proactive investment of both eggs and capital. In this sense, frozen eggs can be used to meet a set of dominant singlehood and family ideologies through the specter of the potential future conception. Yet in doing so, egg freezing in fact often functions as a pathway to alternative family forms.

When frozen eggs are thawed in the attempt to make a family, the OC process introduces a new course of fertility gains and losses. The second phase of egg freezing entails all the familiar ups and downs of IVF. In addition, if the frozen eggs do not result in a child, there is the loss of not only a failed cycle but also a cryopreserved, distributed sense of fertility, often culminated after years of physical, financial, and affective investment in the frozen eggs. This loss may be further intensified through constructions of retrospective regret at not freezing more eggs earlier in life. As the counterpart of women's earlier investment in freezing their eggs, egg freezing extends both fertility and its loss.

Lastly, OC creates a tension between the body's mortality and the cryo-egg's temporary immortality, from which the technical possibility of posthumous motherhood follows. Although as yet an unrealized possibility, its consideration in informed-consent procedures nevertheless has world-making effects by requiring patients to set posthumous reproductive intentions and reclassifying eggs as future research, reproductive, or waste material. In the speech act of informed consent to posthumous reproduction by specific "named recipients," the egg functions as a node for the discursive construction of *intended kinship* relations prior to conception. Through the possibility of posthumous conception with cryopreserved eggs, the reproductive process becomes recognizable not only in earlier stages but also later on in life, beyond the limits of mortality.

In the next, and final, chapter I explore how the egg further complicates the limits of mortality and the linearity of aging in regenerative medicine and address the unprecedented global mobility of eggs now that they may be frozen.

6

Oocyte Futures

The Global Flow of Frozen Eggs

Thus far we have followed the egg's journey from the bioprepared body to the freezer and, after fertilization, from the incubator to the womb. However, the egg's journey in OC need not find its endpoint in motherhood, whether older or not. In fact, given the potential for failure at every step of the way—thawing, fertilizing, incubating, implanting, continuing pregnancy—the chances of a single frozen egg resulting in a live birth are as slim as 2–5%.[1] Not only are live birth rates limited, but it appears that most women who freeze their eggs do not return to use them. For example, according to Zeynep Gürtin and colleagues' 2019 study at the London Women's Clinic, one of the major UK fertility clinics specializing in egg freezing, of all "social egg freezing" cycles performed in the 2012–2016 period, the vast majority of eggs (92.8%) remain in storage.[2] A Dutch study of women who underwent OC between 2009 and 2015 similarly showed only a 5% usage rate for the frozen eggs.[3] If, in the long term, a significant percentage of women do not claim their frozen eggs, OC can be considered a new source of eggs that could be circulated in networks of egg donation. More broadly, the freezability of donor eggs radically shifts existing practices of both reproductive and research egg donation.

The remarkable emergence of egg freezing in the last decade is therefore not only transformative as a means of "fertility preservation," but it also has important implications for egg *donation* practices. This final chapter, then, considers how the trajectories of the frozen eggs produced by OC differ from those of their "fresh" counterparts in egg donation. The extended durability of frozen eggs means they may be stored in egg banks—by analogy with the more familiar sperm banks—which collect a repository of donor eggs for third-party use. In the years following the Dutch 2011 legalization of OC, three egg banks were founded in the

Netherlands, and the London Egg Bank was the first to open its doors in the United Kingdom in 2013. Although there is no central registry of egg banks in the United States, the first egg banks were founded much earlier across the Atlantic; the World Egg Bank in Phoenix, Arizona, for example, was freezing eggs as early as 2004. Egg banks function as hubs for the discursive production and material distribution of cryopreserved eggs to fertility clinics nearby or far away. Once frozen, the eggs become as mobile as the liquid nitrogen tanks that contain them and may cross unprecedented distances—as well as a variety of borders—between clinics, countries, and continents.[4] Egg freezing is thus the key condition of emergence for the development of a global flow of eggs, which entails a broader respatialization of reproduction.

This global mobility of eggs should be situated within larger contemporary processes of change pertaining to globalization and aging. On the one hand, global developments—the deregulation of financial markets, the ubiquitous reach of communication and data technologies, the growth of tourism industries, and the outsourcing of labor—are the conditions of emergence for a globalization of biomedicine through transnational "reproflows" and "reproductive pathways" of technologies, people, and cells in cross-border reproductive care (CBRC) and internationalized research networks.[5] On the other hand, global population aging, following from declining fertility and increasing life expectancy, has locally specific sociocultural, political-economic effects on assisted reproduction.[6] The emergence of cross-border flows of cryo-eggs must be positioned in relation to the increasing age of people seeking fertility treatment—and the concomitant demand for younger donor eggs—as well as dominant narratives on "successful aging" that advocate individual responsibility for health and functionality. As locus of both reproductive youth and regenerative potential, the movement, procurement, and (potentially) therapeutic use of eggs is intimately caught up with a politics of aging that gains a global dimension when these eggs become mobile.

This chapter explores the implications of the transnational mobility of frozen eggs for reproductive and research egg-donation practices through two case studies. I first address the US-based World Egg Bank, which ships frozen eggs to intended parents across the world. Focusing on the movement of frozen eggs from the US bank to UK clinics, I consider what factors drive this reproflow and analyze how importing eggs retemporalizes and respatializes assisted reproduction. What is at stake in the movement of eggs—rather than people—in cross-border reproduction is a deterritorialization of egg donation, in which remote regulatory, clinical, and discursive practices govern a different set of localities.

Besides reproductive egg donation, I also turn to the procurement of donor eggs for research. I focus on the case study of the first successful derivation of human embryonic stem cells created through somatic cell nuclear transfer (SCNT), also termed "therapeutic cloning," which relies on donor eggs. This technique radically reconfigures the egg's relation to bodily time, and thereby raises questions about the relation between aging and reproductivity in new ways. The long-awaited success of SCNT technology revives the question of research egg procurement at a time when cryopreservation creates the possibility of shipping and banking eggs. This discussion highlights how the potential clinical applications, marketization, and regulation of SCNT research, along with its dependence on oocytes provided by young women, relate to a broader global biopolitics of aging that intersects with existing reproductive stratifications.

"Eggs without Borders": Transnational Frozen Egg Donation

The US-based World Egg Bank is one of the first companies to turn the global movement of frozen eggs into its core business. Specifically targeting the international demand for donor eggs, the World Egg Bank obtains eggs from American women and transports them to contracted fertility clinics in countries like the United Kingdom, Canada, and Australia. Combining gamete mobility and egg banking, the World Egg Bank offers insight into the transnational trajectories of frozen eggs.[7] As eggs move between countries, they also import and export the regulatory, temporal, and discursive dynamics of egg donation across national borders. The cross-border movements of frozen eggs thereby enable a *deterritorialization* of egg donation, as regulatory, financial, and clinical practices pertain less to a specific locality and more to the distant pathways of the eggs' cold chain.

Many institutions in the fertility industry have based their business models on national disparities in egg scarcity, procurement regulations, and treatment costs, but the World Egg Bank (TWEB) is one of the first to do so by moving eggs—rather than people—across national borders. Founded in 1997, the company originally focused on recruiting and screening egg donors, but in 2004 began to freeze eggs as, self-reportedly, the first commercial egg bank in the world.[8] It has been shipping frozen eggs internationally since 2007, distributing over 3,000 frozen eggs within the United States and abroad, with destinations including five fertility clinics in the United Kingdom. TWEB's roster includes 450 donors, some of whom have eggs frozen for donation, while others undergo stimulation and provide eggs only when selected by intended parents. In both cases, eggs can be frozen, transported, and subsequently fertilized and implanted at the recipient's clinic.[9]

In order to create transnational egg flows, egg banks like TWEB rely on international courier companies that provide a global infrastructure for moving frozen eggs through bio-cryogenic "cold chains," which are largely already in place given the existing transport of various cell and tissue cultures for clinics and laboratories globally.[10] Catherine Waldby notes that such cold chains combine innovations of storage and spatial distribution, and are shaped by regulatory landscapes that constrain and protect egg donors and recipients through "trail[s] of documentation, licensing arrangements, and compliance procedures that meet the ethical criteria set out by the importer jurisdiction."[11]

Traveling in the opposite direction of egg recipients seeking donor eggs abroad, frozen egg trajectories are developing along existing pathways between wealthy nations with egg shortages and popular donor-egg IVF destinations with relatively permissive egg-procurement regulations. A case in point is Ovobank Spain, the first European egg bank shipping frozen eggs across national borders. Its location reflects the popularity of Spain as a destination for donor eggs. Spain is responsible for over half the donor-egg IVF cycles in Europe and is particularly popular among intended parents in the United Kingdom, for whom local gamete shortage—particularly eggs—is the top motivation (71%) for traveling to overseas clinics.[12] By shipping eggs, Ovobank Spain now allows international patients to partake of the Spanish availability of eggs without leaving their home country. Whereas Spain's relative proximity and available travel options are attractive to many UK patients, once eggs can be shipped, limitations on the distances people are willing to travel need no longer be a primary consideration. Consequently, frozen egg transfers could raise the popularity of egg banks further afield, such as TWEB, thereby globalizing the donor egg market more than is currently the case.

Indirect Financial Inducement

The disparities in the regulatory frameworks governing egg donation and its remuneration—and the concomitant differences in the availability of donor eggs—play a key role in motivating TWEB's US-UK egg trade. In contrast with the relatively unregulated US fertility industry, the HFEA, which licenses all UK fertility clinics, sets limits on the payments for egg procurement.[13] These limits have risen steadily over the last two decades—in part in response to the increasing popularity of purchasing eggs abroad to circumvent UK waiting lists. The HFEA has increased maximum payments from £15 per cycle in 1998 to £250 in 2005 and £750 in 2011.[14] The maximum payment for donors of imported eggs was, however, maintained at £250 in loss of earnings per cycle.[15] Testifying to the influence of financial compensation in motivating egg donors, the number of egg donors increased by 35% in the two years after 2011.[16] Although around half of the UK clinics reported an increase in egg donations after 2011, donor shortages remained—particularly for Black and minority ethnic intended parents seeking eggs from "phenotypically similar" donors—and British patients continued to travel abroad to seek treatment with overseas donor eggs.[17]

Notably, the HFEA regulations only seek to avoid the financial inducement of potential egg donors. Meanwhile, other parties, such as TWEB, international courier companies, and the recipient's clinic, may operate on a commercial basis—i.e., be financially induced to engage women in egg procurement. This disparity suggests a regulatory emphasis on egg freezing and egg donation as an individual's consideration, rather than a focus on the socio-institutional contexts that frame and promote egg donation. In other words, it governs direct but not *indirect* financial inducement.

When the business models and profit margins of fertility companies are not governed by regulatory limits, they may provide an indirect financial inducement to promote specific treatment choices or patient recruitment practices. One example of such financial inducement comes from the Australian market leader Virtus Health, the world's first publicly listed fertility business, which owns—among many other clinics across the world—the Queensland Fertility Group, a partnership clinic of TWEB.[18] Virtus Health directly financially induces its clinicians to deliver high numbers of IVF cycles through its High Performer Share Incentive Scheme. This scheme financially rewards fertility specialists who "consistently deliver more than 400 cycles per annum for a consecutive three year period" because "the Board recognises those fertility specialists that achieve a high level of fresh cycles over a defined period acknowledging the value they generate for shareholders."[19] Situated within a regime of financialized capitalism, which Nancy Fraser describes as authorizing finance capital to discipline publics in the immediate interests of investors, the fertility company here becomes beholden not only—or even primarily—to its patients but also to its shareholders.[20] While regulations governing individual patients' and donors' reproductive decision making abound, the business practices that affect patients and their treatment choices by financially inducing their doctors to "deliver" more cycles are not subject to similar regulatory scrutiny.

In the case of frozen egg donation and TWEB, the modes of indirect financial inducement differ from those governing the Virtus example—or, for that matter, fresh egg donation. In UK and US fresh egg donation, intended parents typically pay for the donor to undergo a cycle, irrespective of the number of eggs produced. This arrangement reflects the ethical justification upheld by both the HFEA and the ASRM—if with different monetary standards—that women are compensated for their time, inconvenience, and expenses, rather than for their bodily tissue.[21] However, in frozen egg-donation practices, such as TWEB's, the recipients order a specific number of eggs at a fixed price, instead of linking payment directly to the donor's cycle. Consequently, the number of tradeable eggs a woman produces per cycle directly affects her profitability for the organization.

TWEB's egg donors receive $3,000 to $6,000 compensation per cycle, and on average the company "retrieve[s] 12–18 mature eggs per donor."[22] Frozen eggs are sold in batches of six for $16,500, plus $1,600 for international shipping and, where applicable, a $3,000 "Asian fee" for eggs from Asian donors. Provided the eggs are selected by intended parents, the average donor cycle could therefore generate between \$36,200 and \$54,300 revenue. The difference between retrieving 12 or 18 eggs from a donor can thus translate to an \$18,100 difference in revenue for the Egg Bank. By charging for a specific number of eggs rather than a cycle, TWEB's sales model commodifies the individual eggs rather than the egg donor's labor and expenses.[23] This model links capital accumulation directly to the outcome of the donor's cycle and thereby creates a financial incentive that favors donors and stimulation protocols that produce more eggs per cycle.

This is not unique to TWEB; frozen eggs are typically not sold by cycle, but as a particular number of eggs. Major US egg banks such as Donor Egg Bank USA (part of Generate Life Sciences) and Fairfax Egg Bank sell "lots" or "cohorts" of five to eight eggs. Cryos, the world's largest sperm bank, known for its Danish "Viking sperm," also has an egg bank in Florida, which sells individual eggs for \$2,300–\$2,500 each. My Egg Bank, part of the Prelude Network, similarly ships lots of six to eight eggs to affiliate clinics and offers guarantee programs for the creation of one or more embryos after a partner or donor ships sperm to the egg bank. These embryos can then be shipped to the intended mother's clinic.[24] When the remuneration of donors is organized per cycle, and the resultant eggs are sold in a set quantity, donors producing more eggs per cycle become more profitable for the egg bank. While egg banks may or may not adjust their practices accordingly, it is nonetheless important to note that this particular business model sets up financial incentives that reward exactly that. So while regulations and bioethical discussions focus on limiting remuneration to limit egg donors' financial inducement, the indirect financial inducement resulting from the financial incentives in for-profit egg banks remains unchecked.[25]

Deterritorializing Egg Donation

The question of financial inducement takes on a different character when the donor eggs are intended to be shipped from the United States to the United Kingdom. Taking up the UK's donor egg shortage as a business opportunity, TWEB's home page includes a prominent "Welcome UK" section, which links to a page explaining that a selection of TWEB egg donors complies with the UK's HFEA's Code of Practice.[26] Accordingly, each TWEB donor has to decide whether to become an international donor, which entails agreeing to the release of identifying information when the child turns 18 and receiving less financial compensation—a consideration situated in a US cultural context that favors altruistic donations and encourages donors to downplay financial motivations.[27] While the compensation to so-called international egg donors is curtailed, the price of the frozen eggs remains the same for UK patients. By catering to the HFEA requirements, TWEB demonstrates how the international movement of eggs affects local egg-donation practices, thereby extending UK regulations to new territories—along the pathway of the eggs' cold chain. Emerging with the transnational cryo-egg flows is, then, a deterritorialization of egg donation, pertaining to the regulations, remunerations, and specific donation practices they engender.

This deterritorialization of egg donation works in both directions and is propelled by the cross-border movement of eggs. Besides the introduction of UK remuneration practices into the US clinic, the movement of cryo-eggs into the United Kingdom also imports at least two important aspects of US egg-donation practices. Firstly, frozen egg banking changes the temporal dynamic of international egg procurement; whereas fresh egg donation is characterized by a degree of uncertainty about the outcome of the donor's treatment, which may take up to three months, cryopreserved eggs are available for immediate shipment and do not require synchronization between the two women's cycles. Because there is no need to await a match between recipient and donor to start a stimulation cycle, egg banks can accommodate both a continuous supply of eggs by donors and a continuous demand for "high-quality" eggs in anticipation of a diverse group of future intended parents not limited to the local population. If there are enough donors and recipients available, egg banks can thus speed up the egg-donation process by stalling the eggs' cellular time. TWEB's specific transatlantic egg flows likewise may speed up egg-donation procedures by making the more abundant bioavailability and variety of donor eggs in the United States accessible for local treatment of UK intended parents. For those patients seeking to avoid waiting lists, this speeding up of the reproductive process may be a key motivator for purchasing eggs abroad.

The second key element that frozen US oocytes import into the United Kingdom is the particular discursive framing of the eggs by

TWEB and the concomitant choice for a specific donor by the intended parents. In the United Kingdom, the choice for an egg donor is anonymized and typically made by the fertility clinic, rather than by the intended parent. The clinic normally controls "all aspects of the matching process," including the classification of donors, the range of preferences recipients can specify, and the allocation of donors to intended parents.[28] Priya Davda's research into matching in UK egg donation highlights some of the issues that may arise with this practice. She found that the matching process "singled out 'race' as a primary indicator of kinship and 'racial difference' as a primary 'kinship risk.'" She describes how "clinicians sought to curtail BME [Black and minority ethnic] recipients' reproduction of racialised white features whilst maintaining the reproduction of racialised white features of white British recipients."[29] Instead of clinicians allocating donors to recipients, the London Egg Bank allows intended parents to do their own matching through an online catalogue.[30] This catalogue includes donor characteristics such as weight, height, eye, hair, and skin color, and categorizations of "race" and "religion" along with medical test results and keywords on "personality" and "hobbies." The London Egg Bank explicitly foregrounds its use of individualized—if anonymized—donor presentation in its marketing with slogans like, "The choice is yours. You are in control."

TWEB nevertheless introduces a much more specific donor choice in the United Kingdom through its detailed online catalogue. While the frozen donor eggs cross a greater spatial distance for UK egg recipients, TWEB offers a closer encounter with the donor through profiles that include photographs as well as donor statements about their talents, reasons for donating, favorite books, future goals, and exercise habits. The profiles also feature a detailed medical history, including birth control method, abortions, plastic surgery, and diagnosed conditions—from dwarfism to near-sightedness—of the donor and her (biogenetically related) family members. TWEB's profiles are carefully constructed to meet widespread preferences for healthy donors who physically resemble the intended parents, but they also invite selection based on traits like beauty, intelligence, and athleticism through photographs of graduation ceremonies, beauty pageants, and cheerleading. Similarly, the textual descriptions of the donors convey gender-specific positive traits that intended parents are expected to be looking for, such as caring qualities, altruism, or maternal solidarity with infertile people. The profiles thereby attest to the importance of not only the eggs' bioavailability but also their "biodesirability" in cross-border reproductive care.[31] By extension, the introduction of these biodesirability markers to people receiving donor-egg IVF treatment in the United Kingdom may be a driving factor for transnational egg movements.

TWEB website's interface is organized around this more detailed type of reproductive decision making for the most biodesirable egg donor. Rival international egg and sperm bank Cryos has designed its website with donor profiles specifically "to resemble Match.com, a dating site," because, according to its founder, "finding a donor should be as close to finding a natural partner as possible."[32] TWEB's website similarly facilitates such a search by offering the option of arranging profiles in "ascending" or "descending" order based on organizing categories like "weight" and "height," thereby inviting a comparison between the donors. Likewise, filters allow recipients to only show blue-eyed or French-ancestry donors, thereby presenting racialized categorizations as key considerations to potential egg recipients.

The interface and metrics of these online platforms demonstrate how transnational egg donation is embedded in systems of social organization based on race, class, and nationality. There is a prevalent preference among intended parents for egg donors who look like themselves, in order to invisibilize the donation process. This leads to a demand for egg donors who reflect the racial and class disparities in the take-up of these technologies; in the United States, the vast majority of patients are middle- or upper-middle-class, and white women are more than twice as likely to access fertility services as Hispanic or Black women.[33] In keeping with this, Catherine Waldby notes that the availability of donors of "Caucasian" appearance, "which matches that of [the majority of] the North European purchasers," explains the popularity of Spanish and Eastern European clinics in transnational egg donation.[34]

Beyond resemblance, Carolin Schurr emphasizes the importance of (post)colonial imaginaries of white desirability in her study of transnational assisted reproduction in Mexico, where higher value is ascribed to white eggs and egg donors, while the differential selection of egg donors and surrogates reflects how the genetic traits of nonwhite women are devalued.[35] In her study of US egg donation, Anne Pollock similarly writes that "most of those with the means to use the technology are seeking white eggs, and it is likely that even among those Black egg consumers dark skin is undesirable."[36] Daniels and Heidt-Forsythe found that dominant cultural norms of white femininity were overrepresented in gamete databases, as "egg donors [we]re racially whiter, taller, thinner, and more highly educated than the national average of women their age."[37] While Rene Almeling's research into the egg-donation industry found that clinics have trouble "recruiting diverse donors" and therefore may pay African American women more for their eggs, Diane Tober's study of hundreds of US egg donors found that Black egg donors were paid significantly less for their eggs than white or Asian donors.[38] At TWEB, intended parents pay an additional "Asian fee" for eggs from donors with an Asian background, probably reflecting the increased demand for donor eggs following China's shift to a two-child policy.[39] Through these varying dynamics of supply and demand in egg-donation practices such as TWEB's, "race/ethnicity is genetically reified to the degree that it serves as the basis for program filing systems."[40] The mobility of frozen eggs moreover accommodates a wider range of nationally specific and racialized origin stories for eggs that may be accessed from the comfort of one's home.

Otherwise unavailable to British intended parents, these particular presentations of the egg through visual and textual representations of donors introduce new dimensions of consumer choice to the recipients. As a result, the intended parents choose not *whether* they would like to receive a donor egg preselected by a medical team but *which* donor egg would suit them best. This choice introduces a higher degree of patient agency over the reproductive process that may reposition conventional anonymous egg donation as lacking in comparison. From the UK perspective, frozen egg imports thus enable a move from a system in which the clinic is trusted to match intended parents to egg donors to one in which patients adopt a more agentic role in the donor-selection process. The TWEB donor catalogue, in turn, functions as an instrument of fostering trust in spite of its distance from intended parents by means of its detailed disclosure of donor characteristics. And in doing so, the online donor-selection system enables choices that at once reify, reflect, and reproduce the very social hierarchies of race, class, and cultural privilege that shape the direction of the transnational egg flows in the first place.

Cryo-egg Cold Chains and the Stratification of Reproductive Aging

While the speedy bioavailability and the choice for biodesirability drive these US-UK egg movements, the underlying demand for egg donation—both for donors and recipients—emerges from age-specific social realities. In a majority of cases, eggs move from fertile younger women to older women with age-related infertility. TWEB donors only qualify if they are between 18 and 29 years old, while UK women seeking donor eggs abroad are on average around 40 years old.[41] Furthermore, reproductive youth tends to have an inverse relation with financial means, and many young women—especially those who bear the expenses associated with their own "proven fertility"—are attracted to egg donation for the financial compensation.[42] As described on their *Eggs without Borders* blog, TWEB specifically focuses on recruiting students—targeting campus newspapers and handing out TWEB flip-flops and sunglasses—given that they are typically young and their education levels are a selling point. One blogpost announces that "ASU's [Arizona State University] Spring Semester will soon be underway. . . . With thousands upon thousands of qualified young women moving back into the area, The World Egg Bank is giving them the resources they need to learn more about egg donation."[43] Such recruitment drives coincide with a time in which US students are in an increasingly precarious financial situation as university tuition and living costs rise and available grants and scholarships fall.[44] Moreover, at times of financial recession, young American women who are not students are particularly vulnerable to unemployment, making the option of donating eggs financially attractive.[45]

On the other side of the ocean, and the other side of the donor-recipient relation, British women approaching 40 are relatively well-to-do compared to younger age groups.[46] Women who turn to overseas egg donation as a second option after failed treatments with their own eggs are typically older than women who try IVF for the first time—averaging around 40 years compared to 35.[47] As reproductive youth becomes a transferable quality that may be "outsourced" to women across the world, these intersections of age, gender, fertility, and economic means drive the international movements of eggs.

A variation on the distribution of reproductive aging between bodies and eggs in OC, transnational egg flows likewise distribute reproductive aging in a heterologous fashion between bodies and eggs across the globe. Now spanning a much larger spatial scale, it intersects the physicality of cellular and physical reproductive age with broader political-economic structures. As a form of distributed reproductive aging, the reproductive youth materialized in the egg gains a transferable quality, and its production may be outsourced to women across the world.

While cross-border egg donation was previously geographically limited by the distances intended parents and donors were willing to travel, the mobility of frozen eggs allows the extension of international egg-donation networks across the globe. Although TWEB's egg transfer discussed above occurs between two relatively privileged national contexts, future flows of eggs—following the logic of the existing cross-border trade of fresh eggs—may follow a trajectory from poorer donors to wealthier intended parents, from less regulated national contexts to more restrictive health systems, as well as from younger to older women. These cross-border egg flows emerge in the context of global patterns of inequality in which re/productive labor moves along "transnational hierarchies that are the legacy of colonial, imperial and diasporic 'non-flat world' routes."[48] Situated in systems of oppression, Dorothy Roberts argues, global ART markets tend to reproduce racial hierarchies, as they are prone to benefit people who have higher social status and exploit those who do not.[49] Research on specific routes of more established forms of third-party cross-border reproduction, such as fresh egg donation and surrogacy, highlights how they reproduce global inequalities organized around gender, capital, and race.[50] The conditions are in place for global cryo-egg flows to recreate these patterns in which the reproductive choices of privileged global biocitizens require the "clinical labor" and reproductive substances of those who become implicated through structural economic, racialized, and gendered stratification.[51] Because eggs, rather than people, move in this practice, it is more subject to the logic of outsourcing, whether through price differentials between the eggs' origin and destination countries, through regulatory discrepancies, or through "racialised notions of the world" that guide intended parents' choices in global reproductive trajectories.[52]

As the fertility industry has expanded beyond Europe, North America, and Oceania to the Middle East, Asia, Africa, and Latin America, institutional infrastructures are in place that could be employed to further extend transnational transfers of cryopreserved eggs. Numerous Asian and Latin American countries, including India, Malaysia, Thailand, and Cuba, have actively encouraged—and, in some cases, subsequently discouraged—medical and reproductive tourism; they illustrate that government policies can play a key role in further encouraging the growth of a more globalized ART circuit for egg donation.[53] Meanwhile, contemporary global IVF is experiencing a significant merger and acquisition cycle, resulting in the creation of ever larger transnational fertility corporations spanning several continents. For example, the abovementioned Virtus Health operates 46 IVF clinics in Australia, Ireland, Denmark, and Singapore; Spanish IVI and US RMANJ have merged to create the world's largest fertility network; and Korean CHA Fertility (see below), which owns local and US clinics, has recently bought majority stakes in large Australian and Singaporean fertility groups, thereby aiming to jointly create the largest Asian-Pacific reproductive healthcare network in order to "address the rapidly growing demand" for IVF amid "trends of diminishing fertility."[54] The investments required for these global fertility corporations are in part motivated by demographic trends towards later reproduction, while the emergence of transnational fertility companies creates the infrastructures for streamlining egg flows between countries and across borders. Both market developments and government regulations provide the infrastructures for the distribution of global egg flows. The stratified nature of these distributions according to the age-specificity of both the demand and provision of donor eggs highlights how Shellee Colen's classic notion of stratified reproduction is also organized by a global biopolitics of aging.

In these global flows of frozen eggs, the "cold chain" may start to function like the "global care chain."[55] The latter references "the international transfer of caretaking" by the commodification of care work through the employment of lower-waged migrant women.[56] Rather than the migratory displacement of women as a result of the marketization of domestic care work, the marketization of technologically assisted reproduction may result in the displacement of the cryopreserved gametes of relatively lower-paid egg donors. From the example of TWEB, it may be extrapolated that a global cold chain of distributed reproductive aging would flow from sites in which women's reproductive youth intersects with forms of indirect or direct financial inducement in a national context characterized by high biotechnological development and permissive regulations. This flow would be directed to the places where an increased age of reproduction—or reduced fertility for other reasons—meets relative wealth, high biotechnological development, and limited or expensive supplies of eggs.

While biodesirability plays a key role in shaping these reproflows, as became apparent in the discursive constructions of TWEB's eggs, the political implications of the irrelevance of biodesirability in egg procurement for research are a central concern of the following section.

Embryonic Stem Cell Research and the Remaking of Egg Donation

In 2013, Shoukhrat Mitalipov's research group at Oregon Health and Science University (OHSU) made a historic announcement: they managed, for the first time, to derive stem cells from human embryos produced through somatic cell nuclear transfer (SCNT), popularly known as "cloning" technology.[57] This nuclear transfer approach is the human equivalent of the "Dolly technique" that was used to create the famous sheep in 1996 and, more recently in 2018, two big-eyed macaques called Hua Hua and Zhong Zhong, who were the first primates to be cloned.[58] In keeping with the global moratorium on human cloning, however, Mitalipov's Oregon group did not seek to create offspring, but instead used the cloned embryos to extract stem cells.

SCNT techniques require eggs—but not sperm—to create embryos. The Oregon group's embryos were created by merging an egg with a somatic cell—in this case a skin cell.[59] The group removed the egg's nucleus, which contains its DNA, and replaced it with the nucleus of a skin cell donated by a patient with Leigh syndrome. The resulting egg was subsequently stimulated to divide into an embryo that has the same nuclear DNA as the skin cell donor.[60] The Oregon team extracted stem cells from embryos produced in this way and reprogrammed them into contracting heart muscle cells. They thus used an egg to create very young, embryonic cells that match the DNA of the—by definition older—skin cell donor. In this way, the egg is at the heart of a cellular reconfiguration of aging in stem cell science.

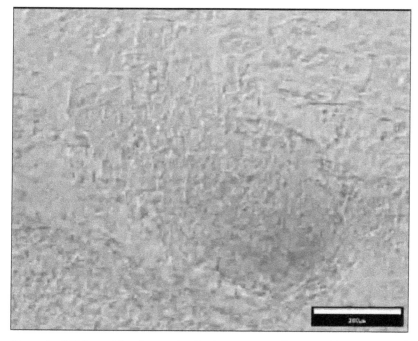

Figure 6.1. Still from video *Contracting Cardiomyocytes Differentiated from NT-ESCs.*[61]

In the *Cell* article announcing their results, the Oregon scientists included a video of rhythmically pulsing heart muscle cells. It showed a blurred figure made up of two round shapes positioned diagonally above one another, which contracted roughly every two seconds. The video visualized both the "remarkable ability to reprogram our body cells back into an embryonic state" and their potential to differentiate into functioning specialized cells.[62] The symbolism and dramatic visual impact of heart muscle cells pulsing in the petri dish were recognized as early as a century prior to this publication, when the famous French biologist Alexis Carrel cultured the contracting cells of an embryonic chicken heart. They were kept alive in culture for over 30 years and ended up outliving him. Given the "connotation of the heart [and its beat] as the seat and sign of life," Carrel used the visibly contracting muscle cells to make a claim about the nature of bodily time *in vitro*.[63] In his 1912 paper "The Permanent Life of Tissues outside of the Organism," Carrel proposed that these disembodied cells could become immortal under the right culturing conditions. In other words, he suggested that the cells' aging process was contingent on its environment and thereby dramatically extendable outside of the body.[64] In Mitalipov's parallel visual strategy, the heart cells visualize a type of aging that does not extend indefinitely but rather regenerates and begins anew *in vitro*. Underlining this regenerative model of aging, Mitalipov's contracting heart cells are reminiscent of the quintessential first encounter with new life in the image of the heartbeat in a fetal ultrasound—but instead of the fetus *in utero*, they present the *in vitro* generation of a new type of cellular human life that may be conceived from oocytes.

Significantly, these successes in human stem cell science rely on the availability of human donor eggs. This section extends the previous discussion of the transnational mobility of frozen eggs for reproductive purposes to a consideration of the relevance of cryopreservation for research egg procurement. The first three scientific studies that successfully obtained SCNT-derived human embryonic stem cells (hESCs) function as case studies: the work of Mitalipov's Oregon group,[65] Dong-Ryul Lee's collaboration of Korean CHA Health Systems, and US biotech Advanced Cell Technology[66] and Dieter Egli's collaboration of Columbia University, the New York Stem Cell Foundation, and the Hebrew University of Jerusalem.[67] Given that they are the first to successfully create these stem cells, the three studies may set a precedent not only for future stem cell research and protocols but also for the acquisition of the required eggs; I therefore use them as a starting point in considering the possibilities for the remaking of research egg procurement. The regulatory, infrastructural, and discursive contexts of the studies' emergence are indicative of the factors that can drive the movement of eggs across state and national borders. Reading SCNT research as a rearrangement of biological time, these studies point to a new role for the egg in a global politics of aging, in which age is reconceptualized at the cellular and molecular level, and its regeneration becomes dependent on the reproductivity of young women.

All three studies emphasize the clinical potential of their work, which follows from the possibility of differentiating embryonic stem cells (ESCs) into specialized cell types like skin, nerve, or muscle cells. The SCNT technique is presented as a way to reprogram body cells (in the US-Korean study, those of a 75-year-old man) "back into an embryonic state" in order to generate personalized replacement cells, which would exactly match the DNA of the patient.[68] The studies thus point to the promise of generating personalized, DNA-matched (stem) cells that could be transplanted into the patient's body with a decreased risk of immune rejection. The Egli team proposes that the studies' successes "raise the possibility that 'therapeutic cloning,' as it was originally called, will become a reality."[69] SCNT is thus framed as a key promissory technology in regenerative medicine that may one day treat human tissue damaged by accidents, disease, or aging.[70]

As these achievements provide an incentive for further research and potential future clinical application, they also drive increasing demand for human eggs—and for women to provide them. The study and the creation of ESCs requires a significant number of oocytes; for example, Egli's study created four stem cell lines out of 71 eggs and received a total of 512 mature oocytes.[71] The research teams suggest that the procedures can become more efficient in the future, but such improvements could nevertheless raise interest and investment in this technique and thereby still increase demand for women's eggs.

Donor Eggs and Hwang's Legacy

Egg donation is so important to these three SCNT studies because they achieved what was previously falsely claimed by the South Korean scientist Woo-Suk Hwang. Hwang not only fabricated evidence in his two *Science* publications but also incorrectly reported that his studies used, respectively, only 242 and 185 eggs from donors who received "no financial reimbursement."[72] The Korean National Bioethics Committee later found that over 2,000 eggs were sourced from 119 women, of which more than half were commercially obtained. Hwang's junior colleagues were also among the egg donors, and, according to Jin Sook Myung's research, IVF patients who agreed to receive discounted treatment in exchange for their "surplus" eggs unwittingly donated their best-quality eggs to research.[73] Following the Hwang scandal, a backlash against stem cell research resulted in a stricter Korean regulatory regime on research egg donation.[74] Significantly, this included specific restrictions that prescribed that only leftover eggs could be used for SCNT research. And because fertilization would typically be attempted with good-quality eggs in IVF treatments, frozen eggs are far more commonly left over than fresh ones are.[75]

The Hwang case highlights two important aspects that inform the relationship between stem cell research and the geopolitics of transnational egg mobility: first, the mobilization of bionationalist discourses in shaping these egg trajectories and, second, the interplay between transnational egg donation for reproduction and research. Hwang's research, and the local unpaid "altruistic" egg donations that supported it, drew on a highly bionationalist discourse. Hwang's stem cell research developed in the context of major and concentrated government investments in biotech—$18 billion over the course of 14 years—that sought to make Korea a leading nation in the field. Hwang was bestowed the status of "Supreme Scientist" and the large, $65 million investments in his laboratory were recognized as a way of securing "prestige" and "symbolic and economic capital," while asserting independence from—if not global scientific leadership over—former Western colonial powers.[76] Hwang asserted that "science knows no border, but a scientist has his homeland," and that with his stem cell research, he "stuck the Korean national flag into the heights of biotechnology, America."[77] Against the backdrop of international scientific competition, the idea of the nation was thus highly effective in generating government investment for SCNT.

With the research framed in an "ethos of competitive nationalism," egg donation became "an act of 'good citizenry.'" Hwang claimed in public media that the egg donors were "not paid and were motivated by a desire to help sick people and national pride."[78] In December 2005, hundreds of women supporting Hwang held a ceremony, in which they sang the South Korean national anthem, declared their intention to donate eggs, and left a trail of azalea flowers leading to Hwang's laboratory.[79] Egg donors also contributed to www.ilovehwang.net, where some described their motivation for donating as a "sacrifice" to the nation: "I'm very happy that I can add my tiny self to support him. . . . Please give me a chance to be a patriot."[80] A variation on the traditionally politicized relation between women's reproductivity and the reproduction of the nation, this bionationalist framing of egg donation positions eggs, rather than children, as symbols of the nation's successful future.[81]

Yet alongside the local egg donors, Hwang's team also sourced a significant proportion of its oocytes from the international for-profit egg broker DNA-Bank. This broker initially focused on reproductive egg donation and procured eggs from Korean women for intended parents from Japan, where commercial egg donation was prohibited. For Hwang's project, DNA-Bank allegedly recruited not only Korean but also Chinese and Malaysian women to provide eggs for research. According to Gottweis and Kim's research into the scandal, the Hwang team paid Mr. "K," DNA-Bank's CEO, $1,537 per woman.[82] As Catherine Waldby notes, DNA-Bank's role in Hwang's research demonstrates that existing transnational reproductive egg donation networks can be employed to enable a supply of eggs for research purposes.[83] If reproductive and research egg donation thus begin to approximate one another, the current establishment of transnational cold chains to move donor eggs to fertility clinics should also be considered in the light of their potential use to supply ova to research labs. In theory, transnational egg donation for research could approximate existing cross-border reproductive egg movements if frozen eggs could be used for this work—and the post-Hwang regulation of SCNT research prescribed exactly that.

Following the Hwang scandal, it took three years before the Korean National Bioethics Committee approved another SCNT study involving human eggs, in 2009; a second was approved in 2016—both were based at CHA Medical Group.[84] The latter was directed by Dong-Ryul Lee, who also led one of the three SCNT studies, and the project could use 600 leftover eggs, of which the majority (500) were frozen.[85] This reflects the post-Hwang revisions of the Korean Bioethics and Safety Act, which limited SCNT research to the use of "residual"—typically frozen—eggs to avoid ethical concerns about direct egg donations.[86] These residual eggs are described as eggs that are left over after fertility treatment and are required to be provided free of charge by "medical institutions for producing embryos."[87]

Conveniently, the CHA Medical Group is such an institution—and one that is also a major player in egg freezing for age-related infertility. It claims to be responsible for the first birth of a baby conceived from a vitrified egg in 1999, established the world's first publicly accessible egg freezing clinic in Los Angeles in 2002, and now owns the three hospitals that currently store the largest number of cryo-eggs in Korea.[88] CHA is investing in infertility in Korea, where late pregnancies and age-related infertility are on the rise while the birth rate has hit a record low of

0.98.[89] But CHA also recently acquired majority shares in major international fertility groups, with numerous clinics and frozen egg banks in Australia and Singapore. It aims to become the world's largest IVF group, with 50,000 cycles annually by 2022.[90] Meanwhile, in Korea, CHA's dual focus on stem cell research and fertility treatments creates the institutional infrastructure required to access residual eggs for research.

Notwithstanding CHA's investments in an infrastructure that incorporates both OC and SCNT, the Korean regulations that limit SCNT research primarily to frozen eggs have also attracted criticisms that once again draw on a bionationalist discourse. In the *Korea Times*, scientists argue that stem cell research could be "one of our future growth engines," but that strong government support is needed so "our researchers can get ahead of their overseas competitors." According to the newspaper, "Leaders of stem cell research like the United States, Britain and Japan allow the use of fresh human eggs for therapeutic cloning. By contrast, we have been prohibited from doing so for the past 10 years after the 2005 scandal and that's why we are lagging behind. . . . A lot of scientists went abroad, frustrated by the government's tougher regulation following the Hwang scandal."[91] Hwang's case illustrates how, in the face of international research collaborations, the nation may still be mobilized in framing the scientific breakthroughs, the donors' bodily sacrifices, and the subsequent government regulations restricting embryonic stem cell research primarily to frozen eggs.

US Stem Cell Bionationalism

Notwithstanding Hwang's ethical transgressions, both aspects of the egg-donation practices—the bionationalist discourses on stem cell research and the close relation between research and reproductive egg procurement—are also at play in the US context of the three SCNT case studies by Mitalipov's, Lee's, and Egli's groups. In the United States, the nation is mobilized both to discourage and to promote egg-based research with reference to, respectively, anti-abortion and pro-innovation agendas, which set the stage for changing research egg-donation practices.

In 2001, President Bush famously restricted federal funding for embryonic stem cell research, including SCNT. Encouraged by future vice president Mike Pence, Bush maintained these restrictions on the use of embryos for research by repeatedly vetoing attempts by Congress to lift them—a decision he celebrated with dramatic White House press conferences in which he surrounded himself with children born from "embryo adoption" programs.[92] The limitations on stem cell research provoked fears about a "brain drain" of scientists to other, more permissive regulatory contexts—including those that came to be known as the "Asian Tigers," such as Singapore and South Korea—thereby "fuel[ling] nationalisms" in the United States and elsewhere.[93] Although the primary ethical concern lay with the role of the embryo in stem cell research—informed by its controversial status in the politics of abortion—the US stance on paying women for eggs was also relatively restrictive. While the reproductive egg-donation industry flourished and routinely offered donors $2,500–$10,000 per cycle, influential national bodies such as the US National Research Council and National Academy of Sciences advised against paid research egg donation—a position that was also adopted in various state laws, including Massachusetts's and California's.[94]

However, later that decade, President Obama removed some of Bush's restrictions on federal funding for stem cell research, referencing concerns with national competition in statements like, "We will ensure America's continued global leadership in scientific discoveries and technological breakthroughs."[95] Trump subsequently won the 2016 presidential election on an anti-Obama platform that has consistently "opposed federal funding for embryonic stem cell research" as part of its anti-abortion agenda. After entering office, Trump has focused on restricting federal funding for fetal tissue research—rather than stem cell research—in an attempt to show that "promoting the dignity of human life from conception to natural death is one of the very top priorities of [his] administration."[96]

The ongoing, politicized changes in US federal regulation of stem cell research are complicated by state-based regulations, which may both reinforce and counteract the bionationalist innovation or pro-life federal agendas. For example, when Bush halted new human embryonic stem cell research, California passed the Stem Cell Research and Cures Initiative, which has provided millions of dollars in stem cell research in the state and is understood to have contributed to a recognition of

California as "the national leader in stem cell research."[97] Differing state regulations of egg procurement opened up a "new stem cell geopolitics where not only other countries, but some individual states . . . claimed or were feared to have a new competitive edge."[98] While paid egg procurement within permissive states functioned as a condition of possibility for research projects like Mitalipov's, its successes, in turn, increased pressure on other states and research institutes to reconsider their egg-procurement regulations.[99] For example, in 2013, the year Mitalipov's study was published, California sought to follow Oregon's and New York's precedent with a bill aimed at lifting the prohibition on paid research egg procurement, which passed the Senate but was vetoed by Governor Jerry Brown.[100] The differing state-specific regulations are moreover instrumental in shaping flows of cellular material across the nation and beyond, as is the case in negotiations of "material transfer agreements" for shipping the Oregon stem cell lines between Mitalipov's and other research labs, which may be governed by conflicting egg-procurement regulations.[101] For example, Mitalipov's stem cells could not be sent to and studied by the California Institute of Regenerative Medicine, because the institute's funds could not be used for studies that rely on cell lines produced using paid egg donation.[102] International regulatory differences could similarly play a role in directing the global flow of frozen eggs for research purposes.

At this specific historical moment, a series of factors—the geographically specific relaxation of restrictions on financial compensation for egg procurement, the popularization of OC technology, the mushrooming of egg banks within a general trend of bio-banking, and the availability of cryoshipping infrastructures—paves the way for a transnational flow of eggs. Although strict regulations and bioethical guidelines limit the feasibility of such flows for research projects at present, the global movements for reproductive egg donation provide a model for a more transnationalized research egg-procurement practice. The possibility of shipping eggs could fundamentally shift the spatial dynamics of egg procurement for a research sector that is characterized both by intensive cross-border cooperation in what Charis Thompson calls "stem cell internationalism" and strong pressures of scientific competition, commercial research investments, and politicized regulations linked to local and national identity.[103]

Relating Research and Reproductive Egg Donation

In keeping with this, the three SCNT studies also point to the close regulatory, discursive, and clinical relation between research egg procurement and its more transnationalized reproductive counterpart. Firstly, in the US context of the studies under scrutiny, research egg-donation practices are regulated with reference to their reproductive counterpart. As Waldby has noted, egg donation for stem cell research operates "alongside a transactional reproductive market" in which women are routinely paid up to $10,000 per cycle.[104] Although bodies such as the National Research Council advised that egg donors should only be reimbursed for direct expenses, in 2007, the American Society for Reproductive Medicine (ASRM) adopted the position that financial compensation for egg procurement for stem cell research may be acceptable. The ASRM stated that its compensation guidelines applied to all egg donors "regardless of the ultimate use of the oocytes (e.g., fertility therapy or research)."[105] As mentioned above, states such as California do not permit reimbursement beyond direct expenses for research egg donation. Yet where compensation is allowed, the egg-donation practice is modeled on reproductive egg donation.

In the New York context of Egli's SCNT study, for example, the Empire State Stem Cell Board overseeing the $600 million state-funded stem cell research program permitted its funded researchers to compensate its egg donors "in amounts proportional to those allowed by the state for donation of oocytes for *in vitro* fertilization."[106] In its 2009 decision, the board referenced the ASRM guidelines for donor payment up to $10,000 and cited principles of "justice" and "equity" to argue that the same terms and conditions should govern egg provision for reproductive purposes and scientific research.[107] Over the course of the subsequent nine years, the Egli research lab in New York procured over 1,500 mature oocytes, the majority of which were used for SCNT studies.[108] In these studies, including the abovementioned 2014 SCNT study, egg donors were screened and paid $8000 per cycle with explicit reference to the ASRM guidelines.[109] The team notes that these egg-donation cycles were made possible through a collaboration with "a large, academic-affiliated reproductive endocrinology clinic."[110] The bioethical consensus, clinical practice, and screening and compensation guidelines for reproductive egg donation were thus of direct influence on egg donation for stem cell research.

Secondly, the employment of reproductive healthcare infrastructures has effects on the discursive framing of research egg donation. For example, the OHSU Women's Health Research Unit, which "recruited" the egg donors for Mitalipov's study, frames its research with reference to values of altruism and women's solidarity: "OHSU research has begun to illuminate some of the vast overlooked difference between the genders that influence a woman's overall health" and "This research is vital to the women of Oregon and to women everywhere. You can help."[111] Its Facebook page juxtaposes announcements of clinical trials with quasi-feminist links to Buzzfeed posts on #doublestandards. Many feminist scholars and activists have objected to paid research egg procurement out of concern for women's exposure to significant health risks in the stimulation and extraction procedures.[112] Ironically, it is precisely an identity politics of female solidarity that is employed when egg donors are mobilized by an appeal to, in Charis Thompson's words, a "procures" narrative that frames stem cell research as a contribution to women's health.[113] This discursive framing of egg donation for research thus appeals to notions of "sisterhood" and altruism, which also characterize discourses of reproductive egg donation and surrogacy.[114]

Notwithstanding their close relation, an important difference between reproductive and research egg donation is the fact that sociocultural biodesirability is irrelevant in donor selection for research. As a result, a different group of women can become potential donors, thereby shifting the dynamics of egg-procurement practices—especially so when frozen eggs can be used for research studies.

Cytoplasm Politics: The Egg in the Global Biopolitics of Aging

As egg freezing for fertility preservation was in part motivated by changing societal trends in timing reproduction, so the interest and investment in regenerative medicine relate to a politics of aging in which global, cultural, and cellular scales meet. Most obviously, SCNT research for regenerative medicine must be positioned in the context of profound changes in the age distribution globally—and most dramatically in the so-called aging societies in Europe, North America, Japan, and Australasia. The proportion of older people living in these regions is relatively large—and growing. In Western Europe, for example, by 2030 half the population will be over 50 years old and will have a life expectancy of another 40 years.[115] These changes result from a decrease in birth rates—global fertility almost halved from 5 to 2.6 average lifetime births per woman in the 1960s–1990s period—along with the last century's increase in life expectancy of about 30 years.[116]

These age-related demographics provide the backdrop for the renewed interest in SCNT research, which holds the promise of treating age-related diseases—if not the aging process itself. More precisely, SCNT studies explore the possibility that "the aging body would partake of the embryonic tissue vitality of the very young body" and, in doing so, implicate women's reproductive bodies within a globalized "biopolitics of ageing."[117] Whether or not such a scenario is realized, the magnitude of the capital investments in this promise of regenerative medicine points to a model of aging characterized by an "uneven distribution of longevity throughout the world, and the corresponding polarization of power and wealth derived from these same biotechnological investments."[118] This section positions the abovementioned SCNT studies in relation to this global biopolitics of aging to highlight the key role of the egg's cytoplasm—rather than its nucleus—in political-economic, cultural, and cellular reconfigurations of 21st-century aging practices.

These radical changes in aging patterns over the last decades are, according to sociologist Céline Lafontaine, "surely one of the most profound and sustained revolutions marking the history of humanity." She argues that the widespread increase in life expectancy is "totally redefining our relationship with time and death, . . . which now appears in relatively new forms, as the rapid increase in degenerative diseases such as cancer, Parkinson's disease and Alzheimer's illustrates." Rather than the relatively quick major causes of death prior to the 1950s— namely, war, childbirth, and infectious diseases such as tuberculosis— contemporary deaths tend to occur more slowly and typically follow a stage of prolonged illness.[119] The proliferation of life-prolonging medical technologies for these illnesses also creates a new cultural perspective on the timing of the end of life in which most deaths are considered premature. Sharon Kaufman's study of this phenomenon shows that, in the face of ever more treatment options, death increasingly becomes reconceptualized as the result of a "failure of medicine *regardless of the patient's age.*"[120] As part of the growing medical-industrial complex that is geared towards aging populations, it is precisely this last stage of life that is the focus in stem cell–based regenerative medicine. And to the extent that these efforts rely on SCNT, it is the egg that is recognized as holding the promise of counteracting age-related diseases and prolonging life.

Yet the rise of regenerative medicine does not simply reflect the changing needs of aging populations but is itself an effect of 20th-century social transformations from welfare to neoliberal state models, which are founded on contrasting approaches to aging. While the former sought to guarantee support "from cradle to grave," the neoliberal state withdraws from public healthcare programs for "the extremes of childhood (education, child care, child protection) and old age."[121] Melinda Cooper describes how US cuts in healthcare services were accompanied by government and private investments in biotechnological innovations resulting in medical products that are speculative, individualized, and may only be affordable to a small section of the public.[122] Propelled by the promise of future applications and highly expensive in execution, SCNT studies appear as a case in point of this approach, in which the future potential of patient-specific cures manifests the speculative and individualized qualities of the neoliberal project.

Rather than constituting a welfare crisis, aging and age-related pathologies thus become the occasion for investing in new markets for technologies that "retard or obscure the effects of aging," which are growing both "in size and overall share of the economy."[123] SCNT aligns with a reconceptualization of aging away from a model of homogenous and irreversible decline towards a view of the body as an unevenly aging entity in which specific parts may be replenished and rejuvenated.

A Cytoplasmic Fountain of Youth

Underlying SCNT research, and the commercial investments into this technology, is a reconceptualization of the aging process in which the egg takes center stage. In SCNT, it is the egg that has the potential both to reconfigure the linearity of cellular aging and to develop cell-based therapies for age-related diseases. In an article titled "The Reversibility of Irreversible Ageing," Galkin and colleagues propose that the egg's cytoplasm can be used to "set a genome age to zero." The embryo created from this egg may then "produce embryonic stem cells with the age apparently erased."[124] In other words, the egg's cytoplasm is presented as a cellular fountain of youth.

The potential profitability of this reconceptualization of aging is reflected in the involvement of the Massachusetts biotechnology company Advanced Cell Technology (ACT) in the SCNT study by Dong-ryul Lee's team. Prior to this study, ACT attracted large multi-million-dollar investments to intensify its research and development activities in order to secure its "intellectual property position in the drive towards commercialization of embryonic stem cell and SCNT technology."[125] ACT had grown from a small agricultural cloning research facility into a large corporation using embryonic and adult stem cells for "therapeutic innovations."[126] Stem cell research provided a means of gaining "ownership rights to critical technologies in regenerative medicine" through patents, of which ACT alone held over 50 in the field of SCNT technology. Following several mergers and acquisitions, ACT is now the Astellas Institute for Regenerative Medicine (AIRM), a biotechnology company that aims to develop and commercialize new therapies in regenerative medicine, particularly in the field of age-related eye diseases.[127] A subsidiary of the Japanese Astellas Pharma, AIRM and its investors are motivated by the "potential size of this market and its projected growth rate largely as a consequence of an increasing aged population."[128] Irrespective of whether clinical applications will emerge from this research, the financial stakes in stem cell technologies reflect the speculative value ascribed to the potential profitability of age-related pathologies in global biotech industries.

Significantly, in the SCNT approach, the egg is positioned as the key tool for "reset[ting] the clock of aging." This idea is expressly stated in ACT's press release on studies with cows that were concerned with

the feasibility of reversing the aging of cells by SCNT and transplanting young cells back into the old animal. . . . [T]hese studies suggest that medicine may one day be able to *reset the clock* of aging in aged human cells by SCNT and then use the resulting young cells to regenerate the immune and vascular system of older patients.[129]

Here the biological clock does not denote time running out, as it did in egg freezing discourses, but rather symbolizes the agency that may be exerted over the passage of bodily time via the egg. Contrasting with the rather passive role that has traditionally been ascribed to the egg in fertilization, the report on the first successful SCNT stem cell derivation describes the egg's cytoplasm's "unique *ability* to reset the identity of transplanted somatic cell nuclei to the embryonic state."[130] This approach foregrounds the egg's cytoplasm as "the only system that can reprogram a somatic nucleus to a full extent," thereby shifting a cell nucleus from the adult to the embryonic state.[131] In other words, researchers recognize the egg's cytoplasm as an active mechanism that can erase aging and "set the genome age to zero" once the somatic cell's nucleus is submerged in this cellular fountain of youth.[132]

This reconceptualization of the hitherto irreversible process of aging as newly plastic at the molecular and cellular level entails a key shift in perspective in which the egg is valued not for its genetic content—as it was in egg freezing and reproductive egg donation—but for its cytoplasm, which interacts with the nucleus of the donated somatic cell. While the somatic cell's nuclear genome is key to the stem cells' desired histocompatibility, the egg's cytoplasm replenishes this genome with embryonic youth. In other words, in SCNT the egg's cytoplasm is the "biological tool" that holds the potential to return the adult cell to the youngest pluripotent state.[133]

It is also possible to bypass the egg and create stem cells directly from somatic cells, such as skin cells, with a technique called "induced pluripotency." The Nobel Prize–winning achievement of inducing pluripotent stem cells (iPSCs) from somatic cells in the mid-2000s initially shifted the research focus away from SCNT because this relatively simple process did not require eggs.[134] However, the subsequent successes in SCNT research have revived interest in a technique that had been on its "death bed" after repeated failures, the Hwang scandal, and the iPSC discovery. The three SCNT studies represent a "remarkable comeback" of the nuclear transfer technique and have led to renewed interest in these technologies and their potential clinical translation.[135] While the creation of stem cells through induced pluripotency (iPSC) is technically less complicated and does not rely on donor eggs, the SCNT stem cells may have several advantages, especially for aging potential patients.

Wolf and colleagues highlight that, over the years, some limitations of iPSCs have become apparent that are especially significant for age-related regenerative medicine. When researchers are working with older somatic cells, induced pluripotency has a distinct disadvantage over SCNT precisely because there is no young egg involved. The main difference between the two stem cell types is concerned with mitochondrial DNA (mtDNA), which is found in the egg's cytoplasm. While in iPSCs the mtDNA comes from the donor somatic cell, in SCNT stem cells it is derived from the donor egg. Because mtDNA mutates more rapidly over time than nuclear DNA, the frequency of mtDNA mutations in iPSCs increases with the somatic cell donor's age. In SCNT stem cells, the mtDNA is unaffected by the somatic cell donor's age because it is determined by the young donor egg.[136] As a result, the researchers specifically note "the limitations of iPSCs derived from elderly patients destined for clinical applications" and propose SCNT stem cells as an alternative that counteracts these age-related limitations with the aid of younger donor eggs.[137] Irrespective of the future development of SCNT-derived therapies, the promise of nuclear transfer for regenerative medicine itself provides the rationale for a renewed interest in this type of research, which is reliant on women providing their eggs.

Chimeric Eggs and Recombinant Fertilities

Beyond regenerative medicine for age-related pathologies, nuclear transfer techniques are also used to regenerate fertility. The possibility of nuclear transfer that the SCNT studies demonstrated can also be used for mitochondrial replacement therapy. This treatment fuses the intended mother's egg nucleus with a donor egg's cytoplasm and subsequently fertilizes this merged egg with sperm.[138] The resulting embryo contains nuclear DNA from the intended mother and father (or sperm donor) as well as mitochondrial DNA from the egg donor. While this treatment allows people with severe mitochondrial diseases to have genetically related children without passing on the condition, the technique has also been used in attempts to treat age-related infertility.

The UK Parliament legalized this so-called three-parent technique for carriers of mitochondrial diseases in 2015. In the same year, it was banned in the United States as a result of an anti-abortion Republican congressional amendment forbidding the FDA from reviewing clinical trials that involve the genetic manipulation of embryos.[139] Circumventing the ban, US doctor John Zhang, founder of the popular New Hope Clinic in New York, decided to fly to Mexico to treat one of his patients there. This was a woman who had already lost two children aged eight months and six years to a mitochondrial disorder called Leigh Syndrome—the same syndrome carried by the skin cell donor in the Oregon team's aforementioned SCNT study. In 2017, Zhang's patient gave birth to the world's first baby following mitochondrial replacement, which ensured that the newborn avoided the risk of inheriting this debilitating condition.[140] The number of women who would be potential candidates for this treatment is relatively small; the estimated number of births per year among women at risk for transmitting mtDNA disease is 152 (out of 680,000) in the United Kingdom and 778 (out of in 3,850,000) in the United States.[141] However, this potential patient group would be dramatically expanded if the technique also worked as a means of treating age-related infertility.

The abovementioned Oregon team responsible for the first SCNT stem cells relates its work to the "current trend toward delayed childbearing in the Western world." They propose that the cytoplasm plays a key role in the egg's aging and therefore "mitochondrial replacement therapy could be considered [an] ART technique to solve cytoplasmic defects due to aging."[142] The nuclei of low-quality older eggs, they suggest, could be combined with the cytoplasm of young donor eggs to create an egg with improved chances of fertilizing and developing. Jose Cibelli, a former ACT researcher and current university professor in biotechnology, suggests that this would be an attractive alternative for the many women opting for donor eggs for age-related reasons because then "older women could have children carrying their own DNA thanks to the cytosolic contribution of a healthy, young surrogate egg."[143] In other words, this approach reframes reproductive aging as differently distributed between the nucleus and the cytoplasm within the cell. If age-related infertility is understood to be located in the cytoplasm, these researchers suggest that mitochondrial transfer could provide a solution by creating a *chimeric egg*, which retains the intended mother's nuclear DNA, but benefits from the reproductive potential of the donor egg's cytoplasm.[144] In this way, this approach constitutes a recombinant fertility at a cellular level.

This application of mitochondrial transfer has already found its way to the clinic.[145] In 2019, a woman gave birth to a baby in Greece after receiving mitochondrial replacement treatment. She received this treatment not because of any mitochondrial disease but specifically to improve her fertility after repeated IVF failures.[146] The Institute of Life, the Athens clinic where the woman was treated, subsequently stated that it intended to continue using the mitochondrial transfer technique "to help even more couples facing fertility issues to have children with their own DNA, without having recourse to egg donors."[147] Like Mitalipov's Oregon group, the researchers working on the development of the Athens mitochondrial transfer protocol suggested that "faulty mitochondria" could be the main culprit in poor egg quality, one of the main reasons why IVF fails. They resolved this by moving the nuclear DNA of the intended mother into a donor egg with healthy mitochondria.[148]

Sensing a business opportunity for this extended indication for mitochondrial transfer, John Zhang started a company called Darwin Life to commercialize mitochondrial replacement therapy for infertility in older women, which was branded H.E.R.—Human Egg Reconstitution—IVF. Although the FDA warned Zhang against his practice, the US-Ukrainian team at Darwin Life-Nadiya in Kiev recently claimed the birth of several more babies after mitochondrial transfer.[149] A study by the Nadiya team itself found that the technique offered little benefit to women of "advanced maternal age," but the clinic's director does maintain that the technique remains promising for women with failed IVF cycles, and the Darwin Life-Nadiya website states that they "hope in the near future to be able to help many women under the age of 42" achieve "the birth of a healthy native child without donation of eggs."[150]

The suggestion that donor egg cytoplasm could improve IVF outcomes is also the basis for research into a new approach to generating extra eggs through nuclear transfer. When an egg is formed, a small cell forms alongside it called the "polar body," which, like the egg, only has a single pair of chromosomes (haploid). Normally these cells cannot fertilize, but Mitalipov's group found that they could if the polar body nuclei were transferred into donor eggs' cytoplasms. Harnessing nuclear transfer as an "alternative route for oocyte formation," the researchers have patented this technique as a means to create an additional "source of oocytes for fertility treatment."[151] They suggest that this could be particularly helpful for "patients of advanced maternal age, who have a low oocyte yield or are poor responders, commonly observed in ART cycles."[152]

While it remains uncertain whether mitochondrial transfer will in fact clinically aid infertility, research interest in the possibility of combining "genomes from older women with young donor cytoplasts" certainly does require young women to provide gametes in order to create a new kind of egg that combines the reproductive youth ascribed to the cytoplasm and the biogenetic connection to its nucleus.[153] The interest in this work suggests that "the need for human eggs for research is back. It seems like it never left the stage after all."[154]

This renewed reliance on egg donation to explore the regenerative potential of youthful cytoplasms once more reconfigures the relation between fertility and aging. A postfertile cell par excellence, the chimeric egg, created by merging the intended mother's and the donor's eggs, materializes both fertility and infertility in new ways that hold the promise of shifting the temporal limits of reproductive finitude. Yet unlike autologous oocyte cryopreservation, this cytoplasmic regeneration implicates the bodies of egg donors. And because this process mirrors conventional egg donation, but relies only on the egg cytoplasm, it transfers the logic of research egg donation to reproductive egg donation, thereby expanding the group of potential egg donors as well as the risk of a concomitant stratification in donation practices.[155]

OC as Ethical Instrument: Direct and Indirect Egg Donation

The three SCNT studies under scrutiny all used "fresh" egg donation. However, if human frozen eggs could also be used for stem cell studies, the effects of the renewed demand for eggs may be felt far away from the lab. Given that a limited egg supply is one of the key practical constraints for SCNT research, the logistical advantages of banking eggs have been recognized by the biomedical research community.[156] Back in 2009, researchers in reproductive and regenerative biomedicine—including those at RBA, the fertility clinic acquired by egg freezing company Prelude—predicted that "in the future, if the efficacy and efficiency of cryopreserved oocytes are comparable to those of fresh oocytes in human therapeutic cloning, the use of cryopreserved oocytes would be invaluable and generate a great impact to regenerative medicine."[157]

These possibilities are coming closer to reality; Dong-Ryul Lee and colleagues write that the "production of cloned embryos using cryopreserved human oocytes and derivation of their SCNT-ESC lines was not achieved until recently."[158] Cryopreserved eggs have yielded embryonic stem cells (ESCs) after SCNT in various species, and several recent Korean studies have proposed more efficient methods for using frozen eggs to create SCNT-stem cells.[159] In Korea, the tightening of egg-procurement regulations after the Hwang scandal has become a driving force for investing in stem cell research with cryopreserved eggs because they "could provide a steady source of eggs for research, such as SCNT, and its use also reduces ethical concerns."[160] This is particularly relevant in a context where payments for egg donations are curtailed and regulations prescribe the use of "residual" eggs that are "intended to be discarded"—typically low-quality or frozen eggs.[161] In this way, egg freezing functions as an *ethical instrument* that both shifts the regulatory permissibility of egg donation and drives future research directions in stem cell biology that accommodate cryopreservation.

A similar prospect of broadening egg donation underlies further Korean research by Dong-Ryul Lee's team into new egg-manipulation protocols that suggest that "low-quality" eggs, which are of limited clinical value in IVF, may also yield nuclear-transfer stem cell lines.[162] In response to these protocols, Mitalipov and his colleagues express that "it is exciting to think that oocyte quality may become a less dramatic factor [in SCNT]," and "fresh or frozen" eggs from IVF programs could become an alternative source for human SCNT. He proposes that "perhaps we are at the stage where all oocyte donors produce functional oocytes and rejected patient oocytes from IVF programs could be recovered, if not for fertility purposes then for the production of NT-ESCs."[163] The new protocols suggest that low-quality eggs, which would normally be discarded in IVF procedures, could provide valuable material for creating embryonic stem cells.

In the context of the growing popularity of egg freezing, these new possibilities pave the way for a model of egg donation in which the categories of patient and donor begin to overlap more. If frozen eggs could also be used, the increasingly widespread preservation of eggs could similarly provide the material for stem cell generation and research. Given that the vast majority of women who freeze their eggs never return to use them, and given the fact that the leftover eggs may not be suitable for reproductive donation due to testing protocols required for third-party reproduction, donation to research could become a rational alternative to destroying the cryo-eggs when they are no longer needed. This would then lead to a situation in which those who provide eggs for research studies also pay for the stimulation, extraction, and cryo-preservation procedures, thereby becoming self-financed egg donors.[164] This model, in which women freeze eggs for their own future use and indirectly become donors if their eggs are no longer needed, is under-stood to "reduce ethical concerns" because it circumvents ethical issues pertaining to donor recruitment and financial inducement, while still providing a "steady source" of eggs.[165] Indirect egg donation after egg freezing may thus be upheld as a solution to the ethical concerns sur-rounding direct egg donation; cryopreservation thereby becomes itself an ethical instrument that renders egg donation more acceptable.

The future potential of using frozen eggs for stem cell research could also shift direct egg-donation practices, given that the mobility of frozen eggs could remove the need for spatial proximity between research labs and egg-procurement sites. As is the case for its reproductive counter-part, the use of frozen eggs allows for research egg donation to become more spatially dispersed. The possibility of shipping eggs could then fundamentally shift the dynamics of global egg procurement in ways that intersect with local gender- and age-specific social realities, as is now happening in transnational reproductive egg procurement. In fact, existing infrastructures of (cross-border) reproductive healthcare could be employed for research purposes; TWEB, and its advanced infrastruc-ture for handling large egg repositories and creating a transatlantic egg flow, give an indication of how similar biomedical and logistic technolo-gies could be used to move eggs for research purposes.

Because the donor's biodesirability is irrelevant in research egg pro-curement, Widdows contends that stem cell research may lead to a situ-ation in which "women from lower socioeconomic strata would be more likely to become the providers of eggs . . . because the genetic content of the enucleated egg . . . is irrelevant."[166] This is particularly pertinent if eggs become movable between different national and economic con-texts. If this were to become the case for egg procurement for research, the concerns raised in scholarship on CBRC that the "international economic imbalances" that make "underprivileged women in poorer countries an especially vulnerable population" would become newly relevant.[167] As global care chains create "a series of personal links between people across the globe based on the paid or unpaid work of caring" for both children and the elderly, so global cold chains of frozen eggs may develop to redistribute both reproductive youth and regenerative potential across borders and bodies, creating new relations of dependency that shift what it means to age for donors and recipients alike.[168]

Conclusion

Once frozen, eggs become mobile and thereby change the dynamics of egg donation for reproductive and research purposes. Transnational reproductive egg donation is exemplified by the World Egg Bank's flow of frozen oocytes from the United States to the United Kingdom, which is limited to those eggs that meet the HFEA restrictions on donor payment. Although the HFEA regulations seek to protect women from "financial inducement," the focus on the payment of egg donors does not address the *indirect financial inducement* resulting from the wider marketization of reproduction through practices of procuring and transporting eggs by for-profit parties. TWEB's transatlantic movement of eggs introduces new discursive practices in UK donor-egg IVF through the online donor profiles and the form of (consumer) choice they represent. TWEB thus illustrates the feasibility of creating transnational egg flows motivated by the speedy availability and detailed discursive framing of the eggs. By analogy to the global care chain, global cold chains are developing in which eggs, and the reproductive youth they represent, travel from local cryobanks to intended parents worldwide.

Breakthroughs in SCNT stem cell research have increased interest in technologies that position the egg—and its cytoplasm—at the center of regenerative approaches to healthcare. Nuclear transfer technologies become particularly relevant to (reproductive) aging in the scenarios envisaged for (future) clinical application, in which young women's reproductive bodies hold the regenerative potential for both age-related pathologies and infertilities. Researchers proposed that the SCNT technique could use eggs to create stem cells "with the age apparently erased"—positing the egg as a cellular fountain of youth.[169] However, both SCNT research and its potential clinical applications rely on the provision of donor eggs. The Hwang scandal rendered this supply particularly contentious, and subsequent Korean regulations restricted research egg donation to "residual," typically frozen, eggs as a more ethical alternative. If leftover frozen eggs could be more widely used in stem cell research, egg freezers could become *indirect egg donors*, who pay for the hormonal stimulation and egg extraction themselves. Because the vast majority of women who freeze their eggs do not return to use them, there is a growing pool of potential research eggs frozen across the world. In both direct and indirect egg-donation arrangements, the lack of specific biodesirability requirements opens up this research egg donation to a broader group of young women—and attendant forms of reproductive respatialization and stratification.

Both in reproductive egg donation and in nuclear transfer techniques, eggs are cast as the medium through which age may be reconfigured— whether through the transfer of reproductive youth to women with age-related infertility or through the regeneration of older cells to counteract age-related pathologies and infertilities. The concomitant increased "need for human eggs" following from the clinical use and scientific development of these technologies coincides with the availability of OC.[170] Egg freezing enables frozen egg flows and a concomitant respatialization of oocyte procurement, characterized by an increased geographical distance between the young women who provide the eggs and those who receive them. Within the context of the internationalization of fertility treatment and stem cell research, the global regulatory and economic disparities pertaining to egg procurement, increasing demands on egg supplies, and the neoliberalization of both biomedicine and "successful aging," OC thus creates the conditions of emergence for a far-reaching reconfiguration of egg donation within a broader biopolitics of aging.

Conclusion

When I imagine my eggs again, I feel a weightlessness hovering unmoored. My eggs have been called a thousand times by new and ancient names of loss and promise. I hear the quiver in the voice of a woman at a Q&A. I smell the brochure of a new technology. I breathe in the lives of women whose books are many. I call to the graves of my grandmothers. I see a parliament of owls; their eyes are round and soulful. I feel the storm of a planet whose roar is growing louder. I hold up my sign and my drum at injustice. I lie in the arms of a woman who is a teacher of life and death. She says, not all paths are those of our choosing. I listen in the night for her quiet breath. I imagine again trillions of cells lit-up and awake, and how life is held silently within each one—whether haploid or not.

As IVF has become normalized over four decades after the birth of Louise Brown (1978), procedures like egg freezing—essentially a variation of IVF with a period of cryostorage—continue to capture the public imagination and raise controversy. Beyond a clinical procedure that a growing, but relatively small, group of women undergo, egg freezing both reflects and enables a broader gender politics of reproductive aging. Both celebrations and criticisms of OC appeal to changing normative ideas about when people should (not) use reproductive technologies. National regulations and insurance guidelines reinforce maximum age limits to accessing treatment with reference to the "normal reproductive years," while egg freezing start-ups are redefining the ages at which younger women are encouraged to freeze their eggs, whether for their own or another's use. In *Freezing Fertility*, I have analyzed the changing relations between reproductivity and aging at each stage of the OC procedure by following the journey of the egg as it moves from the body to the freezer, the incubator, and the womb, into wider reproductive infrastructures and across the world. Through these movements, egg freezing expands the scope of thinkable and actionable reproductive potentialities later in life, and after death.

The current popularity of OC reflects a historically specific reality in which there are few biotechnological alternatives for female "fertility preservation," but future technologies may render egg freezing obsolete. As research is ongoing into other approaches to decoupling bodily aging and reproductive ability, new technologies may find their way to the clinic in the coming decades, including ovarian cryopreservation, *in vitro* maturation of immature eggs, mitochondrial transfer, and the more distant possibility of creating artificial gametes, or *in vitro* gametogenesis.[1] For the moment, however, egg freezing remains the most popular technology for circumventing future age-related infertility.

Egg freezing has emerged in the wake of the dramatic social and technical changes associated with the timing of reproduction that characterized the 20th century. The introduction of the contraceptive pill, expanded access to safe abortion, and women's increased participation in waged labor coincided with a trend of increasing maternal ages at first birth. As women were having children later in life, the possibility of "leaving it too late" and "having it all" raised widespread public concern. Since the late seventies, reporting on women's "biological clock" has remained newsworthy, often serving as a reminder of a biological limit to "liberation" in the face of ongoing gendered social change.[2] With the introduction of IVF and egg donation, the biological clock became relevant once again. Age-related infertility no longer necessarily signaled the end of the reproductive life span. Rather, it could become an indication for infertility treatment, as expressed in IVF patients' experience that they "have to try IVF" in order to reach "the end of the road" of fertility's finality.[3] As the emergence of egg donation gave rise to media coverage of both celebrities having children later in life and exceptional cases of women becoming pregnant in their sixties and seventies, the temporal limit to female reproduction once more became hotly debated.

Whereas the 20th century saw the rise of numerous biotechnological and biopolitical modes of family planning, the postmillennial introduction of egg freezing offers a means of *fertility planning* that revolves around timing not only when to have children but when to be fertile.

We are now at the cusp of a shift in ART practices from reproduction to fertility. And egg freezing is the first major technology to popularize IVF treatment for making fertilities, rather than primarily making babies. As OC has become widely known as the primary technology for circumventing age-related infertility, its introduction has once again politicized female reproductive aging. When the temporal limits to female fertility become, at least potentially, agentically alterable with new reproductive technologies, the reestablishment of such limits becomes the result of sociocultural renegotiations, rather than a biological given.[4]

My initial interest in egg freezing developed in response to such a negotiation, when the Dutch government barred the introduction of OC in the Netherlands in 2009. I was living in Amsterdam at the time and was struck by the restrictive gender- and age-specific norms expressed in public debates about egg freezing, which often revolved around what reproductive choices women ought to make at different points in their lives. As egg freezing practices were established across various national contexts, specific ages and time periods for freezing, storing, thawing, and implanting eggs, and the gendered chrononormativities underlying them, became institutionalized. Meanwhile, the promotion of egg freezing—particularly in the US context, and especially after the ASRM lifted OC's experimental label in 2012—intensified, whether at my students' career fairs, where they were encouraged to freeze their eggs if they chose to train as lawyers or doctors, or in the rising popularity of corporate egg freezing insurance in many more companies than only the highly publicized pioneers Apple and Facebook. Both the restriction and the commercialization of egg freezing are indicative of the ongoing changes in what it means to be fertile, and to age, in the 21st century. This book has traced these changes, which are also often continuities, by following the egg from the ovary to the freezer and beyond.

Emergent Fertilities

Contemporary egg freezing practices have shifted the logic of reproductive aging both for younger and for older women. As a technology that is used to counteract reproductive aging, egg freezing uniquely implicates fertile women, who are confronted with the clinical possibility of anticipating future infertility at increasingly early ages. Conversely, unlike existing technologies of IVF and egg donation, egg freezing offers a chance of not only birthing but also conceiving later in life with one's own frozen eggs. The possibility of egg freezing thus produces emergent modes of being fertile and infertile as, on the one hand, infertility may be lived prior to its arrival and, on the other, the onset of age-related infertility need not signal the end of the reproductive life span.

In this way, new groups of fertile and infertile people have become potential candidates for treatment. It is now common to read statements suggesting that you are never too young to freeze your eggs because "you'll never be more fertile than you are today" and "the younger you freeze eggs the more fertile they are."[5] Equally, once you have frozen your eggs, reproductive aging does not preclude the possibility of having a child at a later time, as suggested in one fertility company's mission to ensure that "everyone can have the opportunity to be a mom or dad when they are ready."[6] This opens up new possibilities and uncertainties about the assumption of fertility earlier in life and the closure of infertility later in life.

Becoming Infertile Earlier in Life

Egg freezing is by definition an infertility treatment for the fertile life phase. Because, unlike most IVF patients, women who freeze their eggs are typically not trying to conceive and need not experience any symptoms of infertility, the indication for undergoing this treatment is much more flexible in nature. Accordingly, different moments in the life cycle can become associated with the fertility precarity or fertility potential that warrants undergoing an egg freezing cycle.

One increasingly popular approach—touted by celebrities such as singer Rita Ora—is freezing eggs in the twenties to preserve "peak fertility." The promotion of OC to maintain the optimal fertility of early adulthood became part of the UK news cycle when an influential fertility specialist suggested that egg freezing "should be every dad's graduation present for his daughter," who could then keep "20 beautiful eggs" in the freezer.[7] Reflecting a host of class and gender issues by invoking the wealthy father and the youthful beauty of the daughter's cells, this statement points to the tension between the suggested biological optimum age for treatment and younger women's relatively limited access to the financial means to cover the pricey procedure. It is this tension that new US egg freezing companies seek to mitigate by offering financing and discount packages while heavily promoting OC to increasingly younger women. By shifting to earlier freezing, they are banking on appealing to larger numbers of women—literally so, given the substantial private equity investments in egg freezing companies.

By contrast, Dutch fertility clinics have set 30 years as the minimum age for egg freezing in order to avoid unnecessary treatment of younger women. This regulation favors an alternative approach of freezing in the early to mid-thirties, which is also rationalized in relation to the widespread association of 35 years with intensified fertility decline. Yet, so far, most women who have frozen their eggs are in their late thirties and early forties.[8] This trend reflects a last-minute approach to egg freezing that preserves a chance of genetically related motherhood when people expect they will soon lose that ability.

In all these instances, the possibility of "preserving fertility" is matched with new forms of preemptive fertility loss. Whether one is 24 or 38, fertility can be rendered precarious, in the sense that it is understood to be at risk in new ways. The precariousness of fertility may be linked to the imminent loss of peak fertility, cost-efficient fertility, last-minute fertility, or significant moments in life, such as a graduation, a relationship break-up, or a particular birthday. As a result, fertility loss may arrive as a clinically and culturally relevant notion much earlier in life—if not throughout the adult female reproductive life span. Because the indication for egg freezing is less straightforward than for traditional IVF, the discursive framing of reproductive aging in medical and public discourses plays a crucial role in establishing when the ongoingness of fertility may be assumed, and when it becomes perceived as precarious.

Indeed, egg freezing has become such a culturally significant technology because the widespread public coverage of OC transforms conceptualizations of fertility for much wider audiences. Beyond a procedure that only a very small proportion of women undergoes (OC comprises only 1.5% of all UK IVF cycles), the stories that circulate about frozen eggs and frozen fertility provide influential interpretative frameworks for understanding female reproductive aging and its (im)mutability in the context of cryopreservation.[9] Whether in newspapers, advertisements, celebrity stories, or patient information, OC's introduction has provoked both a rearticulation of natural time limits to conception in

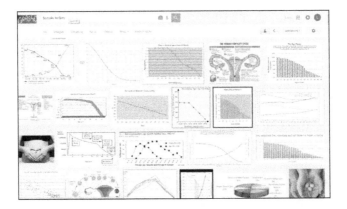

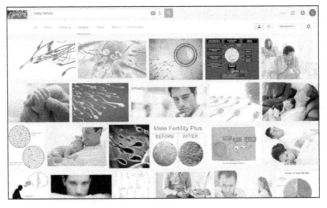

Figure C.1a and b. A Google image search illustrates the dominance of the decline frame for "Female Fertility," which contrasts with representations of "Male Fertility".

the face of their potential transgression and a redefinition of these time limits to fertility as something over which one can exert agency at specific moments in the life course.

Whether they are celebrating or dismissing egg freezing, one common element in these public discourses is the emphasis on the importance of *being informed* about female reproductive aging. Yet in the context of OC, efforts to inform and educate often position female fertility not as a locus of potential generativity but as effectively synonymous with loss and decline.

Rather than simply presenting a biological reality, the rhetorical framing of female fertility failure can be particularly effective in perpetuating underlying ideas about individualized responsibilities for reproduction, the desirability and importance of motherhood, the value of genetic relatedness, gendered differences in age-specific parenting abilities, and temporal limits to "normal reproductive years"—as well as the presumed access to the capital and care required to circumvent fertility concerns.

In what appears to be a pedagogical turn in the egg freezing industry, OC marketing efforts are increasingly focused on education as a means of addressing new audiences. Rather than directly promoting egg freezing, major fertility companies instead invest in fertility education— whether through websites, apps, trade shows, cocktail parties, or sponsorships. While it is of course important to be well informed about reproductive aging, it is equally important to note when the rhetorical framing of "fertility facts" aligns with a treatment logic that indicates OC to a large new target group. Normal physiological development—such as the loss of large quantities of eggs from birth onwards—can easily be reframed in an alarmist way ("you'll never be more fertile than you are today") to render fertility in need of treatment at earlier points in the life course.[10] What is at stake is not so much the truthfulness of these claims but the normalization of an alternative model of reproductive aging that associates a wide variety of life course stages with fertility precarity—a fertility that is at once fragile and freezable—as an effective means of creating demand for treatment.[11]

New marketing initiatives moreover promote *fertility testing* as a means to personalize the indication for egg freezing. The major US egg freezing networks—Extend Fertility, Prelude, Progyny—all combine their information campaigns with fertility testing as the first step in the egg freezing process. Kindbody goes one step further and has introduced fertility vans in the streets of US urban centers that offer passersby hormone tests to check their ovarian reserve. Suggesting that their customers "deserve to know the facts" about fertility, the stories told through these facts set up a dynamic between knowing and not knowing, between gaining statistical information and raising questions about one's own reproductive embodiment. Although fertility tests are presented as a resolution to these uncertainties, it appears that ovarian reserve tests have limited predictive value for the time to pregnancy and can have significant negative psychological effects.[12]

Fertility tests do, however, create a personalized pathway to treatment. By undergoing a fertility test, women adopt the position of the patient and develop a familiarity with the fertility clinic and its treatment rationales. Subsequently, the test results provide a personalized indication for treatment through a more specific, individualized address to the potential patient. This functions so well as a marketing tool because both below- and above-average outcomes can become an indication for treatment—whether to salvage declining fertility or maintain optimal fertility.

In these ways, women can be rendered individually responsible for managing the future finality of their fertility at earlier points in life. A heightened awareness of predictable and testable but nevertheless uncertain fertility futures can easily be coupled with a moral injunction to anticipate reproductive aging as a sign of responsible citizenship. As fertility information and testing expand the scope of risk associated with reproductive aging, they provide a rationale for services that promise to counteract these risks and provide a degree of biopreparedness for future fertility decline.

This move towards responsibilizing women for counteracting fertility precarity is embedded in a broader neoliberal political trend of governments devolving their responsibilities onto individual citizens by shrinking spending on public services for the well-being of people while—as Laura Briggs puts it—"keep[ing] corporate taxes low and profits high."[13] The political legacy of neoliberalism, Melinda Cooper reminds us, entails the withdrawal from the state in favor not only of the individual but also of the family as a "privileged site of debt, wealth transfer and care."[14] As women are encouraged to take individual responsibility for maintaining the futurity of fertility and the family form, it is in fact what Briggs calls a "structural infertility" that creates the conditions for which egg freezing is a coping mechanism. She writes that for a growing swath of the middle class, reproductive technologies are "how people are coping with the structural infertility of the long period of education and economic insecurity that is the price of the ticket these days to the middle class but that virtually requires delayed childbearing."[15] This structural infertility is furthermore positioned in a "financialised capitalist regime" characterized by a steep rise in the amount of waged labor required to support a household.[16] The popularization of OC thus occurs at a time when the widespread socioprecarity of late capitalist labor, housing, education, relationship, and financial insecurities all contribute to trends of later childbearing, in relation to which the bioprecarity of ongoing fertility becomes an intensified concern.[17]

An important counterpart to these precarious social conditions of late capitalism that likewise results from diminished spending on public services is the devolvement of state responsibility for reproductive healthcare to the private IVF market. The neoliberal divestment of public spending that Briggs and Cooper describe, then, entails a twofold intensification of reproductive bioprecarity. On the one hand, increased socioprecarity contributes to a trend of later reproduction in relation to which reproductive bioprecarity becomes a concern. On the other, corporate investment in OC services does not simply meet a preexisting demand but plays an active role—and has a stake in—reframing female fertility as precarious in nature at various points in the life cycle.

With the move of serial entrepreneurs into the fertility industry, and the rise of private equity driving IVF clinics, the very understanding of fertility becomes itself entrepreneurialized as the site of ongoing personal investment into reproductive futures. As a result, fertility becomes liable to being enlisted in a logic of investment, indebtedness, and capital accumulation—both for individual women and for the fertility companies that serve them.[18] When egg freezing becomes a means of individual self-investment in a reproductive future—matching a corporate investment in future demand for counteracting fertility precarity—it not only creates individual responsibilities but also produces new dependencies.

These dependencies follow in part from the fact that egg freezing relies on an egg-based model of reproductive aging that requires a clinical infrastructure to become legible. Although reproductive aging can be conceptualized as occurring throughout the body, the focus on the egg reflects an IVF-based model of reproduction, in which the extracorporealized egg both takes center stage in its iconic imagery of fertilization in the dish and presents the main bottleneck in the treatment of female age-related infertility.[19] With this focus on the egg, which remains hidden in the body, embodied fertility becomes accessible and measurable primarily through the fertility clinic and the tests on offer. This presents a very different relation to embodied fertility than the fertility awareness approaches of the 1970s and 1980s women's health movements or the current mobile apps that render fertility legible by self-observing body temperature and cervical fluid. Instead, the clinic becomes the main point of access to counteract the uncertainty, the opacity, and the finitude of fertility. In this way, fertility becomes precarious in the older sense of the word, which the *OED* describes as being "vulnerable to the will or decision of others" and inhabiting a "condition of dependency."

Becoming informed, testing, and freezing are all presented as strategies for rendering fertility legible and extendable; yet, through these strategies, fertility becomes newly reliant on clinical infrastructures built around the intensified bioprecarity of women's reproductive bodies. The precariousness of fertility, then, follows not only from the threat of its decline but from novel relations of dependency that emerge in the context of new norms of technologized fertility management—both earlier and later in life.

Staying Fertile Later in Life

As a counterpart to becoming infertile earlier, egg freezing also enables new ways of *staying fertile* later in life. Cryo-eggs offer the possibility— albeit a slim one—of conceiving and bearing children after the onset of age-related infertility with a chosen partner or donor. Irrespective of the technique's efficacy, the notion that women can stay fertile in this technologically mediated way destabilizes biological age limits to reproduction. As became clear in the critical responses to older motherhood—whether in Schellart's or Buttle's stories—the possibility of "extending fertility" may provoke the rearticulation and regulation of these reproductive age limits in the face of their potential transgression.[20] Yet equally, the promise that freezing eggs will allow women to "extend fertility," as one of the major networks is called, gives rise to a more flexible, agentic, and distributed model of reproductive aging, which straddles both the freezer and the body, and is embedded in broader reproductive infrastructures.

Encompassing both the lived, aging body and the cryopreserved, timeless egg, this model of reproductive aging is distributed across divergent trajectories of *in vivo* fertility decline and *ex vivo* fertility accumulation. The tension between these reproductive counterpoints was evident in the story of Eggfreezer, who described her cryo-eggs as "quite literally frozen in time" and her body as the place where "many millions [of eggs] die off."[21] Her account staged a life-death dyad between the ongoing egg death in her ovaries and the continued reproductive potential ascribed to the eggs in the freezer. She nevertheless recognized the cryo-eggs as "part of [her]" and therefore an integral part of her ongoing fertility. What is at stake in this egg-based distribution of reproductive aging is thus the reconfiguration of the reproductive body as a locus of fallibility and decline that contrasts with the cold freezer, which holds the promissory value of timeless reproductive potential.

Nevertheless, the distribution of reproductive aging across the body and the freezer does not necessarily suffice to attain a sense of bioprepared fertility. After the first egg freezing cycle, the question quickly arises whether one has frozen enough eggs to "stay fertile." Because OC yields eggs, rather than babies, the measure for "reproductive success" is much more flexible than it is in traditional IVF cycles. When reproductive success becomes a matter of degree measured by the number of cryo-eggs, the egg freezing process becomes an ongoing course of *fertility accumulation*, the endpoint of which is organized by new and flexible norms.

Clinics set such norms by recommending a wide variety of egg quantities for a reasonable chance to have a child. Particularly the larger private UK and US fertility clinics tend to couple such specific recommended egg quantities with prepackaged treatment and financial plans. These plans can rationalize a multicycle approach to OC with discounts on repeat cycles, guarantee packages for freezing a specific quantity of eggs, and loans to cover the associated high up-front payments. In this way, medical considerations of potential future success with a particular number of eggs are coupled with financial considerations of cost efficiency; the plans thereby set up a *calculus of fertility* for deciding how many OC cycles to undergo. So while the value of frozen eggs follows from their potential to shift the uncertainty associated with precarious fertility into a more bioprepared fertility, the variable quantities associated with reproductive success can equally extend fertility precarity beyond the first freezing cycle and set up a multicycle norm through this egg-based calculus of fertility. Egg freezing may thus be characterized by a series of *incremental steps*, in which fertility tests represent the first encounter with the clinic and the basis for a personalized indication for egg freezing, while subsequently multicycle or guarantee packages provide the rationale for further cycles after the first one.

These developments point to a shift that reframes egg freezing from a single anticipatory gesture to the basis for an *ongoing technologized fertility management* throughout the life course. In other words, staying fertile with frozen eggs entails a longer-term engagement with the clinic. When used to circumvent age-related infertility, egg freezing is by its very nature a long-term arrangement that spans an extended time between the eggs' extraction and their intended fertilization. Yet the flexibility of fertility accumulation with frozen eggs opens up possibilities for repeat treatments and multicycle norms that extend the time of active engagement with the clinic. In these ways, the OC process sets up a long-term, future-oriented relation with the clinic that differs from the dynamic of a set of fresh IVF cycles that promptly succeed or fail. While the eggs remain in the freezer, distributed reproductive aging is enacted through a two-way flow of monetary and reproductive value exchange between women and fertility companies. This ongoing value exchange couples long-term storage and loan payments for the cryo-eggs with an affective investment in their continued reproductive value. In this way, egg freezing enables a capitalist reconfiguration of reproductive aging, in which value exchange lies at the foundation of the postfertile relation between the cell and the self.

The distribution of reproductive aging thus stretches beyond the body and the freezer, into the reproductive-industrial complex of IVF.[22] Beyond an individual or clinical treatment option, efforts to mainstream and promote egg freezing have integrated fertility preservation in existing infrastructures of labor, finance, data, and insurance, to name but a few. One salient example of the infrastructural integration of distributed reproductive aging is corporate egg freezing insurance, in which assisted reproductive life course management becomes entangled with workplace human resource management. Now that leading fertility insurance company Progyny has a strategic alliance with Mercer, the world's largest HR consultancy firm, over 10% of large US companies offer egg freezing as a perk to their staff, covering an estimated 1.4 million people. This fertility insurance frames egg freezing as, on the one hand, a tool for employees to self-invest in future fertility and, on the other, a tool for employers to increase ROI (return on investment). Here the question of fertility and its ongoingness is played out in the organization of labor, in which egg freezing functions as at once a reproductive and an HR technology to recruit and retain female staff. In this arrangement, the merit of egg freezing is reinforced through the employer and the fertility company alike. The distribution of reproductive aging is, then, not confined to the body and freezer but is equally propelled by the financial-institutional infrastructures through which investment in egg freezing is rationalized, promoted, and financed.[23]

Yet frozen eggs allow women not only to maintain fertility later in life but also to *lose* it over prolonged periods of time. Most women do not return to use their eggs, either because they are not trying to conceive or because they have not needed the frozen eggs to become pregnant. For example, a recent study in a Dutch clinic showed that only 5% of all the women who froze their eggs returned to use them.[24] For the majority of women who will not use their eggs, the continued existence of these cryo-eggs after the onset of age-related infertility will require agentic decision making about the ongoingness and loss of a latent, frozen fertility later in life. Complementing embodied fertility loss, egg freezing will moreover give rise to new modes of regulatory fertility loss—or, as Emily Jackson calls it, a "non-biological clock"—as a result of ten-year storage limits or specific age limits that preclude the use of the cryo-eggs.

The accounts of women who do decide to use their frozen eggs highlight how the second phase of egg freezing can involve a cascade of fertility gains and losses—rather than a straightforward extension as such. If women decide to thaw the frozen eggs, the return to the clinic is itself contingent on a degree of embodied fertility loss— whether expected or experienced—to motivate the use of frozen eggs over those in the ovaries. As is the case in traditional IVF, each step of the procedure—fertilization, incubation, implantation, etc.—presents a moment of potential success and failure. Yet there is also the additional possibility of an OC-specific loss of extended fertility that has been shaped by a prolonged period of physical, financial, and affective investment in the frozen eggs. When frozen eggs fail, as Brigitte Adams's story suggested, age-related infertility can moreover gain an agentic and preventable character as the outcome of an earlier decision not to freeze more eggs.[25] Egg freezing thus multiplies the arrival of infertility in the lived body and the freezable eggs; it thereby extends not only fertility but also its loss.

Beyond the finitude of fertility, the prospect of the finality of life itself is encountered through the frozen egg. The case of A., whose frozen eggs outlived her, highlighted how the possibility of posthumous motherhood with the cryo-eggs can deeply impact experiences of living and dying—irrespective of whether the intended conception in fact occurs. The possibility of a posthumous reproductivity is highly relevant to the growing group of women who undergo OC in the context of a serious diagnosis. But also for healthy women freezing their eggs, the informed-consent procedure is a reminder that the end of life does not equal the end of reproductivity. The continued existence of frozen eggs after the intended mother's death permits the establishment of *intended kinship relations* with those who may fertilize and gestate the eggs and parent the children born from them. OC thus allows people to grapple with mortality through the manipulation of the egg, which is now no longer only the locus of a potential beginning of life but also holds the key to confronting its end.

The temporal stretch between egg extraction and fertilization in OC not only enables staying fertile later in life and after death, but it also creates a new proximity between autologous and heterologous donation—between donation to a future self and donation to a third party. The period of cryostorage introduces a flexibility in rerouting the frozen eggs' destinations—whether to the original egg freezer, another intended parent, or a research project. Although the shift from autologous to heterologous reproductive donation is not straightforward, the redirection of cryo-eggs is a new possibility that women currently encounter in consent forms.[26] Because the majority of women who freeze their eggs do not return to use them, the growing popularity of OC may also result in a greater availability of donor eggs, which would be particularly significant for (future) research projects that rely on frozen eggs.[27]

More broadly, egg freezing introduces a temporal and spatial flexibility in IVF treatment that benefits egg-donation and fertility-preservation practices alike. Now as mobile as the liquid nitrogen tanks that contain them, frozen eggs can enable a transnational reproduction that does not require any cross-border movements of the egg donor or the intended parents. By stretching the reproductive process across nation-states, new regulatory proximities between distant, but now intimately connected, jurisdictions shift egg-donation practices for all parties involved. This deterritorialization of egg donation particularly highlights differential regulations that seek to curtail financial inducements, which focus primarily on the compensation of egg donors but leave the *indirect financial inducements* resulting from fertility companies' business models unchecked. The transnational flows of eggs across global cold chains, wider socialities, and reproductive infrastructures thus render fertility transferable across borders and time.

Becoming Postfertile

Whether through guarantee plans or fertility vans, consent forms or multicycle norms, the introduction of egg freezing has enabled new ways of both anticipating infertility at increasingly early ages and maintaining fertility later in life. Through this double movement, egg freezing complicates a linear trajectory from fertility to infertility in the adult female life course. Both freezing eggs to prepare for future infertility and thawing eggs to tap into their latent reproductive potential give rise to new states of being that are neither exactly fertile nor exactly infertile, but rather *postfertile*. This is enabled by, on the one hand, the temporal plasticity of the freezable eggs and the fertility ascribed to them, and, on the other, the future-oriented nature of OC, which allows for a wide variety of ages and egg quantities to be posited as markers of fertility or infertility. The concomitant temporal flexibility of recognizing both fertility and infertility at different points in the life cycle gives rise to the postfertile condition. Postfertility, then, refers to a state in which fertility and infertility are not discrete phases but become meaningful in relation to one another through such temporal orientations as anticipation, retrospection, latency, and acceleration.

The temporal plasticity of cryopreserved eggs provides the material counterpart to the conceptual flexibility of fertility within the postfertile condition that is enabled by these temporal orientations. It has become clear that the possibility of cryopreservation has introduced new ways of anticipating and living future infertility in the present. Equally, retrospection and hindsight can reframe age-related infertility as the result of not having frozen (more) eggs. A focus on the latency of the cryo-egg's continued reproductive potential diffracts reproductive aging into multiple embodied and disembodied fertile temporalities. Acceleration of time to live birth—now acronymized as TTLB by Merck as a parameter for reproductive success—provides a wider indication for undergoing IVF-based infertility treatments, as opposed to trying less technologized approaches for a longer amount of time. Each of these examples is indicative of a broader postfertile condition, within which fertility and infertility become increasingly fluid and entangled categories as reproductivity and aging relate to one another in new ways.

The conceptual fluidity of postfertility permits egg freezing to be adopted in a wide variety of repropolitical projects. The Japanese city Urayasu, for example, seeks to address its low birth rate by subsidizing egg freezing for women between 20 and 34 years. As a treatment for "fertility at risk," egg freezing functions as a reproductive act, which is expected to increase the number of births by expanding the fertile life span.[28] The Chinese government likewise considers egg freezing to be a reproductive act, but instead bans single women from doing so because it is understood to encourage single motherhood. Here the future reproductivity assigned to the cryo-eggs comes to bear on the present, given that egg freezing is thought to preemptively transgress family planning policies that require women to be married before they have children.[29]

By contrast, until recently, women in France could not access egg freezing because the technology was understood to *discourage* reproduction. The national ethics committee, CCNE, considered OC to be "hardly defensible," in part because it could cause women to feel "obliged to postpone motherhood" and would be a poor substitute for "providing the kind of [social] organization that enables women . . . to have children naturally and earlier in life."[30] The 2018 CCNE advice on the revision of the French bioethics law cautiously suggests that egg freezing could be adopted, but specifies a number of temporal regulations—e.g., permitting freezing only for women aged 30 to 35 and thawing up until 43 years—in the face of an evolving and uncertain "dividing line between 'normal' and 'pathological'" reproductive aging.[31] Amid similar postfertile uncertainties, the Dutch Parliament was initially likewise concerned about the potential conflict between OC's introduction and government policy to reduce female childbearing ages. Age limits of 43 for IVF insurance coverage and 45—later, 50—years for the use of frozen eggs provided a regulatory resolution to the unclear biological boundaries to female reproductive aging in the face of cryopreservation. Against the specter of an unnatural older motherhood, Denmark similarly approaches OC as a "technology to be tamed" and limits the use of frozen eggs to 45 years in order to discourage women from postponing pregnancy.[32]

Yet what is also at stake in the postfertile condition is the expansion of fertility markets that both meet and create demands for these emergent modes of (dis)embodying fertility. In the absence of federal regulatory age limits in the United States, for example, the postfertile condition enables an intensification of concerns about reproductive aging in ways that align with market incentives for increasingly widespread indications for treatment. Egg freezing is, then, not simply the result of later childbearing trends and the various sociodemographic drivers underlying them, but is itself actively constructed as a good solution to conflicting pressures of increasing work hours, unstable relationships, financial insecurities, and a neoliberal self-responsibilization for future (reproductive) health. Notwithstanding women's capability of intelligently navigating these complex markets and new reproductive choices, it is crucial to note how the self-investment logic underlying dominant egg freezing rationales matches the investment of hundreds of millions of dollars of private equity in egg freezing enterprises, which are reflected in the emergence of specialized fertility insurance companies, online egg freezing platforms, and large new chains of fertility clinics that specialize in egg cryopreservation. These massive capital investments in egg freezing reflect the financial stakes in mobilizing affects of anxiety and empowerment to reframe fertility as in need of information, tests, and freezers, as precarious but extendable, as something that requires a course of action and, indeed, is itself in need of proactive investment.

In order to create returns for these large-scale investments, fertility companies reach out to new, larger, and younger target groups of women to promote egg freezing—and the treatment logic that rationalizes it— on the streets, in hotels, at work, and through social media. The rise of fertility insurance, web-based OC services, and consolidating (inter) national chains of fertility clinics all create new institutional contexts for rationalizing, mainstreaming, and streamlining egg freezing in ways that affect not only the women who opt for OC but the public at large.

Fertility Literacy

As egg freezing is becoming a more mainstream procedure, it is important to also mainstream a critical approach to understanding fertility that not only focuses on biological facts, treatment success rates, and the pervasive association of female aging with failure and decline but also calls attention to the new modes of postfertility emerging today, along with their biopolitical and biocapitalist dimensions. Being aware of the temporal limits to fertility is important for making informed reproductive decisions, especially when both men and women are having children later in life. Yet rather than a general fertility education focused only on women's declining conception rates, what we need is a *fertility literacy* for analyzing the rhetorical framing of fertility facts, situating one's experiences within sociocultural and political-economic systems, and positioning oneself in relation to structures of power, whether organized by nation-states or by global markets. Fertility literacy requires a critical reflection on the production, distribution, and mediation of female fertility. This also includes a consideration of both the social inequalities that are naturalized through its presentation and the power relations and cultural systems that govern its social and technological management. Fertility literacy involves considering what cultural normativities, whether of idealized motherhood or successful aging, inform experiences and representations of fertility. When fertility becomes distributed beyond the body, who is affected by the eggs' movements? Which parties benefit, and who suffers as a result? What systems do emergent postfertilities reproduce?

Freezing Fertility has aimed to provide some of the critical reflections on these aspects of fertility literacy through the figure of the egg. This is where I return to the opening paragraph of this book, where I imagined my eggs as lit-up and awake. My intention was to find a language for a nonanxious fertile embodiment that resists the will to youth and the telos of loss—in the face of the narratives of precarity and opacity that so powerfully fuel new (and old) reproductive imperatives. Throughout the book, I have sought to foreground how to critically assess relations of dependency and constructions of need in fertile and infertile bodies alike. I have highlighted how frozen eggs reflect social inequalities, aging ideologies, government policies, and business philosophies in the complex cellular trajectories enabled by their new temporal and spatial flexibilities. Fertility literacy, accordingly, requires a consideration of the biopolitical and biocapitalist projects mobilized in the reframing of female fertilities—at each step of the egg freezing procedure. In *Freezing Fertility*, I have attempted to offer such a consideration by following the freezable egg across time and space, infrastructures and discourses, institutions and regulations, within and without the body, as priceless currency in timeless suspension, as the small cell in which global regimes collide, as barely visible yet ubiquitously reproduced sign of a contemporary gender politics of reproductive aging.

The egg that, having been vitrified *in vitro*, remains viable bears a complex and contradictory relation to aging. The frozen egg has been described as defying the biological clock, yet in OC's public representations this very notion, its naturalizing effects and anxious affects, are actively produced and abundantly reiterated. Paradoxically, the extraction of eggs brings their embodiment into discourse. Their frozen stasis renders them globally mobile. The frozen egg, seen to embody the promise of new human life and reproductive futurity, also entails a confrontation with finality. These complex counterpoints of OC, of fertility, and of finitude meet in the figure of the egg. The egg, frozen, its age suspended, has become the locus for grappling with the beginning and end of life, and the mortal passage from one to the other.

ACKNOWLEDGMENTS

Barbara Katz Rothman wrote that acknowledgments are "like a will you don't have to die to have read: a public thank-you, a wrapping-up, a final gesture of appreciation." I have so much to be grateful for and so many to appreciate. I celebrated my PhD defense as a wedding to scholarship and feminism, complete with dramatic white train and fallopian tube dress. Let this, then, be my living will—a celebration of the lives of many that contributed to this book.

What a wonderful, extraordinary time it has been. First and foremost, I would like to acknowledge my mentors Sarah Franklin, Mieke Bal, José van Dijck, and Esther Peeren, who have so generously supported this work. Sarah, I cannot thank you enough for the trust, the time, and the encouragement you have offered me over the years. It is a true joy to work with someone who has such an intellectual sense of adventure, feminist commitment to care, and boundless curiosity about reproduction. Thank you for the years of advice, inspiration, humor, and golden-hearted honesty. Mieke, thank you for always making time, offering such careful, detailed readings of my work, and celebrating all the good moments with such joyous spirit. José, thank you for your enthusiasm, encouragement, and inspiring reflections. After speaking with you I always feel more motivated and energized. Esther, thank you for your lightning-speed, ever-precise, and insightful feedback, and the wise and energetic support you have offered me all these years. I am deeply grateful for your generosity, and it is an honor to have worked with all of you.

The Reproductive Sociology Research Group (ReproSoc) at the University of Cambridge has been my intellectual home for the last four years. ReproSoc is a delicious combination of rigor and refuge; I am so grateful to Sarah, my colleagues, and all the students who make it such a stimulating and inspiring place to research eggs and everything reproductive. My ReproSoc colleagues know how much I appreciate them, of course for their feedback on earlier versions of this book, but mostly for the close academic companionship we all share. Thank you, Noémie Merleau-Ponty, Robert Pralat, Marcin Smietana, Katie Dow, Karen Jent, Kathryn Medièn, Sigrid Vertommen, Mwenza Blell, Janelle Lamoreaux, Zeynep Gürtin, Nitzan Peri-Rotem, Yuliya Hilevych, and Lea Taragin-Zeller. I am also grateful for the input of all the ReproSoc visitors and students, particularly of Jarrah O'Neill and Elisabeth Sandler, who provided very helpful research assistance. The Changing In/Fertilities collaborative project has offered me the invaluable opportunity to develop my research in dialogue with a global network of reproductive scholars, including Marcia Inhorn, Aditya Bharadwaj, Daphna Birenbaum-Carmeli, Trudie Gerrits, Sandra González-Santos, Tsipy Ivry, Venetia Kantsa, Sebastian Mohr, Michal Nahman, Sharmila Rudrappa, Charis Thompson, Soraya Tremayne, Ayo Wahlberg, and Andrea Whittaker. Chantal Nowak and Lois Gibbs deserve much appreciation for making it all happen. I have also greatly benefited from the many reproductive projects at Cambridge, including IVF Histories and Cultures, Generation to Reproduction, CIRF, and the SRI Reproduction. I am very grateful for the support and recognition offered by the Wellcome Trust (100606/Z/12/A; 209829/Z/17/Z), the Alan Turing Institute, the Praemium Erasmianum Foundation, U21, Newnham College, and the University of Cambridge. The Wellcome Trust has also generously supported the open access publication of this book.

I would also like to acknowledge the Amsterdam School for Cultural Analysis (ASCA) at the University of Amsterdam for making this research possible through its generous financial support and lively research community. Eloe Kingma and Jantine van Gogh run ASCA with such joy and dedication and I am so grateful to them. At the beautiful, sunny ASCA offices at the PC Hoofthuis, there were always kind colleagues to share thoughts and drinks with, many of whom have become my dear friends. It was a pleasure to be part of such a vibrant and interdisciplinary community and get to know Blandine Joret, Alexandre Poulin, Selçuk Balamir, Simon Ferdinand, Annelies Kleinherenbrink, Lara Mazurski, Thijs Witty, Tim Yaczo, Erin La Cour, Peyman Amiri, Uzma Ansari, Marie Beauchamps, Birkan Tas, Adam Chambers, Pedram Dibazar, Enis Dinç, Moosje Moti Goosen, Penn Ip, Noam Knoller, Melle Kromhout, Aylin Kuryel, Flora Lysen, Niall Martin, Miriam Meißner, Judith Naeff, Marjan Nijborg, Nur Ozgenalp, Jeffrey Pijpers, Irina Souch, Eliza Steinbock, Mikki Stelder, Margaret Tali, Irene Villaescusa, and

Vesna Vravnik. Mireille Rosello, thank you for all the energizing discussions, your stimulating questions about mammals, your openness, and warmth.

I cannot begin to thank everyone who has inspired me and offered me opportunities to share ideas about eggs over the years and across the world. However, some special thanks go to Diane Tober, Hannah Gibson, Risa Cromer, Carrie Friese, Rene Almeling, Anne Pollock, Joyce Harper, Charlotte Krøløkke, Olga Loblóvá, Stuart Hogarth, Anindita Majumdar, Victoria Boydell, Gina Glover, Susan Pickard, Nick Hopwood, Martin Johnson, Philip Kreager, John Dupré, Emily Jackson, Wendy Sigle, Sarah Douglas, Amanda Gore, Caroline Humphrey, Martin Rees, Natasha Tanna, Amade M'Charek, Nelly Oudshoorn, Jules Sturm, Fran Bigman, Merete Lie, Nina Lykke, and Laura Briggs. Carrie Hamilton, thank you for reading the manuscript so carefully and for sharing your uplifting insights and editorial suggestions. I would also like to thank Marieke Schellart, Sjoerd Repping, Sebastiaan Mastenbroek, and Roger Gosden for sharing their professional reflections on various reproductive technologies.

I am very grateful to New York University Press, and especially to Ilene Kalish, Sonia Tsuruoka, Lisa Jean Moore, and Monica Casper for all their work. It was also a pleasure to work with Sarah Bode, Alexia Traganas, and Martin Coleman. Emily Wright, thank you very much for your careful copyediting. And I would especially like to express my gratitude for the exceptionally inspiring reflections offered by the four anonymous reviewers, which were very helpful in the revision process.

My friends have offered me comfort, encouragement, and pleasure throughout this endeavor, for which I am grateful. Mark Robinson and Take Lijftogt are as close as kin, ever kind and welcoming. Rebecca Gomperts, bright light, you move the world and you move me, with the generosity of your open arms, your strength and vulnerability, with a life of adventures, and precious quiet moments. Abital and Amun, thank you too for all the fun times (let's do wat leuks!), honest questions, and enthusiastic stories; it is so lovely to see you grow up into such great people. Thank you, Jennifer Mathews, for showing me your kindness, hydration, and the vast expanse of the world's edge. And Diane Barlee, what a joy to live with you. I warmly appreciate the company, distractions, and life lessons from Barbara Knapper, Wanda Klein, Rachel O'Reilly, Eva

Reijman, Margaret Kruszewska, Úna Monaghan, Cohl Furey, Sophie Seita, Kat Buchmann, Marguerite Rigoglioso, Esther Beek, Monica Germino, Isis Maakestad, Filippa Barfvestam, Shanti Freed, Goxwa Borg, Sigrid Merx, Carmen Ket, Rebecca Marshall, Jane Levi, Esther Ending, Ray Malone, Boukje Cnossen, Lisa Clayton, and Tashina Blom. I would like to celebrate the people who have taught me about birthing: Soraya Soebhag, Merlijn Kamps, Bea van der Put, Jennifer Walker, Jacky Bloemraad-de Boer, Ina May Gaskin, Michel Odent, Liliana Lammers, Anija Dokter, and Carolyn Cowan. I cherish the memory of Fenne Bordat, Sandy Hayes, Layne Redmond, and Lois Tonkin.

I thank my dear parents for making, raising, and cherishing me. Thank you for providing the egg and sperm, the blood and milk from which I grew. Thank you, Astrid, for carrying and birthing me so many years ago. Thank you also for teaching me how to learn, for celebrating each step with genuine joy, for passing on your strength and determination, for giving me books and self-confidence, for always forgiving me, and loving me more. Thomas, thank you for reading your dermatology books with me when I was 3 years old, for saving the medical records of when I was 3 cm. long, for making it your life's work to tenderly show me the world, for encouraging my curiosity, for taking me for a walk when there was too much work. Thank you both for your smiles, for your kindness. I am increasingly aware of the magnitude of the gift of your unwavering, continuous love.

I give thanks to my grandparents, especially my grandmothers, whom I have had the honor of knowing, and my extended family of aunts, uncles, cousins, nephews, and nieces across the world who have always received me with a smile and open arms.

Then there are those who become kin not by blood, or by choice, but by the heart's compass. Caroline Smart, otherworldly sister of shining spirit, I thank you. For love, for music, for laughter, a thousand times over. For walking this life path with me, for seeing the birthing of an idea into a book, for enriching me with other knowledges, for bearing witness, for holding, for being held. You are my home and I love you. Lesley Gamble, thank you for whirling into my life all those years ago, luminous and liquid, from the hot and humid land of swaying trees and icy, breathtaking waters. Across the oceans, heart-sung gratitude for our wild, precious, entangled lives. Thank you both for being my guardians on this journey.

ASRM: American Society for Reproductive Medicine

Autologous: Autologous donations are donations for a person's own (future) use.

CBRC: Cross-border reproductive care

Cytoplasm: The cell's cytoplasm consists of all the contents of the cell besides the nucleus.

ESHRE: European Society of Human Reproduction and Embryology

hESCs: Human embryonic stem cells. These stem cells may be derived from the inner cell mass of the embryo and can differentiate into various cell types.

Heterologous: Heterologous donations are donations from one person to another.

HFEA: Human Fertilisation and Embryology Authority (UK)

ICSI: Intra-cytoplasmic sperm injection. An embryological technique for fertilization in which the embryologist inserts a single sperm cell into an egg through micro-injection. This differs from conventional IVF, in which an egg is placed in a petri dish with sperm.

iPSCs: Induced pluripotent stem cells. These stems cells are generated from somatic cells without the use of eggs and can differentiate into various cell types.

IVF: *In vitro* fertilization

IVM: *In vitro* maturation

Nucleus: The nucleus of a cell is a structure that holds the cell's DNA, RNA, and nuclear proteins. A membrane called the nuclear envelope separates it from the cell's cytoplasm.

OC: Oocyte cryopreservation, technical term for egg freezing

OHSU: Oregon Health and Science University

SCNT: Somatic cell nuclear transfer, a technique for creating an embryo from an egg and a somatic cell, also known as "cloning."

Somatic cell: A somatic cell is any cell of the body that is not a sperm or egg cell.

TWEB: The World Egg Bank

NOTES

1 See West 1994, 289–90; Valk 2000, 148; Leeming 2005, 82. The figure of the cosmic egg also occurs in Egyptian, Chinese, Vedic, Greek, Phoenician, Finnish, Polynesian, and medieval Christian mythology.

2 The frontispiece references the Greek myth of Leda and the swan, in which Zeus disguises himself as a swan and rapes Leda, who bears two eggs from which the demigods Helen and Polydeuces hatch (Maguire 2009).

3 Landecker 2007.

4 Squier 1994; Huxley 2007 [1932], 2–3.

5 An estimated further 32 million attempted cycles of IVF have not resulted in the birth of a child.

6 Gosden and Lee 2010, 973.

7 Franklin 2013b. In conventional IVF, egg and sperm cells are combined in a petri dish to allow spontaneous fertilization. ICSI (intracytoplasmic sperm injection) may be used if there is reduced sperm quality or quantity or if the egg no longer allows fertilization, as is the case when the egg has been frozen and thawed.

8 Franklin 2000, 189.

9 Nowak 2007.

10 Reflecting the wider discourses on egg freezing that are the subject of this study, I use the term "women" throughout. Of course, not all women experience age-related infertility; some were never fertile, lose their reproductive ability due to causes that are not age-related, or do not live long enough. Also, some people who do not identify as women may experience pregnancy, birth, and age-related infertility. It is important to note that egg freezing technology also opens the way for people of various gender identities—including nonbinary people and transmen—to explore different paths to pregnancy and childbirth. Although the focus in this book lies specifically on egg freezing to circumvent age-related infertility, some of the other indications for OC are particularly relevant for gender-variant people. As I discuss in chapter 1, egg freezing is routinely recommended to transgender men who (intend to) use hormone treatment. Because hormone treatment can affect fertility, egg freezing can help maintain the possibility of having biogenetically related children in the future (HFEA 2019a).

11 Richards 2013, 74.

12 Bunge et al. 1954; Zeilmaker et al. 1984.

13 Chen 1986.

14 Gosden 2011, 266.

15 Inhorn and Patrizio 2012.

16 Franklin 2019, 26; Harris 2013, 201.

17 Harris 2013, 201.

18 Harris 2013, 201.

19 Italy is a case in point as a country that, in the late 1980s and 1990s, had one of the world's "most cutting-edge" fertility industries. It came to be known as the "wild west" of European IVF and developed "the beginning of an industry intended for career women who had delayed conception into their 40s and beyond" (Inhorn et al. 2010, 850). In line with this focus on later reproduction, doctors in Bologna started working on frozen eggs in 1997 (Gosden 2011, 266). This intensification of research into OC anticipated the legal restrictions on embryo freezing and egg donation in Italy's prohibitive 2004 IVF Law, and proved useful when egg freezing became the only legal alternative to embryo freezing (Benagiano and Gianaroli 2004, 118; Gook 2011, 284; Martin 2010, 527). Reflecting the Italian focus on OC, the first live birth with the—currently dominant—vitrification technique for egg freezing occurred in Italy: on June 20, 1999, a girl was born to a 47-year-old mother who had used vitrified donor eggs (Kuleshova et al. 1999).

20 Kuwayama et al. 2005, 76. The Cryotop system consists of a plastic holder and a thin film strip onto which the egg can be laid in only a minimal volume of fluid. The Cryotop system has been applied in over 1.2 million clinical cases in 90 countries (Kitazato 2019).

21 Although these calves are referred to as fetuses, they have been removed from the uteri of their slaughtered mothers and briefly live independently from her.

22 Van der Valk et al. 2018.

23 E.g., Chen 1986; Yoon et al. 2003.

24 Haraway 2010; Kowal and Radin 2015, 70; Merleau-Ponty 2019.

25 HFEA 2018b.

26 In the United States, the permissive attitude to reproductive technologies stands in sharp contrast with the strict regulatory control over nonreproductive technologies. The current rise of insurance coverage and promotion of egg freezing coincides with a severe curtailing of abortion rights. Increasingly restrictive state regulations all but outlaw abortion, while the FDA attempts to prevent women from accessing medical abortion on politically motivated "safety" grounds (Dyer 2019; Aiken et al. 2019). While the Trump administration politicizes reproductive rights with renewed vigor to mobilize the conservative Christian electorate—whether with White House prayers for "the unborn child" or through antichoice Supreme Court appointments—the IVF sector, in spite of its frequent introduction of new technologies, operates relatively unconstrained and unregulated.

27 Spar 2005; Mladovsky and Sorenson 2010.

28 See chapter 3 and Van de Wiel 2020.

29 Gerrits 2016, 316–17.

30 Franklin 2019.

31 Franklin 2019, 26.

32 HFEA 2017.

33 Inhorn et al. 2018.

34 Witkin et al. 2013.

35 Waldby 2015a.

36 Prior to egg extraction, OC requires one–two weeks of hormone injections, which can cause discomfort and side effects. This hormonal stimulation can result in ovarian hyperstimulation syndrome, a potentially serious condition that may cause pain and inflammation and, in extreme cases, can be fatal; it may have additional as-yet-unknown long-term risks for later reproductive health. Once matured, the eggs are surgically removed, which causes internal bleeding or infection in 1% of cases (Waldby 2008, 20–21; NVOG 2010).

37 Carbone and Cahn 2013.

38 Roberts 2017a, xviii. Nonetheless, as Dorothy Roberts has noted, reproductive technologies are no longer only marketed towards white women (2017a). Financing and decreased pricing make egg freezing more widely accessible—albeit by enlisting those who can least afford it into a debt relation with lenders (see chapter 3).

39 Smietana et al. 2018, 117.

40 Bhatia and Campo-Engelstein 2018, 872. ESHRE is the European Society for Human Reproduction and Embryology.

41 Balkenende 2018.

42 Goold and Savulescu 2008; 2009.

43 Inhorn 2013.

44 Harwood 2009; Carbone and Cahn 2013; Browne 2018.

45 Ikemoto 2015, 114.

46 Cattapan et al. 2014, 239.

47 Goold and Savulescu 2008, 47–48.

48 See, for example, Goisis and Sigle-Rushton 2014 on the socioeconomic advantages of having children later in life.

49 See Hanson 2003 for a challenge to the association between maternal age and infertility.

50 Daniluk and Koert 2013.

51 Spivak 1996, 27.

52 Franklin 1997, 175.

53 It is not unusual that specific groups of fertile people undergo infertility treatment. Fertile heterosexual women may undergo IVF to have children with their subfertile male partners. Single people and same-sex couples may access gametes, embryos, or surrogacy arrangements, whether or not they experience infertility. People with diagnosed pathologies may access treatment to avoid passing on heritable diseases. As Franklin notes, fertility "has always been biologically relative," given that it is both a shared and an individual condition and contingent

on external factors (2013b, 224). Therefore, people considered to be fertile may undergo treatment in the context of a particular partnership or desired kinship arrangement. Egg freezing is, nevertheless, unusual as a treatment for future infertility aimed at people who are presumed to be fertile at present.

54 WHO 2019.

55 Franklin 1997.

56 OED 2019.

57 Butler 2006.

58 Spar 2006, 63.

59 Berlant 2011, 192.

60 This egg-based model of fertility reflects an IVF treatment logic that is primarily reliant on the egg for *ex vivo* fertilization or fertility preservation.

61 Here I use "bioprecarity" to refer to the discursive constructions and sociocultural effects of positing certain bodies and bodily abilities as precarious. The dynamic of epistemic uncertainty and biotechnological interdependency is particularly pertinent with the emergence of new technologies for predictive testing and cryo-preserving that render the body differently (il)legible in the face of anticipatory interventions.

62 Foucault 2003, 241.

63 Kowal and Radin 2015, 68–70.

64 Smirnova 2012, 1240.

65 See, respectively, Vincent 2009; Lock 1995; and Segal 2013.

66 Neilson 2003.

67 This focus is in keeping with a Foucauldian reading of biopolitics in which power structures within a "normalizing society" maintain and manage life through the logic of the norm (Foucault 2003, 252–53; Lemke 2011, 39).

68 A performative understanding of normative (cis)gender positions the construction of the subject's consistent categorization as "male" or "female" throughout the life course as the effect of a repeated enactment of norms, thereby "'freezing' masculin-ity and femininity into timeless truths of being" (Freeman 2010, 4; Butler 1997a, 14). Age identities can similarly be considered as performatively constituted (Biggs 2004), but whereas gender normativity entails the maintenance of a stable category of "female" or "male" throughout the lifetime, age normativities necessitate timely changes in accordance with culturally specific temporal schemes. At their intersec-tion, normative expressions of "female" or "male" differ at various life stages, as, vice versa, those of any particular age are inflected by gender norms.

69 Moscucci 1993; Friese et al. 2008; Van de Wiel 2014b.

70 Freeman 2010, 3.

71 Freeman 2010, 3. The ideal of domestic femininity associated with the separate spheres was particularly associated with the middle and upper classes; i.e., the idea of gendered time was—as it is now—linked to class-specific constructions of normative womanhood.

72 Heath 2009, 15; Freeman 2010, 5.

73 Luciano 2007, 125–27.

74 Thompson 2005, 9–10.

75 Similarly, the discovery of sexual hormone production reinforced the temporal gender binary as the female reproductive body became "characterised by its cyclic hormonal regulation and the male body by its stable" counterpart (Oudshoorn 1994, 146–47).

76 Freeman 2010, 3.

77 Friese et al. 2006, 1551.

78 Harter et al. 2005, 84.

79 Amir 2006, 64–65. See chapter 1 for a more extensive discussion of the biological clock trope.

80 Schwartz and Mayaux 1982; Menken et al. 1986.

81 Friese et al. 2006, 1550–51.

82 Stephenson 2010, 11.

83 Bos et al. 2012.

84 The journey is a familiar metaphor in discourses of fertility clinics, where the experience of undergoing treatment may be described as one's "IVF journey." *In vivo* conception is conventionally presented as the sperm's journey through the female reproductive tract towards an egg waiting in the fallopian tube. By structuring the chapters according to the egg's journey, I intend to draw attention to the egg's mobility in OC and the site-specific meanings ascribed to this cell.

85 Bal 2002, 4; Peeren 2007, 3.

86 Schellart 2010.

1. MAKING FERTILITY PRECARIOUS

1 However, contraceptive and nonreproductive technologies have also widely been used as tools for "reproductive oppression." In the US context, Dorothy Roberts demonstrates that the growth of a fertility industry that facilitates the reproduction of affluent, educated, disproportionately white women contrasts with policies and stereotypes that penalize poorer and Black women's childbearing (2017a, xviii).

2 HFEA 2018e, 37.

3 The AMC had offered egg freezing for "medical" reasons since 2006.

4 Schippers 2011a. The Dutch government consisted of the CDA (Christian Democratic Appeal), PvdA (Labour), and ChristenUnie (Christian Union) parties.

5 NVOG 2010.

6 Boseley 2000.

7 HFEA 2000.

8 J. Harper et al. 2018. There are, however, NHS regulations, insurance policies, and clinical guidelines that identify maximum ages for fertility treatment and distinguish between cancer-related and other motivations for egg freezing; see, for example, NICE 2013.

9 CHA 2019a.

10 In 2003, Extend Fertility launched its website, announcing that it "give[s] women the chance to take control of their fertility" through "revolutionary science and service" (Extend Fertility 2003). Likewise, the Florida Institute for Reproductive Medicine offered egg freezing through a dedicated savemyeggs.com website from 2002 onwards.

11 ASRM 2004.

12 ASRM Practice Committee 2013, 42.

13 ASRM Ethics Committee 2018.

14 All three newspapers have a broad readership in their respective countries; the *Guardian* (digital and printed) has the third largest reach of all UK newspapers, the *New York Times* has the largest print circulation of all US daily newspapers, and the *Volkskrant* has the third largest circulation in the Netherlands (Mediatique 2018; The New York Times Company 2018; NOM 2019).

All three newspapers are generally considered to be center-left publications. This inquiry addresses what implicit normative messaging is perpetuated, reinvented, or resisted within relatively progressive publications that have a history of "plead[ing] for the oppressed and those whose rights are violated" (Gutteling et al. 2001, 232).

The *Guardian* targets "a progressive audience" of "forward-looking individuals who are curious about the world and embrace change and technology" (Guardian.co.uk 2012). The *New York Times* describes its readers as "educated, affluent and influential audiences" (The New York Times Company 2018, 26). *Volkskrant* readers are similarly presented as "well-to-do, curious and well-informed" (De Persgroep Advertising 2012). All three newspapers advertise that their audiences are well educated, with high socioeconomic status, thereby matching the demographic of egg freezing candidates (Gold et al. 2006).

The *Guardian* has the most progressive readership in the United Kingdom, with 67% Labour support and only 2% Conservative (Fahmy and Kim 2008, 448). *Volkskrant* readers have an outspoken voting preference for left and center-left political parties (Van Cuilenburg et al. 1999, 88). About two thirds of the *New York Times* audience (65%) have political values that are left of center, and only 12% are conservative (Pew Research Center 2014).

15 I have included all articles on egg freezing in the 2000–2018 period, with a focus on the 2007–2014 period. I include news articles, feature articles, opinion pieces, editorials, and columns. I searched in the databases of the newspapers and in the Lexis Nexis database. Search terms were "egg freezing," "oocyte cryopreservation," "frozen eggs," "frozen egg," and "eicellen invriezen," "eicel invriezen," "oocyte cryopreservatie," "ingevroren eicellen," "ingevroren eicel," "bevroren eicellen," "bevroren eicel," "eitjes invriezen," "eitje invriezen," "ingevroren eitjes," "ingevroren eitje," "bevroren eitjes," and "bevroren eitje."

16 An earlier version of sections of this chapter appeared in the special issue on "Non-Reproduction: Politics, Ethics, Aesthetics" of *Studies in the Maternal*. See Van de Wiel 2014a.

17 Sample 2006a.

18 Sawicki 1999, 194.

19 Briggs 2018, 126.

20 Sample 2006a.

21 Faludi 1991, 12.

22 Faludi 1991, 118.

23 Faludi 1991, 103.

24 Oliver 2010, 776.

25 Campbell 2009; Richards 2014.

26 Geelen 2010. The CDA (Christen Democratisch Appèl) is a Dutch Christian Democratic political party.

27 ANP 2009.

28 Bos et al. 2012, A4145.

29 Gillian Lockwood treated Helen Perry, who gave birth to the first British frozen-egg baby in 2002.

30 Groskop 2006.

31 The focus on the absent partner is crucial because it links the physical necessity of sperm for conception with a set of social relations associated with reproductive partnership. The positioning of singlehood as a "social indication" for medical treatment naturalizes a set of norms, including life-course conventions about when to have a long-term partner and preferences for having an "own child" who is also genetically related to a partner (Lesnik-Oberstein 2008; Carroll and Krøløkke 2018).

32 See chapter 2 for a discussion of egg freezing and willfulness.

33 Batty 2006; emphasis added.

34 Groskop 2011.

35 Bewley qtd. in O'Kelly 2005.

36 The subject position of the "lifestyle freezer," and the life course trajectory associated with it, have unspoken class assumptions that particularly pertain to middle-class, highly educated women. For a further discussion on egg freezing, class, and the life course, see Carbone and Cahn 2013.

37 The opposition between single and lifestyle freezers is a subdivision of the main medical-social opposition along which women's subject positions are organized in egg freezing news coverage.

38 As part of a cancer treatment plan, egg freezing costs are covered by both the British National Health Service and the Dutch basic insurance [basisverzekering]. The first phase of egg freezing for so-called social reasons is not covered by national insurance in either country. The subsequent use of these frozen eggs may be covered, depending on existing IVF regulations.

39 Herderscheê 2011a.

40 Sample 2009.

41 Shaw and Giles 2009.

42 Bos et al. 2012, 192.

43 As the medical indications for egg freezing expand, so the number of women who become "candidates" for fertility preservation may rise over the coming years.

44 Gürtin et al. 2019.

45 See, respectively, Hildingsson 2008; Abraham-Van der Mark 1996; Viloria et al. 2011.

46 Stoop et al. 2014, 594.

47 Stoop et al. 2014.

48 Knill et al. 2014, 852. In the *Volkskrant* the phrase "social indication" is used in coverage of both egg freezing and abortion debates (Effting 2011; Herderscheê 2011b).

49 Linders 1998, 500.

50 Linders 1998, 499.

51 McGee 2014; Ridley 2014; Eggbanxx 2015.

52 Campbell 2009.

53 The Observer 2009.

54 With the exception of celebrity coverage, media analyses suggest that older motherhood is predominantly negatively framed in terms of accusations of reckless postponement, selfishness, and "violations of the 'natural order'" (Shaw and Giles 2009; Campbell 2011). See chapter 5 for a discussion of OC and older motherhood.

55 Swanson 2015.

56 R. Cohen 1978.

57 R. Cohen 1978.

58 Wiegel 2016, 218–20.

59 R. Cohen 1978.

60 Groskop 2006.

61 Anam 2008.

62 Boseley 2009.

63 Sample 2006b.

64 Kasperkevic 2016.

65 Groskop 2011.

66 Groskop 2011.

67 These numbers may be compared to two studies into age-related fertility decline among heterosexual couples attempting to conceive without diagnosed fertility problems. Rothman and colleagues analyzed 2,820 couples and concluded that 87% of women within the 30 to 34 age group became pregnant within one year, compared to 72% in the 35 to 40 age group (2013). Dunson and colleagues examined 770 European women and found that 86% of women between 27 and 34 years became pregnant within a year, compared to 82% in the 35 to 39 age group (2004). Although these studies affirm that there is a decrease in pregnancy rates over time, these figures do not evoke the notion of a "deadline" or "no exit" at 35, as described in some of the articles above (Twenge 2013).

68 The figures for the woman in her twenties would sound even grimmer if the comparator were not the one to two million eggs present at birth, but the seven million she had as a four-month-old fetus.

69 Martin 2001, 45.

70 Sample 2011.

71 Sawicki 1999, 194.

72 Sample 2007.

73 Sometimes the news coverage responds to these studies, notably with the publication of Marcia Inhorn and Daphna Birenbaum-Carmeli's study of egg freezers, which confirms that singlehood is a key motivator and calls attention to the sociodemographic deficit of educated men with whom they can pursue childbearing. News outlets report that "Lots of Successful Women Are Freezing Their Eggs. But It May Not Be about Their Career" and that absent partners are the "Real Reason Women Freeze Their Eggs" because "the issue that drives the success of the egg freezing industry has never been employers' attitudes to motherhood, but instead, men's" (Wiseman 2017; Gürtin 2017; H. Murphy 2018). Notwithstanding the fact that these articles discuss the intertwining of the relational and professional realms—as is evident in the fact that these single women freezing their eggs are overwhelmingly highly educated and occupy high-status jobs—the disavowal of the career motivation as a false assumption is a key element in these news reports.

74 Kindbody 2018.

75 Depmann et al. 2017.

76 Richards 2014. Bartasi was also director of Progyny, the fertility benefits company that is a market leader in corporate egg freezing insurance. Eggbanxx is part of Progyny.

77 Cavanaugh 2014.

78 Hafer et al. 2018.

79 Kindbody 2018.

80 Barbey 2017, 201.

81 Mulkerrins 2017.

82 McGee 2014; Richards 2018.

83 Richards 2018.

84 Ferla 2018.

85 Ferla 2018.

86 Campo-Engelstein et al. 2018, 186–87, 192.

87 Boseley 2014.

88 Minter 2014.

89 Miller 2018a.

90 See chapter 3 for an extensive discussion on egg freezing benefits and fertility insurance.

91 Qtd. in Fraser and Jaeggi 2018, 40, 86.

92 Miller 2018b.

93 Qtd. in Fraser and Jaeggi 2018, 87.

94 Blell 2018.

95 As discussed above, corporate egg freezing benefits have also been celebrated as a means of responsibilizing employers to cover reproductive costs, rather than externalizing these to the state or the private sphere.

96 See chapter 3 for a discussion of the investment models and treatment rationales underlying fertility insurance.

97 Waldby 2015a.

98 Franklin 2013b.

99 See chapter 2 for a further discussion of this age limit and its subsequent revision.

2. FREEZING IN ANTICIPATION

1 Adams et al. 2009, 246–48.

2 Adams et al. 2009, 246–47.

3 Luijt 2010.

4 Berlant 2007, 664.

5 An earlier and shorter version of this chapter appeared in *Women's Studies International Forum*. See Van de Wiel 2015.

6 Martin 2010, 529–30.

7 See Mills and Lavender 2011; Budds et al. 2013, 134.

8 HFEA 2018b.

9 Sample 2011; Mertes and Pennings 2011.

10 Freeman 2010, xv.

11 Shaw and Giles 2009.

12 Schellart 2011.

13 See Carbone and Cahn 2013 for an analysis of the class dimensions of egg freezing practices and later first-time reproduction. Both in the Netherlands and in the United States, white, highly educated women have their first child at significantly later ages than women of other racial backgrounds (Martin et al. 2017; Boschman 2012). For example, US women with a college degree have their first child on average seven years later than those without (Bui and Miller 2018).

14 Harris 2006, 9.

15 Ahmed 2010, 183.

16 Adams et al. 2009, 249.

17 Ahmed 2010, 222–23.

18 Waldby 2015a.

19 Z. Williams 2010.

20 McAuliffe 2012.

21 In this sense, Silber presents a "diagnostic expansion" of infertility as a condition that can be treated prior to its emergence (Loe 2006).

22 Adams et al. 2009, 249.

23 Extend Fertility 2016. By contrast, Dutch fertility clinics do not permit egg freezing below 30 years of age because, they argue, younger women cannot predict whether they will need the frozen eggs and may be treated unnecessarily.

24 Prelude Fertility 2017a.
25 Prelude Fertility 2016.
26 See chapter 3 for a discussion of egg quantities and multicycle norms in OC treatment packages.
27 Adams et al. 2009, 254.
28 Lafontaine 2009, 67.
29 Gill 2007, 149.
30 B. Rothman 1993.
31 Powell 2010, 121.
32 Ahmed 2006, 555.
33 Van Dijck 2004, 262, 273–74.
34 Kuhn 2010, 298.
35 Van Dijck 2007, 144.
36 Edelman 2004, 30–31.
37 Van Dijck 2007, 132.
38 Edelman 2004, 31.
39 Bos et al. 2012, 193.
40 Ahmed 2006, 554.
41 Ahmed 2006, 555.
42 Groskop 2006.
43 Herderscheê 2009.
44 Shaw and Giles 2009, 226.
45 Budds et al. 2013, 133.
46 Kelhä 2009, 89.
47 Adams et al. 2009, 257.
48 Ahmed 2010, 181.
49 Betterton 2002, 262.
50 Groenier 2010, 22.
51 Franklin 1997, 94.

3. FROZEN EGGS AND THE FINANCIALIZATION OF FERTILITY

1 The notion that reproductive technologies are also visual technologies has become abundantly clear in the last half-century. The images produced by reproductive technologies have had profound political effects and cultural impact; fetal ultrasound imagery was (and continues to be) at the heart of abortion politics, *in vitro* embryo images were in stem cell debates, and the iconic scene of the egg's micro-injection in ICSI fertilization influenced the popular imagination of the reproductive process and the "helping hand" of ARTs (Franklin 2013a, 25).
2 Although not all clinics offer their patients images of their eggs, it is a familiar practice among UK and US clinics to share egg photographs.
3 Some sections of this chapter overlap with Van de Wiel 2018 and Van de Wiel 2020.
4 Eggfreezer 2008.

5 Sheryl de Lacey studied how IVF patients observe their embryos. Her participants described the impact of the visual as an affirmation of embryonic development as the first stages of a "continuum of human development," from which the growth into the potential future child may be extrapolated (2005, 1666).

The conceptualization of embryos as individuals is epitomized in the reframing of embryo donation into embryo adoption in schemes such as the "Snowflakes" program run by the Nightlight Christian Adoptions agency since 1997. They refer to the embryos as "preborn children" and emphasize their individual personhood: "Each snowflake is frozen. We understand that each snowflake is unique. Each snowflake is a gift from heaven. We hope each donated embryo will become a snowflake baby" (Nightlight Christian Adoptions 2015).

6 Moore 2003, 291.

7 In *The Transparent Body*, José van Dijck traces the techno-cultural history of visualizing the interior body, from the popularization of X-rays to MRI and endoscopy (2005). In the case of OC, the eggs, paradoxically, need to be disembodied in order to become visually recognizable in the cellular photograph as what was "inside of me" (Eggfreezer 2008).

8 Radin 2013, 484.

9 Eggfreezer 2008.

10 Eggfreezer 2008.

11 An early practitioner of cell culturing remarked in 1916 that "through the discovery of tissue culture we have, so to speak, created a new type of body in which to grow a cell" (Uhlenhuth qtd. in Landecker 2007, 12). In a similar vein, Landecker reflects on tissue culturing as a practice in which "the body was not replaced by the cell, but rather this technique substituted an artificial apparatus for the body. As a result, the understanding of the cell and the body as well as their relation to one another was fundamentally altered" (2007, 33).

12 Landecker 2007, 233.

13 For Landecker, the question of what it is to be cellular, or biological, offers a framework through which organic life can be reconceptualized across species.

14 Landecker 2007, 228.

15 Landecker describes the history of tissue culturing as "the realization and growing exploitation of the plasticity of living matter, with interventions in plasticity tightly linked to interventions in the way biological things lived in time" (2007, 31). Egg freezing emerges in the wake of this history and likewise affects how eggs—and bodies—live in time. While the egg's temporal plasticity materializes only at the cellular level, by "becoming biological," the cell's plasticity also affects the meaning of aging.

After all, the egg's temporal plasticity shifts the conceptualization of reproductive aging as not only tied to the "immovable intrinsic age of living matter" but also having "a moveable—plastic—quality" over which agency and intentionality may be exerted (Landecker 2007, 231).

16 Franklin 2013a, 29.

17 Murphy 2011, 23.

18 Murphy 2017, 141.

19 Sharon Kaufman draws on Arnold Relman's definition of the medical-industrial complex as "a large and growing network of private corporations engaged in the business of supplying health-care services to patients for a profit" to explore evidence-based medicine and the clinical trials industry (2015, 54–55). Sigrid Vertommen specifically analyzes the "reproductive-industrial complex" of Israel in "which the interests of a pronatalist Jewish state and a biomedical establishment—consisting of academic entrepreneurs, venture capitalists, biotech companies and pharmaceutical giants—have coalesced" (2017, 286). See also Ayo Wahlberg's notion of the "reproductive complex" (2018, 9).

20 Haraway 2016.

21 CDC 2018.

22 ASRM 2014. A European study suggests that the live birth rate per extracted egg remains remarkably stable between ages 23 and 37 (D. Stoop et al. 2012, 2034).

23 Shady Grove Fertility 2017.

24 CARE Fertility 2016.

25 E.g., see Shady Grove Fertility 2016.

26 Franklin 2014a.

27 Franklin 2013b.

28 For example, Inhorn's study demonstrates an average age of 36.6 in the United States (2018).

29 Waldby 2015a.

30 If 20 or 30 eggs are retrieved within, respectively, one or two cycles, women receive a refund.

31 Extend Fertility 2017a.

32 CARE Fertility 2016.

33 Guarantee packages are often presented as a sign that clinics are confident enough in their success rates to take a financial risk. However, FertilityIQ's survey of 300 US patients enrolled in IVF refund programs found that 67% of patients succeeded on the first egg-retrieval cycle. This is almost twice the national average of a 34% success rate. They conclude that the selectivity of refund programs resulted in the "vast majority" of patients in refund programs overpaying to get a positive result (FertilityIQ 2017b).

34 Robertson and Schneyer 1997; Hawkins 2010.

35 IVF can result in different forms of reproductive success—whether fertilized embryos, chemical pregnancies, ongoing pregnancies, or live births resulting in a "take-home baby"—that may be contractualized in treatment packages.

36 Because egg freezing is in effect an IVF procedure separated in two phases by a period of cryostorage, the endpoint of reproductive success may arrive twice: first as a particular number of eggs representing bioprepared fertility and, second, as a "take-home baby." Accordingly, egg freezing patients may purchase guarantee packages to "assure" themselves of a desirable outcome twice.

37 For example, Shady Grove Fertility recommends freezing 15 to 20 eggs for women 37 or younger with a favorable ovarian reserve and 20 to 30 eggs for women over 37 or for those who have an unfavorable ovarian reserve. Of course, if women aim to have more than one child, the recommended number of eggs accordingly doubles or triples.

38 FertilityIQ 2017a.

39 Thompson 2005, 255; FertilityIQ 2017b.

40 A failed IVF cycle still incurs other expenses, such as costly fertility drugs, which are typically not included in the packages.

41 Thompson 2005, 255; Waldby 2015b.

42 Hawkins 2009, 863; Jacoby 2009, 148.

43 Market Cube 2015. Medical debt for healthcare is a widespread phenomenon in the United States and accounted for over 62% of personal bankruptcies in 2007 (Himmelstein et al. 2009). Over a quarter of Americans report that their households have trouble paying for medical costs. There are clear racial disparities in both the accruement of medical debt and its social consequences, such as home foreclosures (Hamel et al. 2016; Lichtenstein and Weber 2016).

44 Hawkins 2009, 863.

45 For example, as of 2017, majority shares and directorships are shared among Access Fertility, Fertility Finance, the US clinic Shady Grove Fertility, and the major US fertility loan company, CapexMD. Alternatively, clinics may operate independently from lenders, or even pay lenders for taking on their patients, because fertility financing allows sales to increase (Hawkins 2009, 865).

46 Von Hagel 2013, 15.

47 Von Hagel 2013, 16.

48 Jacoby 2009; Hawkins 2009.

49 Stoop et al. 2011. In assisted reproduction more broadly, costs are the largest impediment to treatment (Von Hagel 2013, 15), and complete insurance coverage of IVF is associated with a 277% increase of utilization rates (Jain 2006, 277).

50 AMC 2019; FertilityIQ 2017c.

51 Jain 2006.

52 Carbone and Cahn 2013, 304.

53 Smietana et al. 2018.

54 Of course, the promise of an expanded patient group is still highly selective, and prohibitive costs continue to limit access for many women. Feminist scholarship has demonstrated that class, racial, and gendered hierarchies and histories continue to structure access and marketing of reproductive technologies, and egg freezing is no exception (Smietana et al. 2018; Thompson 2011; Franklin 2011).

55 In the United Kingdom, the number of egg freezing cycles almost doubled between 2014 and 2016 (85% increase) and, in the United States, OC cycles increased 43% in the same period (HFEA 2018e; SART 2018).

56 Dresner Partners 2018.

57 Extend Fertility 2019b.

58 B. Lee 2016; Crunchbase 2019. Other egg freezing companies receiving capital investment include the abovementioned Kindbody, which was founded in 2018 with $6.3 million seed funding and is best known for its promotional "fertility vans" (Kindbody 2019). In 2017, embryologist Colleen Wagner Coughlin founded Ova Egg Freezing in Chicago as part of the four business entities of which she is the sole owner: Gamete Resources, Ova Institute, Cryovault, and Egg Bank Foundation. Ova Egg Freezing is a member of the California Cryobank Donor Egg Bank Network—a major cryopreservation company that combines sperm, egg, and cord blood banking after a larger merger and acquisition deal worth an estimated $1 billion by San Francisco-based private equity firm GI Partners (Ditkowsky 2018).

59 See Van de Wiel 2020 for a more detailed discussion of egg freezing and the financialization of fertility.

60 Qtd. in Robbins 2017.

61 Prelude Fertility 2017b.

62 Extend Fertility 2019a.

63 Prelude Fertility 2018b.

64 These benefits are particularly popular in the tech industry. Companies that confirmed they offer egg freezing benefits include Facebook, Apple, Google, Uber, Yahoo, Netflix, Snapchat, Intel, eBay, Time Warner, Salesforce, LinkedIn, and Spotify (Kerr 2017). In 2016, 10% of US employers with 20,000 or more employees offered egg freezing benefits (Mercer 2016).

65 Prelude Fertility 2017a.

66 Extend Fertility 2017b; Bartasi 2016.

67 Specialized fertility lenders such as Fertility Funds play an active role in reframing fertility. For example, Fertility Funds' representative Carolyn Kim suggests that "all women should consider this [egg freezing] at any age in their life" and that it is "great family planning" before it is too late. She herself wished she "had done it in her early twenties so it would have been taken care of." The loans are meant to give women "the flexibility to do [egg freezing] at an earlier age before they have savings to write a $20,000 check" (Hopewell 2014). By thus providing the financial means to freeze eggs earlier in life, fertility lenders benefit from—and actively promote—a precarious notion of fertility as something that ought to be "taken care of" before it is too late and thereby encourage freezing sooner rather than saving up for treatment later on.

68 The distribution of consumer credit through fertility clinics is widespread. Almost 50% of SART-registered US clinics mention credit and typically claim to help or understand financial stress (Hawkins 2009; Jacoby 2009). Fertility financing may broaden access, but of course, as Michelle Murphy notes, "the loan is both an investment in life and a rejigging of your precarity. The investment comes in the form of a debt" (2017, 140).

69 Christopher et al. 2013, ix.

70 Christopher et al. 2013, ix.

71 Fertility financing charges between 7% and 22% interest rates and 1–6% origination fees, depending on one's credit score.

72 Varsavsky 2016.

73 Varsavsky 2016.

74 Prelude Fertility 2015.

75 Prelude Fertility 2017a.

76 Varsavsky 2016.

77 Sunder Rajan 2006, 167.

78 Varsavsky 2016.

79 Progyny 2017.

80 The UK regulator HFEA advises that "assisted hatching is not recommended because it has not been shown to improve pregnancy rates" and that "more evidence is needed" to support pre-implantation genetic screening—in fact, it "can actually reduce success rates" (HFEA 2018d).

81 Yang 2018.

82 McGinley 2016.

83 Nonetheless, these fertility benefits illustrate reproductive "infrastructures built narrowly in the name of individual choice," which "selectively mitigat[e] conditions, without disrupting them" (M. Murphy 2017, 139).

   Although these insurance arrangements do not posit egg freezing coverage as an alternative to family support policies, they equally do not disrupt the socioeconomic and labor conditions that drive the demand for this technology.

84 Abdou 2016.

85 Progyny 2019b.

86 Progyny 2019a.

87 Beim et al. 2017.

4. AGING EMBRYOS AND VIABLE RHYTHMS

1 BBC 2013.

2 Kbhandal 2013a. Auxogyn was acquired by a fertility and digital health company called Progyny in 2015. See chapter 3 for a discussion of Progyny's egg freezing insurance.

3 Kbhandal 2013b.

4 Walsh 2013.

5 Time-lapse embryo imaging is a noninvasive alternative to pre-implantation genetic screening (PGS), a procedure in which selection is based on a biopsy of embryonic cells, which are genetically analyzed for chromosomal abnormalities. PGS is similarly presented as a technology that links together embryonic chromosomal normality and "ability to develop to term," although the HFEA states that there is no evidence the procedure improves success rates—in fact it may even reduce them (Pavone and Lafuente Funes 2017; HFEA 2018d).

6 Pribenszky et al. 2017.

7 Armstrong, Arroll, et al. 2015; Armstrong, Vail, et al. 2015; Harper et al. 2017.

8 HFEA 2018d.

9 Another system is Miri® Time-Lapse by ESCO Medical.

10 "Embryonic age" is an embryological term that signifies the age of the embryo since fertilization.

11 Earlier versions of sections of chapter 4 appear in Van de Wiel 2017, 2018, and 2019.

12 Presented as part of a press release, this embryonic "baby Eva" and the recording of its first cell divisions are flanked by logos that also associate the Eeva technology and the GCRM clinic with reproductive success.

13 Eva's naming also points to a conflict between Auxogyn's press release, which announced that "Baby Eva [was] Named after Pioneering IVF Test," and her parents, who stated they named their child Eva irrespective of the technology's name (Kbhandal 2013b). The tension over who names and frames the embryo is indicative of how the time-lapse embryo imaging becomes the site of negotiating origin stories in the complex and increasingly visible entanglements of gamete, embryo, machine, and body.

14 Auxogyn 2012.

15 Wegner 2012.

16 Van Dijck 2008.

17 E.g., Rosalind Petchesky argued that fetal imagery blurs "the boundary between fetus and baby; [it] reinforce[s] the idea that the fetus' identity as separate and autonomous from the mother . . . exists from the start" (1987, 272).

18 Franklin 2014b.

19 Van Dijck 2005. Unlike the ultrasound, which visualizes the womb's interior, time-lapse embryo videos position the locus of the beginning of prenatal life in technoculture rather than in the maternal body.

20 Coe and Altman 2012.

21 Williams et al. 2003, 801–3.

22 Lacey 2005, 1666.

23 In the context of OC, the observable development from cell to embryo can particularly be employed to affirm an understanding of the egg as the "building block" for the potential baby (see chapter 3).

24 Auxogyn 2014.

25 Landecker 2006, 129. These scientific videos also allowed "people other than scientists to participate visually in the sights of scientific work and the mode of experimental looking" (Landecker 2006, 123). Now time-lapse imaging technology likewise allows intended parents to partake in the embryologists' gaze and encounter their embryos at this early stage of development.

26 Microwells are small depressions in the culture dish that each contain an embryo.

27 Moore 2003.

28 Armstrong, Vail, et al. 2015.

29 Sunkara 2018.

30 Walsh 2013.

31 Referencing the quintessential Christian and Jewish origin story recounted in Genesis 1–3, the Eeva system's name suggests a correspondence to the biblical Eve, meaning "mother of all the living." This is a telling association, given that the secular creation story told through the embryo videos shifts the locus of life's origin as they stage a first visible encounter with prenatal life while it is enclosed by the machine rather than the mother.

32 Franklin 2013b, 306.

33 Franklin 2001, 348. See chapter 3 for the Nightlight Christian Adoption's Snowflake embryo adoption program, in which embryos are referred to as "preborn children."

34 Auxogyn 2012. This language of risk and success also characterizes the CARE Fertility clinic's presentation of its EmbryoScope and CAREmaps—with "maps" being an acronym for "morphokinetic algorithms to predict success"—as "a whole system designed to maximise the chances of success" (CARE Fertility 2018).

35 In *Liminal Lives*, Susan Squier claims that the two forms of *in vitro* cellular growth of most interest in tissue culture research are organized growth and unorganized growth, which have been accessed with "iconic overdetermination" through the observation of, respectively, embryos and cancer cells (2004, 61). The timing of organized growth finds its clinical application in time-lapse embryo imaging.

36 Franklin 2013a, 40. In time-lapse systems, the observation, translation, and projection of past embryonic populations shape the value and destination of the embryos under current scrutiny, while also potentially affecting future selections. This process makes explicit how "biological knowledge, biotechniques and biology 'itself' reshape each other, and co-evolve" (Franklin 2006a, 168).

37 See Van de Wiel 2019 for a discussion of *in silico* vision.

38 Waldby 2002, 310.

39 Ramsing 2016, 11.

40 Waldby 2002, 310.

41 Wong et al. 2012; 2013.

42 J. Cohen 2013b, 109.

43 J. Cohen 2013b, 109.

44 Reijo Pera 2013.

45 Reijo Pera 2013, 113.

46 J. Cohen 2013a, 115. The 2013 European patent has been opposed by ESHRE, Sigrid Sterckx, and colleagues. They argued that the patent related to a medical diagnosis, which is not patentable under Article 53(c) of the European Patent Convention (EPC). After the European Patent Office (EPO) decided to maintain the patent, the group filed an appeal and also requested the EPO revisit its definition of a medical diagnosis—a process that is ongoing at the time of writing, the result of which will not be known for several years (Sterckx et al. 2017).

47 See Franklin 2013b, 64, for a discussion of the "retooling" of reproductive substance in processes of "bioindustrialization."

48 Montag 2015; Vitrolife 2015a.
49 Lezaun 2013, 481.
50 CARE Fertility 2018.
51 Vitrolife 2015d.
52 Merck 2015.
53 Hogle 2016, 386.
54 Vitrolife 2015d.
55 Lezaun 2013, 481.
56 Vitrolife 2015d.
57 Curchoe and Bormann 2019.
58 Artificial intelligence techniques may be improved when "a great and growing number of image files might be collected in large databases and shared among IVF laboratories, also to improve pattern recognition methodology" (Manna et al. 2013, 48).
59 Martin 2018.
60 LaFrenz 2018.
61 Merck 2018.
62 Vitrolife 2017, 3.
63 Vitrolife 2019.
64 BusinessWire 2011; Vitrolife 2018; 2019.
65 In keeping with the rising number of systems in use, the number of scientific articles citing time-lapse embryo imaging is increasing, thereby suggesting that this development also transforms scientific knowledge creation about embryos.
    The increase of citations on time-lapse embryo imaging from 235 to 1,144 between 2013 and 2019 indicates the impact of this technology on the field. Citation report generated at Clarivate's Web of Science, searching for "(['time-lapse' OR 'time lapse'] AND [IVF OR ICSI OR 'embryo selection'])."
66 HFEA 2018c.
67 CARE Fertility 2015.
68 Vitrolife 2015c, 4.
69 Vitrolife 2015b.
70 Thurlow 2015.
71 HFEA 2018d.
72 Vitrolife 2016.
73 Merck 2016. A German company, Merck has developed its fertility research policy with reference to the German Embryo Protection Act (1990), which prohibits invasive embryo research. Also outside of Germany, the company does not sponsor clinical trials using "invasive biopsy" of the embryo for chromosomal research (Merck 2011, 1–2). Offering a noninvasive alternative, time-lapse embryo imaging adheres to Merck's fertility research policy (Merck 2011, 6).
74 Allahbadia and Allahbadia 2016.
75 GFA 2018.

5. POSTFERTILE CONCEPTIONS

1 The cryopreservation of embryos also allowed women to have genetically related children at a later age.

2 Shaw and Giles 2009.

3 CBO 2003.

4 Health Council of the Netherlands 1997.

5 Kortman et al. 2006.

6 Van Erp 2009.

7 Schippers 2011b.

8 In 2012, Dutch Health Minister Schippers followed the Health Care Insurance Board's (CVZ) recommendation to cut healthcare costs by restricting IVF coverage to women up to 42 years of age. Schippers recognized that the decreased IVF success rates motivating this change did not apply in the same way to IVF with frozen eggs and argued that the policy change would prevent future costs associated with women returning to use their frozen eggs (Schippers 2012). Here 42 was pinpointed as the age at which infertility transforms from an "impairment" to a "natural loss of fertility" (Zorg & Financiering 2012). This change illustrates how the meaning ascribed to the relation between age and fertility is contingent on, and reified through, political and financial practices.

9 NHS Choices 2013. Although the United Kingdom does not set a legal age limit to fertility treatment, it does have a 10-year storage limit for frozen eggs.

10 ONS 2016; CBS 2017.

11 Beets et al. 2013.

12 In 2014, women over 40 accounted for 20% of all UK IVF. 60% of women over 44 used younger women's donated eggs, compared to only 2% of women under 35 (HFEA 2016).

13 HFEA 2018e. IVF is also becoming increasingly reliant on cryopreservation: in 2015, the number of frozen embryo cycles overtook that of fresh ones (HFEA 2018e).

14 CBS 2017.

15 ONS 2016. More children were born to US women over 40 in the 1950s than in the 2010s (P. Cohen 2012).

16 Friese et al. 2008.

17 Ylänne 2016.

18 Ahmed 2011.

19 De Wert 1999, 47–48.

20 Shaw and Giles 2009.

21 Channel 4 is a British public-service television network.

22 Grant 1992, 57.

23 Boyer 2012.

24 Smyth 2008, 96; Bartlett 2005, 84–109.

25 Whitehorn qtd. in Segal 2013, 76.

26 Fleck and Hanssen 2016; De Pater et al. 2014.
27 Pickard 2018
28 Twigg 2007, 293.
29 Vincent 2006.
30 Cardona 2008, 475, 482.
31 In the context of OC, the treatment was less controversial for cancer patients than it was for presumably healthy women seeking to circumvent age-related infertility. The relative acceptance of cancer survivors bearing children in spite of decreased life expectancy illustrates the fact that this factor alone does not account for the rejection of older motherhood.
32 Ylänne 2016.
33 Ahmed 2011, 233.
34 Ahmed 2014, 118–19.
35 Ahmed 2014, 120.
36 Ahmed 2014, 118.
37 Qualtrough 1998.
38 Franklin and Roberts 2006, 33.
39 Smajdor 2009.
40 See chapter 1.
41 NVOG 2010; Schippers 2011b.
42 NVOG & KLEM 2018. Alongside the legal limit, fertility clinics use their own maximum age limits for IVF, varying from 41 to 50 years for women and 55 to 80 years for men (Freya 2017).
43 NVOG 2016.
44 Smirnova 2012.
45 Gow et al. 2012.
46 Wood 2008, 326.
47 I use phrase "maternal genetic relatedness" to refer to a woman's genetic contribution to the embryo through the provision of an egg. Beyond this individualized model, other approaches may "code" genes and gametes for "group inclusion and exclusion," and thereby conceptualize genetic relatedness as extending within familial, racial, or "ethno-national" communities (Thompson 2001, 192)
48 Bordo 2004, 26; Smirnova 2012, 1236–37.
49 Mills et al. 2015.
50 The positive images of donor-egg IVF in this PowerPoint implicitly respond to the "stigma[s] associated with infertility" and "procedures involving donated gametes" by presenting celebrity women as unable to conceive with their own eggs, yet successfully fulfilling normative gender, age, and motherhood roles (Murray and Golombok 2003, 93).
51 Extend Fertility 2017c.
52 Extend Fertility 2018.
53 Mills et al. 2015, 93. In her study of women freezing their eggs, Kylie Baldwin affirms this connection between intensive mothering ideologies and the timing

of readiness for childbearing: "it was women's intentions to mother intensively as well as the perception that motherhood would inhibit other opportunities, which signalled to them that it was not yet the right time to pursue motherhood" (2017, 10).

54 Martin 2017, 97.

55 Inhorn 2017.

56 The dearth of accounts of this crucial stage of the procedure follows from the relatively recent popularity of egg freezing and the fact that the vast majority of women do not return to use their frozen eggs.

57 Gootman 2012.

58 Adams 2017c.

59 Mann 2015a.

60 Mann 2014.

61 Thompson 2001, 177. Assisted reproduction exemplifies the work of "doing" kinship as opposed to simply "being" a particular type of kin. Charis Thompson analyzes the "kinship work" performed by fertility clinics, in which gestational, genetic, or absent biological relations with children are foregrounded and re-crafted to match intended kinship ties (2001, 177).

62 Adams 2017a.

63 Mann 2017a.

64 Waldby 2015a; Inhorn et al. 2018; Baldwin 2019.

65 Brown and Patrick 2018.

66 Carroll and Krcløkke 2018.

67 Inhorn 2017, 7.

68 Lahad 2012, 183.

69 Lahad 2016, 9.

70 Lahad 2014, 241.

71 Lahad 2016, 8.

72 Adams 2016a.

73 Mann 2015b.

74 Chappel 2017, 148.

75 Cooper 2017, 23.

76 Fraser and Jaeggi 2018, 40, 86.

77 Mann 2016d.

78 Adams 2016b.

79 Kopaylopa 2015.

80 Mann 2016a; 2016b.

81 Mann 2016c.

82 Adams 2016b.

83 Adams 2016a.

84 Adams 2016c.

85 Adams 2017b.

86 Adams 2017c.

87 Eggfreezer 2015.
88 Eggfreezer 2008.
89 Mann 2017b.
90 The HFEA's 2018 estimation is that two thousand children have been born from frozen eggs worldwide (2018a).
91 Cook 2018.
92 Pennings et al. 2006, 3050.
93 Mr & Mrs M vs HFEA 2016, 3–4.
94 Mr & Mrs M vs HFEA 2016, 4–5.
95 Mr & Mrs M vs HFEA 2016, 5.
96 Mr & Mrs M vs HFEA 2016, 4–6
97 A.'s conceptualization of her eggs is reminiscent of Eggfreezer's individualization of her egg as the building block of her future child (chapter 3).
98 A Dutch survey shows that almost 30% of women freezing their eggs do so after a cancer diagnosis (Balkenende et al. 2015). Because many women freeze their eggs in these circumstances, the question of posthumous reproduction is more pertinent in OC practices than in other fertility treatments, which women undergo when they are healthy enough to become pregnant.
99 HFEA 2019c, 1.
100 HFEA 2019b; 2019c. The form also mentions that it is possible to donate your eggs for research purposes.
101 HFEA 2015; 2019b. If a woman decides to make her eggs available for posthumous reproduction, she is required to undergo screening tests to ensure their safety for the gestational mother.
102 UMCU 2012, 3; MCK 2014, 3.
103 See chapter 6 for a discussion of the transnational mobility of frozen eggs.
104 Pennings et al. 2006, 3051.
105 Corrigan 2003.
106 Butler 1993, 225.
107 Butler 1993, 2.
108 Butler 1997b, 3, 15.
109 Indeed, consent for posthumous reproduction is referred to as a "biological will" (Sabatello 2014).
110 Monk 2014, 239.
111 Ahmed 2014, 113.
112 Monk 2014, 240. Egg freezing may provide an alternative for women to meet what Ahmed calls the "reproductive duty" by maintaining a futurity of motherhood (2014, 114).
113 Clarke 2012, 1332–34. Under the pressure of public opposition, the family decided to drop their efforts to use Ayah's eggs posthumously (Stewart 2011).
114 Ahmed 2014, 113. This case should be positioned within the context of Israel, a "strongly pronatalist" country characterized by the "extreme medicalisation of reproduction," in which national and religious identity is expressed through

reproductive practices (Shkedi-Rafid and Hashiloni-Dolev 2011, 293). Jewish law, unlike its Roman Catholic and Islamic counterparts, permits posthumous reproduction (Pennings et al. 2006, 3050–51). Israel has the most IVF clinics per capita in the world and extensive state funding for fertility treatments; its endorsement of ARTs reflects "the centrality of future citizenry" in this context (Birenbaum-Carmeli 2009). Indeed, Israeli policy concerning male posthumous reproduction is not based on informed consent, but on the "presumed wish" that all men would want their partner to have their child after death (Hashiloni-Dolev 2015).

115 The UMCU consent form explicitly states that the eggs are not subject to inheritance law (2012, 2). Through mandatory informed consent procedures, Dutch and UK clinics seek to avoid inheritance claims to the reproductive cells after a patient's death.

116 Hashiloni-Dolev 2015.

117 HFEA 2010b, 2; Monk 2014, 239.

118 Roberts and Throsby 2008; Waldby and Carroll 2012.

119 Franklin 2006b, 85.

120 Lock 2003, 166.

121 HFEA 2010a.

6. OOCYTE FUTURES

1 See Stoop et al. 2012. In the United Kingdom, the live birth rate per thaw cycle was 18% in 2016. Because these percentages are based on small numbers, different ages at freezing, and older treatment protocols, these numbers "should be used cautiously" (HFEA 2018b, 14). Because egg freezing was introduced relatively recently, representative success rates will not be known for several more years.

2 Gürtin 2019.

3 Balkenende et al. 2018. A US study similarly showed a 6% usage rate of frozen eggs (Hodes-Wertz et al. 2013).

4 Due to their fragility, fresh human eggs are typically only handled within specialized spaces in IVF clinics and biomedical laboratories (Franklin 2006a, 173). By contrast, frozen eggs can become mobile once they are stored in special dry vapor liquid nitrogen shipper tanks, in which they can safely remain for seven to ten days in cryogenic temperatures below −150°C (Cryoport 2014).

5 See Franklin 2011, 815; Inhorn 2015; Adrian and Kroløkke 2018.

6 Neilson 2003, 161.

7 In keeping with the geographical orientation of the earlier chapters, I focus on the World Egg Bank's US-UK shipments. TWEB has not (yet) shipped eggs to the Netherlands.

8 In 1997, TWEB founder and president, Diana Thomas, started a traditional egg donor matching service called X and Y Consulting. In 2004, she founded Cryo Eggs International (CEI), purportedly the world's first frozen egg bank. These two companies merged in 2009 to form the World Egg Bank, which offers both "fresh" and "frozen" egg donation services (TWEB 2009).

Thomas is highly visible on TWEB's website in videos directed at potential patients, in which her own experience with egg donation is foregrounded to claim authority and build trust. In a video featured on the homepage she states, "Because I was one of the first women in the world to conceive and have children through donor eggs nearly 20 years ago, I still stand for the right for women everywhere to have a chance to hold a baby in their arms" (TWEB 2014a). Thomas is listed as the only shareholder of TWEB (ACC 2016).

9 An earlier, if rare, variation of transnational egg donation is the "mail order" arrangement, which entails shipping sperm to the egg donor's clinic and subsequently transporting the frozen fertilized eggs back to the intended parents for implantation (Heng 2006, 1225). This approach has once again been proposed more recently by researchers at Prelude Fertility (Chang et al. 2018).

10 Various international courier companies specialize in shipping reproductive cells; TWEB uses Cryoport (US). Cryoport's service provides a so-called chain of custody and a chain of condition to transport frozen eggs (BusinessWire 2013).

11 Waldby 2019, 134, 142.

12 Kupka et al. 2014; Culley et al. 2011.

13 In the United States, no legal limits on egg donor compensation exist. The HFEA regulations are in keeping with the European Tissues and Cells Directive, which prescribes that "Member States shall endeavour to ensure voluntary and unpaid donations of tissues and cells," although egg donors may be compensated for expenses. It also explicitly allows member states to require "voluntary unpaid donation" as a condition for importing gametes from abroad (European Union 2004, L102/52–54).

14 HFEA 2011; 2012.

15 Jardine 2012.

16 HFEA 2014.

17 See Waldby 2008, 23; Smith 2012; Taneja 2013.

18 Virtus Health has acquired clinics in Ireland, Denmark, the United Kingdom, and Singapore (Williams et al. 2017).

19 Virtus Health 2017, 36.

20 Fraser 2018, 75.

21 Daar et al. 2016; HFEA 2012.

22 TWEB 2018.

23 In spite of their pricing options, TWEB explicitly distances itself from the notion of commodification: "oocytes are never to be treated as commodities. Recipients do not pay for oocytes; they compensate Donors for their time and effort, as well as provide for care for any discomfort that they may endure as a result of the procedure" (TWEB 2015b). This framing aligns with a "clinical labor" model, in which donors "are paid for [their] time, risk, and expertise," rather than paid for their bodily substances (Cooper and Waldby 2014; Waldby 2019, 179).

24 Reflecting Prelude's focus on egg freezing as discussed in chapter 3, My Egg Bank also offers egg donors a free egg freezing cycle.

25 Although the discrepancy between donor compensation and costs of a so-called egg lot can generate significant revenue, the indirect financial inducement of egg donation is not limited to the surplus value derived from direct transactions among clinics, donors, and recipients; it also has a more financialized character. The case of the California Cryobank illustrates that the creation of large egg-donation networks can itself attract large equity investments. In one of the largest deals in assisted reproduction in recent years, in 2018 the private equity firm GI Partners announced a massive investment worth an estimated $1 billion to create California Cryobank Life Sciences (Ditkowsky 2018). This deal entailed the acquisition of Cord Blood Registry, the largest US cord blood bank, California Cryobank's 40-year-old sperm bank, which advertises more than 500 donor profiles, and Donor Egg Bank USA (DEBU). The resultant California Cryobank Life Sciences thus brings together a number of cryofertility services, including sperm, egg, and cord blood banking (DEBU 2019).

Donor Egg Bank USA was originally incorporated by businesswoman Heidi Hayes in 2011 and funded with an offering of $1.25 million. Unlike TWEB, DEBU functioned as a virtual network of frozen eggs and egg donors working with clinics across the United States. In collaboration with Shady Grove Fertility, the largest US fertility group, DEBU grew to 150 donor profiles by 2016 and was bought by two private equity funds in a deal valued at an estimated $200 million (Ditkowsky 2018; California Cryobank 2016). These acquisitions of DEBU point to the financialization of fertility in frozen egg donation, as the speculative value of donor eggs and egg donors—and the growth potential of their movements—pertains not only to their commodification within the fertility company but also to the valuation of the company itself by private equity markets.

26 TWEB 2014b.

27 Almeling 2011.

28 Davda 2019, 319.

29 Davda 2019, 307–8.

30 The London Egg Bank 2014.

31 Payne 2013.

32 Economist 2017.

33 Chandra et al. 2014, 5–6; Daniels and Heidt-Forsythe 2012, 721

34 Waldby 2008, 23.

35 Schurr 2017.

36 Pollock 2003, 251. By contrast, Daisy Deomampo found that intended parents in India did not seek donors to match their own racial backgrounds, but sought egg donors with darker skins in an attempt to subvert dominant racial hierarchies, which nonetheless reified essentialist notions of racial categorization (Deomampo 2016).

37 Daniels and Heidt-Forsythe 2012, 732.

38 Almeling 2011, 173; Tober 2019.

39 TWEB 2018.

40 Almeling 2011, 57.

41 Shenfield et al. 2010.

42 Almeling 2011, 68.

43 TWEB 2015a.

44 Snyder and Dillow 2013.

45 United Nations 2014a, 2014b.

46 Prothero 2013.

47 Shenfield et al. 2010.

48 Smietana et al. 2018, 19.

49 Roberts 2017b, 617.

50 Vora and Iyengar 2016; Schurr 2017; Nahman 2018.

51 See Cooper and Waldby 2014; Franklin 2011. Andrea Whittaker rightly notes that not all patients crossing borders are elites in their home countries, but nevertheless their access to healthcare is enhanced by crossing borders (2015, 118).

52 Homanen 2018; Kroløkke 2018.

53 Pande 2011. In India, for example, international trade agreements, a large private healthcare sector, and a national health policy that overtly sought to "encourage the supply of services to patients of foreign origin on payment" have played an important role in stimulating the medical and fertility tourism market through measures including "low import duty on medical equipment" and arrangements for special "medical visas" (Mukherjee and Nadimipally 2006, 129–30; De Arellano 2007, 197).

Following its 2002 legalization of international commercial surrogacy, India became the leading global surrogacy provider. Its subsequent ban in 2015 did not cause the practice to disappear, Sharmilla Rudrappa argues, but effectively deregulated the sector and thereby placed women at increased risk (2017).

54 See Williams et al. 2017; BusinessWire 2019. Moreover, investors behind Hong Kong's largest IVF clinic group recently bought Genea, one of Australia's largest IVF chains and producer of the Geri time-lapse system ($510 million) (see chapter 3) (Biospectrum 2018).

55 Global cold chains of eggs do not operate in isolation from other transnational reproductive flows; see Siggie Vertommen and Michael Nahman 2019 for a broader theorization of "global fertility chains."

56 Hochschild 2001, 357; Parreñas 2000, 561.

57 Tachibana et al. 2013. The publication lists Tachibana as first and Mitalipov as last of 23 authors. Stem cells had been successfully extracted from human embryos 15 years earlier, but now this technique was combined with the creation of new embryos through nuclear transfer that perfectly matched the somatic cell donor's DNA (Cyranoski 2013a).

58 See Franklin 2007. Reproductive cloning of large mammals like pigs is now performed routinely in so-called cloning factories like the Chinese BGI, which produces up to 500 animals a year (Shukman 2014).

59 A somatic cell is any cell that is not an egg or a sperm. It has two sets of chromosomes, one inherited from each parent.

60 More precisely, as I discuss below, the resulting embryo has the same nuclear DNA as the somatic cell donor and the same mitochondrial DNA as the egg donor. This is relevant here because Leigh Syndrome can be caused by mitochondrial DNA mutations.

61 Tachibana et al. 2013.

62 Yamada et al. 2015.

63 Landecker 2007, 69.

64 Carrel 1912; Landecker 2007, 71, 106.

65 Tachibana et al. 2013.

66 Chung et al. 2014.

67 Yamada et al. 2014.

68 Chung et al. 2015.

69 Yamada et al. 2015.

70 Matoba and Zhang 2018.

71 Landau 2014; Yamada et al. 2014, 537.

72 Hwang et al. 2004; 2005.

73 See Myung 2006; Gottweis and Kim 2010, 513. Local feminist organizations played a key role in exposing the quantities and methods of egg sourcing. A coalition of 35 women's groups assisted the women who suffered serious health complications after the egg extraction (Dickenson and Idiakez 2008, 127–28; Widdows 2009, 10–11).

74 See Spar 2007, 1291; Dong-seok 2016. The 2008 Bioethics Act included new provisions that required health checks for egg donors and restricted the numbers of cycles and financial compensation they may receive (Republic of Korea 2008).

75 Republic of Korea 2009. Korean regulations specify that these are eggs that are created "for reproductive purposes but are going to be disposed of for such reasons as completion of fertility treatment" (Republic of Korea 2009).

In conventional IVF, good-quality eggs usually do not become spare because intended parents "often want to deploy all of them for reproductive bids" (Waldby and Cooper 2010, 7).

76 Kakuk 2009; Thompson 2013, 123.

77 Gottweis and Kim 2010, 503.

78 Kim 2008, 407; Cyranoski 2004, 14.

79 Gottweis and Kim 2010, 514.

80 Kim 2008, 407–8.

81 In South Korean news media, altruistic egg donors were praised while women receiving payment for their eggs were dismissed as "frivolous" for using their reproductivity to pay for things like "ski holidays" (Kim 2008, 408). See chapter 1 on similar accusations of frivolity in egg freezing and abortion discourses.

82 Dickenson and Idiakez 2008, 128; Paik 2010, 82; Widdows 2009, 12; Gottweis and Kim 2010, 514.

83 Waldby 2008, 24.

84 Baylis 2009; Tae-gyu 2016.

85 Dong-seok 2016.

86 Dong-Ryul Lee's SCNT study, one of the three case studies, was also based in the CHA Group, and illustrates that international collaborations enable work on fresh eggs in spite of Korean regulations (Chung et al. 2014).

87 Republic of Korea 2014.

88 See CHA 2019a. Yoon and colleagues claimed the birth of a boy conceived from vitrified eggs at CHA Fertility in Korea as a world's first. However, he was born in August 1999, while Kuleshova and colleagues report the birth of a girl conceived from vitrified donor eggs on June 20, 1999 (Yoon et al. 2000; Kuleshova et al. 1999).

89 The World Bank 2019.

90 C. Lee 2018; Han-soo 2018; CHA 2019b.

91 Dong-seok 2016; Tae-gyu 2016.

92 At the time of Bush's first veto, in 2005, his press conference included 21 children born from the Christian Snowflakes program, which "saves" leftover IVF embryos through its "embryo adoption" program. He stated that "we should not use public money to support the further destruction of human life" (Cromer 2019; Office of the Press Secretary 2005).

93 Thompson 2013, 115, 123.

94 See Klitzman and Sauer 2009, 604; Spar 2007, 1290. The National Research Council recommends that egg donors providing eggs for "research purposes (such as for nuclear transfer) should be reimbursed only for direct expenses" (2008, 19; 2005).

95 Qtd. in Thompson 2013, 116.

96 HHS 2019.

97 Reno 2017.

98 Thompson 2013, 116.

99 Schubert 2013.

100 Bonilla 2013; Thompson 2013, 35.

101 Cyranoski 2013a.

102 Cyranoski 2013a.

103 Thompson 2013.

104 Waldby 2019, 176. See also pp.175–79 for an extensive discussion of the regulation of egg donation for stem cell research.

105 Klitzman and Sauer 2009, 604; ASRM 2007, 306.

106 Roxland 2012, 397; Waldby 2019, 177.

107 Roxland 397, 402.

108 Safier et al. 2018, 1223.

109 Safier et al. 2018, 1221; Yamada et al. 2014.

110 Safier et al. 2018, 1224.

111 OHSU Center for Women's Health 2015a, 2015b.

112 Pfeffer 2011.

113 Thompson 2013.

114 Pande 2011, 619; Almeling 2011, 36. Notwithstanding their approximation, the SCNT studies also indicate that research and reproductive egg procurement may diverge in the future. Particularly the eggs of younger donors (21 to 26 years) and women with a specific genetic profile resulted in ESCs; if these results are reproduced, future research-specific donor recruitment may become more targeted. Egli's study also experiments with ovarian stimulation of egg donors in SCNT studies, which could lead to differences between ovarian stimulation protocols in research and reproductive donation.

115 Harper 2013, xiii.

116 United Nations 2017; Christensen et al. 2009, 1196; Riley 2005.

117 Waldby 2002, 317; Neilson 2003.

118 Neilson 2003, 181–82.

119 Lafontaine 2009, 54–55.

120 Kaufman 2015, 142.

121 Cooper 2006, 17 n. 4; Franklin 2019, 19.

122 Cooper 2006, 17 n. 4.

123 Neilson 2003, 181.

124 Galkin et al. 2019.

125 ACT 2005; Plunkett 2008; Business Wire 2014.

126 Lijing 2010.

127 ACT was renamed Ocata in 2014 and bought by Astellas Pharma in 2016 for $379 million to establish the Astellas Institute for Regenerative Medicine (AIRM) (GEN 2015).

128 Ocata 2015; Astellas 2016.

129 ACT 2005, emphasis added.

130 Tachibana et al. 2013, 1228, emphasis added.

131 Boiani 2013, 631.

132 Galkin et al. 2019. In a similar vein, Karen Jent has theorized the "stem cell niche," or the "particular microenvironment where stem cells reside" as a tool for manipulating cellular biology. She traces the trend in stem cell science of conceiving stem cells as "relational entities" that develop through the intricacies of "cell–microenvironment interaction" (2019).

133 Franklin 2013b, 28.

134 Takahashi et al. 2007.

135 Yamada et al. 2015; Boiani 2013, 629.

136 Kang et al. 2016; Wolf et al. 2017.

137 Wolf et al. 2017, 31–33.

138 This nuclear transfer technique is not a form of cloning because the donated nuclear DNA comes from the intended mother's egg and therefore is haploid, i.e., it only contains half the number of chromosomes. The resulting embryo is the result of fertilization with another set of chromosomes provided by the sperm. In SCNT,

the donated nuclear DNA is diploid—contains a full set of chromosomes—and identical to the resulting embryo's DNA.

There are a number of different nuclear transfer approaches, including Cytoplasmic Transfer, Germinal Vesicle Transfer, Pronuclear Transfer, Polar Body Transfer, and Maternal Spindle Transfer (Tachibana et al. 2018).

139 Pompei and Pompei 2019; Mullin 2019b. The amendment was introduced by Republican congressman Robert Aderholt from Alabama, whose stated mission is "protecting the innocent lives of the most vulnerable among us." Two months later, the National Academy of Science issued a report advising that it would be permissible to use mitochondrial replacement therapy to avoid passing on mitochondrial diseases, but the policy remains unchanged (Aderholt 2019; Mullin 2019b).

140 Zhang et al. 2017; Tanaka and Watanabe 2019.

141 Gorman et al. 2018.

142 Tachibana et al. 2018; Ma et al. 2017.

143 Cibelli 2009. The cytosol is part of the cytoplasm.

144 The chimeric egg is a variation of Hannah Landecker's "ageing chimera" discussed in chapter 3.

145 The transfer of cytoplasm from one egg to another has a longer history; it first resulted in a live birth in 1997 and was commercialized as a technique for treating age-related infertility by the OvaScience company (see Conclusion) (Tanaka and Watanabe 2019; Herbrand 2019). These earlier techniques injected cytoplasm into the egg; the mitochondrial transfer technique instead replaces the whole cytoplasm by moving the intended mother's nucleus into an enucleated donor egg.

146 Devlin 2019.

147 Institute of Life 2019.

148 Mullin 2019a. The Mitalipov team also suggests that mitochondrial transfer could be particularly relevant for treating cryodamage in the egg after OC by replacing cryopreserved cytoplasm with "fresh cytoplasm from young donors" (Tachibana et al. 2018).

149 Darwin Life 2019; Mullin 2019a.

150 DL-Nadiya 2019; Mullin 2019b; Mazur et al. 2019. Although they write "without donation of eggs," this likely refers to the fact that this method retains maternal nuclear DNA; a donor egg would still be required to provide the cytoplasm and mtDNA.

151 Ma et al. 2017.

152 Tachibana et al. 2018.

153 Ma et al. 2017.

154 Tachibana et al. 2018. Indeed, the authors of the Mitalipov study emphasize that "recent fundamental discoveries were successfully made from indispensable and valuable quality human oocytes, donated for research" (Tachibana et al. 2018).

155 The logic of research egg donation here refers to the fact that social markers of biodesirability are not a relevant factor in the selection of egg donors.

156 Chang et al. 2011, 310.

157 Chang et al. 2009.

158 Lee et al. 2019, 545.

159 Chang et al. 2009; Sung et al. 2010; Baek et al. 2017.

160 Baek et al. 2017; Lee et al. 2019, 545.

161 Republic of Korea 2014. Korea's Enforcement Decree of the Bioethics and Safety Act mentions cryopreserved, immature, and abnormal eggs as examples of oocytes that may be used for SCNT research.

162 Chung et al. 2015.

163 Wolf et al. 2017, 31–32.

164 When the frozen eggs that once embodied promissory value of bioprepared fertility become "spare," they are rendered into "a form of waste" that has the potential to become "a valuable surplus" in the research context (Waldby and Cooper 2010, 6). In keeping with this logic, there is typically no financial compensation for donating "spare" eggs.

165 Baek et al. 2017; Lee et al. 2019, 545.

166 Widdows 2009, 13

167 Franklin 2011, 811.

168 Hochschild 2000, 131.

169 Galkin et al. 2019.

170 Tachibana et al. 2018.

CONCLUSION

1 One alternative to oocyte cryopreservation is ovarian cryopreservation. This entails freezing a slice of ovarian tissue, which contains a far greater number of (immature) eggs than are typically extracted in an egg freezing cycle. Although this involves more invasive surgery than OC, ovarian cryopreservation does not require hormonal stimulation to mature the eggs prior to their extraction. Instead, the ovarian tissue, and the large number of eggs it holds, may be frozen and transplanted back into the body at a later date—a technique called "autografting" (Donnez and Dolmans 2014). Ovarian tissue may be transplanted back to its original position, but also in other parts of the body that would require less invasive surgery and could be monitored more easily, such as the forearm (Oktay et al. 2000; Kondapalli 2012, 67). In this way, the organs would be rearranged in the body to facilitate the visibility and the extractability of *in vivo* eggs. Ovarian cryopreservation has led to the birth of 130 children; it is now considered a "viable option for fertility preservation" and is also used as a method for delaying menopause (Pacheco and Oktay 2017; Amorim et al. 2019). Simon Fishel, director of CARE, the UK's largest fertility group, caused a media hype in 2019 by proposing this technique as a means for healthy women to "preserve fertility and postpone menopause." As part of the effort to mainstream this technique, he started a fertility company called ProFam (Protecting Fertility and Menopause) specifically for offering ovarian cryopreservation (ProFaM 2019).

Alternatively, immature eggs could be matured *in vitro*, frozen, and used at a later point for reproductive purposes (Chian et al. 2009). If *in vitro* maturation (IVM) success rates were to approximate those of *in vivo* matured eggs, hormonal stimulation, with its side effects and risks of ovarian hyperstimulation syndrome, could be avoided in OC and IVF practices. This is particularly relevant for those who cannot undergo ovarian stimulation as easily, such as women with polycystic ovary syndrome (PCOS) or cancer patients (Wang et al. 2016).

Other approaches to fertility preservation were proposed by Jonathan Tilly, whose 2004 study countered the long-standing notion that women are born with all the eggs they will ever have. He claimed that stem cells in the ovarian lining can continue to produce eggs and could provide an alternative source of eggs after age-related infertility (Johnson et al. 2004). Although this technique was highly contentious and controversial, he founded publicly listed OvaScience to move towards clinical application. OvaScience also introduced another fertility treatment in 2014, which consists of injecting mitochondria, energy-producing cellular organelles, into extracted eggs. The underlying hypothesis was that cellular aging entails a decline in "both the number and activity of mitochondria" and that this "is a primary contributor to declining egg and embryo quality with advancing maternal age" (Tilly and Sinclair 2013, 841). Zain Rajani, the first baby conceived with this technique, was born in 2015 (CBC 2015). The uptake and efficacy of these technologies proved disappointing, however. In 2018, OvaScience, once worth $1.8 billion, effectively folded and entered into a reverse merger with Millendo Therapeutics, rendering the future of these technologies unclear as a result (K. Lee 2018). Clinical studies have also focused on nuclear transfer, rather than injection of mitochondria, to "rejuvenate" eggs (see chapter 6).

Artificial gametes (*in vitro* gametogenesis) present an entirely different approach to decoupling age and reproductive ability. Instead of freezing them, eggs could be generated from other cells in the body at any point in the life cycle, thereby rendering the need to preserve existing eggs redundant. However, Hayashi and Saitou, the molecular biologists who published a study that claims to have created viable mice from artificial gametes, expect that the translation of this technique to humans—if it happens at all—could take another "10 to 50 years" (Hayashi and Saitou 2013; Cyranoski 2013b, 394).

2 R. Cohen 1978.

3 Franklin 1997.

4 In this sense, the introduction of egg freezing extends what Ian Wilmut has called the "age of biological control" to the timing of fertility. As Sarah Franklin argues in *Dolly Mixtures*, Wilmut's term functioned as a warning that "the increasing ability to re-engineer life forms poses an ever greater social challenge to set the limits biology 'itself' no longer provides" (Franklin 2007, 11). The controversies surrounding egg freezing illustrate such social renegotiations of the debiologized limits to female fertility.

5 Kindbody 2018; Silver 2017.

6 Prelude Fertility 2018a.

7 Bannerman 2012.

8 In the United Kingdom, the most common age to undergo IVF is 35, compared to 38 for egg freezing (HFEA 2018b, 11).

9 HFEA 2018e, 37.

10 Tiffany 2018.

11 Egg freezing emerges alongside the rise of what Waggoner calls the "zero trimester," which references the expanding reproductive surveillance of individual women's health and lifestyle choices in anticipation of their potential future pregnancies. As pre-pregnancy care has adopted a "neoliberal ethos in the sense that all women of reproductive age are set up as being 'at risk' of experiencing a future adverse reproductive outcome," so egg freezing practices have expanded the scope of risk of future infertility to younger, fertile women (Waggoner 2017, 146).

12 Depmann et al. 2017; O'Brien et al. 2018.

13 Briggs 2018, 8–9.

14 Chappel 2017, 148.

15 Briggs 2018, 111. Inhorn draws our attention to the sociodemographic disparities complementing Briggs's structural infertility by pointing to the fact that university-educated women outnumber university-educated men—a phenomenon that is reflected in the fact that most women freezing their eggs today are highly educated and list an "absent [male] partner" as the reason for freezing (Inhorn et al. 2018).

16 Fraser and Jaeggi 2018, 86.

17 Other factors contributing to trends of later childbearing are the idea that IVF can "reverse the effects of age" (Maheshwari et al. 2008), motivation to have a family, independence, health problems, stable relationships, partner readiness and suitability for childrearing, financial stability, career planning, and extended family influences (Benzies et al. 2006; Tough et al. 2007).

18 These trends resonate with wider debates on the temporality of precarity in which "the present is a series of self-regulatory processes that are supposed to enable the prospect (and fantasy) of one day not being vulnerable" (McCormack and Salmenniemi 2016, 8). Here the temporalities of precarity and preservation align as the notion of "freezing time" is upheld to counteract the vulnerability ascribed to aging.

19 See Van de Wiel 2014b for a historical analysis of alternative models of female reproductive aging.

20 See chapters 2 and 5.

21 See chapter 3.

22 See Vertommen 2017 for a discussion of the reproductive-industrial complex.

23 Capital investments in egg freezing have created new infrastructures for fertility preservation, which both drive the mainstreaming of OC for a larger group of women and create new reproductive stratifications by rendering access to OC

contingent on elite employment, insurance coverage, capital accumulation, or credit score—all of which are rooted in existing social inequalities.

24 Balkenende et al. 2018. Out of the women who became pregnant after OC, 76% conceived "naturally" (Balkenende et al. 2018).

25 See chapter 5.

26 Egg freezers may need to undergo additional tests in order to donate their eggs to other intended parents.

27 For example, the French national ethics committee, in its advice on the legalization of egg freezing, has noted that egg freezing could mitigate the country's significant donor egg scarcity by "increas[ing] medium and long-term stock of oocytes." To achieve this, they suggest it "could be useful to create a condition for access to autopreservation in the form of consent to donating the oocytes if they were not used" (CCNE 2017, 15). In contexts where donors are paid to provide eggs, it would be interesting to track who would benefit from the reduced cost for donor eggs that have become available through self-financing egg freezers.

28 Kikuchi et al. 2018.

29 Chen qtd. in BBC 2017. Tiantian Chen's PhD dissertation (University of Cambridge) discusses the restrictive regulations governing egg freezing in China (Chen 2020).

30 CCNE 2017, 16.

31 CCNE 2018, 119–20. The CCNE describes the postfertile condition as an evolving "dividing line between 'normal' and 'pathological,'" resulting from cryo-gametes that are exonerated "from the passage of time" and create a situation in which women know that "somewhere in a gamete bank is a part of themselves" (2017, 10).

32 Herrmann and Kroløkke 2018.

BIBLIOGRAPHY

Abdou, Jenna. 2016. *How Progyny Is Modernizing Family Planning with CEO Gina Bartasi*. 33 Voices. https://www.youtube.com/watch?v=y5YjDlfBlBs#t=462.808435.

Abraham-Van der Mark, Eva. 1996. *Succesful Home Birth and Midwifery*. Amsterdam: Het Spinhuis.

ACC. 2016. "Corporation Annual Report & Certificate of Disclosure—The World Egg Bank." Arizona Corporation Commission. September 24. https://ecorp.azcc.gov/CommonHelper/GetFilingDocuments?barcode=05597144.

ACT. 2005. "Somatic Cell Nuclear Transfer Gives Old Animals Youthful Immune Cells." Advanced Cell Technology. June 29. http://www.advancedcell.com/news-and-media/press-releases/advanced-cell-technology-acquires-intellectual-property-assets-of-infigen-inc/.

Adams, Brigitte. 2016a. "Challenges of Getting Pregnant with Frozen Eggs." *Eggsurance* (blog). July 20. http://eggsurance.com/getting-pregnant-with-frozen-eggs/.

———. 2016b. "Defrost: Why I'm Finally Ready to Use My Frozen Eggs." *Eggsurance* (blog). July 20. http://eggsurance.com/getting-pregnant-with-frozen-eggs/.

———. 2016c. "Fibroids Derailed My Egg Freezing Journey." *Eggsurance* (blog). September 30. http://eggsurance.com/fibroids-derailed-egg-freezing-journey/.

———. 2017a. "Egg Freezing: A Decade in Review; The Pill of the New Millennium?" *Eggsurance* (blog). February 17. http://eggsurance.com/egg-freezing-guide-decade-review/.

———. 2017b. "Please Don't Rely on Frozen Eggs." *Eggsurance* (blog). March 8. http://www.eggsurance.com/pregnant-frozen-eggs/.

———. 2017c. "My Frozen Eggs Failed Me: What I Would Have Done Differently." *Eggsurance* (blog). April 11. http://eggsurance.com/egg-freezing-risks/.

Adams, Vincanne, Michelle Murphy, and Adele E. Clarke. 2009. "Anticipation: Technoscience, Life, Affect, Temporality." *Subjectivity* 28: 246–65.

Aderholt, Robert. 2019. "Family Values." Congressman Robert Aderholt. https://aderholt.house.gov/issues/family-values.

Adrian, Stine Willum, and Charlotte Kroløkke. 2018. "Passport to Parenthood: Reproductive Pathways in and out of Denmark." *NORA—Nordic Journal of Feminist and Gender Research* 26 (2): 112–28. https://doi.org/10.1080/08038740.2018.1457570.

Ahmed, Sara. 2006. "Orientations: Toward a Queer Phenomenology." *GLQ: A Journal of Lesbian and Gay Studies* 12 (4): 543–74.

———. 2010. *The Promise of Happiness*. Durham, NC: Duke University Press.

———. 2011. "Willful Parts: Problem Characters or the Problem of Character." *New Literary History* 42 (2): 231–53. https://doi.org/10.1353/nlh.2011.0019.

———. 2014. *Willful Subjects*. Durham, NC: Duke University Press.

Aiken, Abigail, Jennifer Starling, Alexandra van der Wal, Sascha van der Vliet, Kathleen Broussard, Dana M. Johnson, Elisa Padron, Rebecca Gomperts, and James G. Scott. 2019. "Demand for Self-Managed Medication Abortion through an Online Telemedicine Service in the United States." *American Journal of Public Health* 110 (1): 90–97. https://doi.org/10.2105/AJPH.2019.305369.

Allahbadia, Gautam, and Akanksha Allahbadia. 2016. "Recombinants versus Biosimilars in Ovarian Stimulation." In *Ovarian Stimulation Protocols*, 71–77. New Delhi: Springer. https://doi.org/10.1007/978-81-322-1121-1_4.

Almeling, Rene. 2011. *Sex Cells: The Medical Market for Eggs and Sperm*. Berkeley: University of California Press.

AMC. 2019. "Tarieven En Betaling van Uw Behandeling." Academisch Medisch Centrum. https://webshare.iprova.nl/6pt9k92zmhhdm89p/Document. aspx?websharedocumentid=0c0c526a-3a57-45d9-afd2-0f05089e7535.

Amir, Merav. 2006. "Bio-Temporality and Social Regulation: The Emergence of the Biological Clock." *Polygraph* 18: 47–72.

Amorim, Christiani A., Ellen Cristina Rivas Leonel, Yousri Afifi, Arri Coomarasamy, and Simon Fishel. 2019. "Cryostorage and Retransplantation of Ovarian Tissue as an Infertility Treatment." *Best Practice & Research. Clinical Endocrinology & Metabolism* 33 (1): 89–102. https://doi.org/10.1016/j.beem.2018.09.002.

Anam, Tahmima. 2008. "'It Seems a Shame to Deny Myself the Most Basic of Human Experiences. But I Need More Time . . .'" *Guardian*, December 12. http://www. guardian.co.uk/science/2008/dec/12/stemcells-reproduction.

ANP. 2009. "Kamer Huiverig Voor Invriezen Eicellen." *Volkskrant*, July 15. http://www. volkskrant.nl/vk/nl/2686/Binnenland/article/detail/347680/2009/07/15/Kamer-huiverig-voor-invriezen-eicellen.dhtml.

Armstrong, S., N. Arroll, L. Cree, V. Jordan, and C. Farquhar. 2015. "Time-Lapse Systems for Embryo Incubation and Assessment in Assisted Reproduction." *Cochrane Database of Systematic Reviews* 2: CD011320. https://doi.org/10.1002/14651858. CD011320.pub2.

Armstrong, S., A. Vail, S. Mastenbroek, V. Jordan, and C. Farquhar. 2015. "Time-Lapse in the IVF-Lab: How Should We Assess Potential Benefit?" *Human Reproduction* 30 (1): 3–8. https://doi.org/10.1093/humrep/deu250.

ASRM. 2004. "Ovarian Tissue and Oocyte Cryopreservation—The Practice Committee of the American Society for Reproductive Medicine." *Fertility and Sterility* 82 (4): 993–98. https://doi.org/10.1016/j.fertnstert.2004.07.925.

———. 2007. "Financial Compensation of Oocyte Donors." *Fertility and Sterility* 88 (2): 305–9. https://doi.org/10.1016/j.fertnstert.2007.01.104.

———. 2014. "Can I Freeze My Eggs to Use Later If I'm Not Sick?" ReproductiveFacts.Org. http://www.reproductivefacts.org/news-and-publications/

patient-fact-sheets-and-booklets/fact-sheets-and-info-booklets/
can-i-freeze-my-eggs-to-use-later-if-im-not-sick/.

ASRM Ethics Committee. 2018. "Planned Oocyte Cryopreservation for Women
Seeking to Preserve Future Reproductive Potential: An Ethics Committee Opinion." *Fertility and Sterility* 110 (6): 1022–28. https://doi.org/10.1016/j.fertnstert
.2018.08.027.

ASRM, The Practice Committees of the American Society for Reproductive Medicine and the Society for Assisted Reproductive Technology. 2013. "Mature Oocyte
Cryopreservation: A Guideline." *Fertility and Sterility* 99 (1): 37–43. https://doi.
org/10.1016/j.fertnstert.2012.09.028.

Astellas. 2016. "Astellas Pharma US, Inc." Astellas. https://www.astellas.us/therapeutic/
rnd/airm.aspx.

Auxogyn. 2012. "Eeva—Early Embryo Viability Assessment Test." Eeva. http://www.
eevaivf.com/.

———. 2014. *Eeva in Action (ASRM 2013)*. https://www.youtube.com/
watch?v=hdLokY5rPbM.

Baek, Ji I., Dong-Won Seol, Ah-Reum Lee, Woo Sik Lee, Sook-Young Yoon, and Dong
Ryul Lee. 2017. "Maintained MPF Level after Oocyte Vitrification Improves Embryonic Development after IVF, but Not after Somatic Cell Nuclear Transfer." *Molecules
and Cells* 40 (11): 871–79. https://doi.org/10.14348/molcells.2017.0184.

Bal, Mieke. 2002. *Travelling Concepts in the Humanities: A Rough Guide*. Toronto:
University of Toronto Press.

Baldwin, Kylie. 2017. "'I Suppose I Think to Myself, That's the Best Way to Be a Mother':
How Ideologies of Parenthood Shape Women's Use of Social Egg Freezing Technology." *Sociological Research Online* 22 (2): 1–15. https://doi.org/10.5153/sro.4187.

———. 2019. *Egg Freezing, Fertility, and Reproductive Choice: Negotiating Responsibility,
Hope, and Modern Motherhood*. Bingley, UK: Emerald Group.

Baldwin, Kylie, Lorraine Culley, Nicky Hudson, Helene Mitchell, and Stuart Lavery.
2015. "Oocyte Cryopreservation for Social Reasons: Demographic Profile and
Disposal Intentions of UK Users." *Reproductive BioMedicine Online* 31 (2): 239–45.
https://doi.org/10.1016/j.rbmo.2015.04.010.

Balkenende, Eva, Taghride Dahhan, Sjoerd Repping, Annemiek De Melker, Fulco van
der Veen, and Mariette Goddijn. 2015. "Eicelvitrificatie: Voor Wie Eigenlijk? | Ned-
erlands Tijdschrift Voor Geneeskunde." *Nederlands Tijdschrift Voor Geneeskunde*
159 (October): A9361.

Balkenende, Eva, Taghride Dahhan, Fulco van der Veen, Sjoerd Repping, and Mariëtte
Goddijn. 2018. "Reproductive Outcomes after Oocyte Banking for Fertility Preservation." *Reproductive BioMedicine Online* 37 (4): 425–33. https://doi.org/10.1016/j.
rbmo.2018.07.005.

Bannerman, Lucy. 2012. "Is Egg Freezing the Future for Women?"
Times, November 26. https://www.thetimes.co.uk/article/
is-egg-freezing-the-future-for-women-b059ztcs32b.

Barbey, Christopher. 2017. "Evidence of Biased Advertising in the Case of Social Egg Freezing." *New Bioethics* 23 (3): 195–209. https://doi.org/10.1080/20502877.2017.1396033.

Bartasi, Gina. 2016. "Gina Bartasi, Chief Executive Officer at Progyny, Inc." Linkedin. December. https://www.linkedin.com/in/gina-bartasi/.

Bartlett, Alison. 2005. *Breastwork: Rethinking Breastfeeding.* Sydney: UNSW Press.

Batty, David. 2006. "IVF Experts Advise Caution on Egg Freezing." *Guardian*, September 7. http://www.guardian.co.uk/lifeandstyle/2006/sep/07/familyandrelationships.health.

Bayefsky, Michelle, Alan DeCherney, and Benjamin Berkman. 2016. "Compensation for Egg Donation: A Zero-Sum Game." *Fertility and Sterility* 105 (5): 1153–54. https://doi.org/10.1016/j.fertnstert.2016.01.019.

Baylis, Françoise. 2009. "For Love or Money? The Saga of Korean Women Who Provided Eggs for Embryonic Stem Cell Research." *Theoretical Medicine and Bioethics* 30 (5): 385. https://doi.org/10.1007/s11017-009-9118-0.

BBC. 2013. "First Baby Conceived with Time-Lapse Imaging IVF Born in Glasgow." *BBC*, June 14, sec. Scotland. http://www.bbc.co.uk/news/uk-scotland-22910864.

———. 2017. "Freezing Your Eggs to Enjoy Life in China." *BBC News*, August 2, sec. China. https://www.bbc.com/news/world-asia-china-40183587.

Beets, Gijs, Arie De Graaf, and Coen Van Duin. 2013. "Bevolkingsprognose 2012–2060: Veronderstellingen over de Geboorte." Centraal Bureau voor de Statistiek. http://www.cbs.nl/NR/rdonlyres/3BA03CC0-F684-4481-946E-BB4338AF1083/0/20131002b15art.pdf.

Beim, Piraye Yurttas, David-Emlyn Parfitt, Lei Tan, Elaine A. Sugarman, Tina Hu-Seliger, Caterina Clementi, and Brynn Levy. 2017. "At the Dawn of Personalized Reproductive Medicine: Opportunities and Challenges with Incorporating Multigene Panel Testing into Fertility Care." *Journal of Assisted Reproduction and Genetics*, October. https://doi.org/10.1007/s10815-017-1068-2.

Benagiano, Giuseppe, and Luca Gianaroli. 2004. "The New Italian IVF Legislation." *Reproductive BioMedicine Online* 9 (2): 117–25. https://doi.org/10.1016/S1472-6483(10)62118-9.

Benzies, Karen, Suzanne Tough, Karen Tofflemire, Corine Frick, Alexandra Faber, and Christine Newburn-Cook. 2006. "Factors Influencing Women's Decisions about Timing of Motherhood." *Journal of Obstetric, Gynecologic & Neonatal Nursing* 35 (5): 625–33. https://doi.org/10.1111/j.1552-6909.2006.00079.x.

Berlant, Lauren. 2007. "On the Case." *Critical Inquiry* 33 (4): 663–72. https://doi.org/10.1086/521564.

———. 2011. *Cruel Optimism.* Durham, NC: Duke University Press.

Betterton, Rosemary. 2002. "Prima Gravida: Reconfiguring the Maternal Body in Visual Representation." *Feminist Theory* 3 (3): 255–70. https://doi.org/10.1177/146470002762491999.

Bhatia, Rajani, and Lisa Campo-Engelstein. 2018. "The Biomedicalization of Social Egg Freezing: A Comparative Analysis of European and American Professional Ethics

Opinions and US News and Popular Media." *Science, Technology & Human Values*, February, 864–87. https://doi.org/10.1177/0162243918754322.

Biggs, Simon. 2004. "Age, Gender, Narratives, and Masquerades." *Journal of Aging Studies* 18 (1): 45–58. https://doi.org/10.1016/j.jaging.2003.09.005.

Biospectrum. 2018. "WeDoctor, Other Investors to Acquire Genea for $510 M." *Biospectrum Asia Edition*. September 3. https://www.biospectrumasia.com/news/30/11612/wedoctor-other-investors-to-acquire-genea-for-510-m.html.

Birenbaum-Carmeli, Daphna. 2009. "The Politics of 'The Natural Family' in Israel: State Policy and Kinship Ideologies." *Social Science & Medicine* 69 (7): 1018–24. https://doi.org/10.1016/j.socscimed.2009.07.044.

Blell, Mwenza. 2018. "Keynote: Remaking Reproduction." Presented at the Remaking Reproduction Conference, University of Cambridge, June 28.

Boiani, Michele. 2013. "Cloned Human ES Cells: A Great Leap Forward, and Still Needed?" *Molecular Human Reproduction* 19 (10): 629–33. https://doi.org/10.1093/molehr/gato54.

Bonilla. 2013. *AB-926 Reproductive Health and Research*. http://leginfo.legislature.ca.gov/faces/billCompareClient.xhtml.

Bordo, Susan. 2004. *Unbearable Weight: Feminism, Western Culture, and the Body*. Berkeley: University of California Press.

Bos, Annelies M. E., Petra Klapwijk, and Bart C. J. M. Fauser. 2012. "Wide Support for Oocyte Donation and Banking in the Netherlands." *Nederlands Tijdschrift Voor Geneeskunde* 156 (5): A4145.

Boschman, Sanne. 2012. "Sterke regionale verschillen in vrucht-baarheid naar herkomstgroepering." Centraal Bureau voor de Statistiek. July 11. https://www.cbs.nl/nl-nl/achtergrond/2012/28/sterke-regionale-verschillen-in-vruchtbaarheid-naar-herkomstgroepering.

Boseley, Sarah. 2000. "Ban on Births from Frozen Eggs Lifted." *Guardian*, January 26. http://www.guardian.co.uk/uk/2000/jan/26/sarahboseley.

———. 2009. "Doctor Tells of First 'Social' Fertility Engineering Cases." *Guardian*, June 29. http://www.guardian.co.uk/society/2009/jun/29/fertility-engineering-social.

———. 2014. "Freezing Eggs for Female Staff Is Great in Theory: But It Offers No Guarantees." *Guardian*, October 15. https://www.theguardian.com/society/2014/oct/15/freezing-eggs-female-staff-apple-facebook-analysis.

Boyer, Kate. 2012. "Affect, Corporeality, and the Limits of Belonging: Breastfeeding in Public in the Contemporary UK." *Health & Place* 18 (3): 552–60. https://doi.org/10.1016/j.healthplace.2012.01.010.

Briggs, Laura. 2018. *How All Politics Became Reproductive Politics: From Welfare Reform to Foreclosure to Trump*. Berkeley: University of California Press.

Brown, Eliza, and Mary Patrick. 2018. "Time, Anticipation, and the Life Course: Egg Freezing as Temporarily Disentangling Romance and Reproduction." *American Sociological Review* 83 (5): 959–82. https://doi.org/10.1177/0003122418796807.

Browne, Jude. 2018. "Technology, Fertility, and Public Policy: A Structural Perspective on Human Egg Freezing and Gender Equality." *Social Politics: International Studies in Gender, State & Society* 25 (2): 149–68. https://doi.org/10.1093/sp/jxx022.

Budds, Kirsty, Abigail Locke, and Vivien Burr. 2013. "Risky Business." *Feminist Media Studies* 13 (1): 132–47. https://doi.org/10.1080/14680777.2012.678073.

Bui, Quoctrung, and Claire Cain Miller. 2018. "The Age That Women Have Babies: How a Gap Divides America." *New York Times*, August 4. https://www.nytimes.com/interactive/2018/08/04/upshot/up-birth-age-gap.html.

Bunge, R., W. Keettel, and J. Sherman. 1954. "Clinical Use of Frozen Semen: Report of Four Cases." *Fertility and Sterility* 5 (6): 520–29.

BusinessWire. 2011. "Vitrolife Is the First Company in China to Receive Regulatory Approval for an Entire IVF Culture Media Portfolio." *Business Wire*, May 5. https://www.businesswire.com/news/home/20110505005795/en/Vitrolife-Company-China-Receive-Regulatory-Approval-Entire.

———. 2013. "Cryoport Expands Logistics Services for Reproductive Medicine with the World Egg Bank." *Business Wire*, August 19. https://www.businesswire.com/news/home/20130819005236/en/Cryoport-Expands-Logistics-Services-Reproductive-Medicine-World.

———. 2014. "Advanced Cell Technology Secures $30 Million Equity Facility from Lincoln Park Capital." *Business Wire*, July 3. https://www.businesswire.com/news/home/20140703005301/en/Advanced-Cell-Technology-Secures-30-Million-Equity.

———. 2019. "CHA Health Systems Subsidiary to Form the Largest Healthcare Network to Provide Premium Comprehensive Suite of Medical Services." *Business Wire*, February 21. https://www.businesswire.com/news/home/20190221005197/en/CHA-Health-Systems-Subsidiary-Form-Largest-Healthcare.

Butler, Judith. 1993. *Bodies That Matter: On the Discursive Limits of Sex*. New York: Routledge.

———. 1997a. "Further Reflections on Conversations of Our Time." *Diacritics* 27 (1): 13–15. https://doi.org/10.1353/dia.1997.0004.

———. 1997b. *Excitable Speech: A Politics of the Performative*. New York: Routledge.

———. 2006. *Precarious Life: The Power of Mourning and Violence*. Reprint edition. London: Verso.

California Cryobank. 2016. "California Cryobank Announces Acquisition of Donor Egg Bank USA." California Cryobank. December 13. https://donoreggbankusa.com/resources/press-releases/california-cryobank-announces-acquisition-donor-egg-bank-usa.

Calmthout, Martijn. 2011. "Mister Right." *Volkskrant*, September 22. http://www.volkskrant.nl/vk/nl/2844/Archief/archief/article/detail/2923055/2011/09/22/Mister-right.dhtml.

Campbell, Denis. 2009. "Fertility Experts in Moral Warning over Egg Freezing." *Guardian*, February 1. http://www.guardian.co.uk/.

Campbell, Patricia. 2011. "Boundaries and Risk: Media Framing of Assisted Reproductive Technologies and Older Mothers." *Social Science & Medicine* 72 (2): 265–72. https://doi.org/10.1016/j.socscimed.2010.10.028.

Campo-Engelstein, Lisa, Rohia Aziz, Shilpa Darivemula, Jennifer Raffaele, Rajani Bhatia, and Wendy M. Parker. 2018. "Freezing Fertility or Freezing False Hope? A Content Analysis of Social Egg Freezing in U.S. Print Media." *AJOB Empirical Bioethics* 9 (3): 181–93. https://doi.org/10.1080/23294515.2018.1509153.

Carbone, June, and Naomi Cahn. 2013. "The Gender/Class Divide: Reproduction, Privilege, and the Workplace." *FIU Law Review* 8: 287–316.

Cardona, Beatriz. 2008. "'Healthy Ageing' Policies and Anti-Ageing Ideologies and Practices: On the Exercise of Responsibility." *Medicine, Health Care, and Philosophy* 11 (4): 475–83. https://doi.org/10.1007/s11019-008-9129-z.

CARE Fertility. 2015. *Jaycie's Journey Using Embryoscope Time Lapse Imaging at CARE Fertility.* https://www.youtube.com/watch?v=vnm56Kiy4Jg.

———. 2016. "EGGsafe—Egg Freezing and Storage at CARE Fertility." CARE Fertility. https://www.carefertility.com/treatments/fertility-preservation/eggsafe/.

———. 2018. "CAREmaps." CARE Fertility. https://www.carefertility.com/treatments/embryology-treatments/caremaps/.

Carrel, Alexis. 1912. "On the Permanent Life of Tissues outside of the Organism." *Journal of Experimental Medicine* 15: 516–28.

Carroll, Katherine, and Charlotte Kroløkke. 2018. "Freezing for Love: Enacting 'Responsible' Reproductive Citizenship through Egg Freezing." *Culture, Health & Sexuality* 20 (9): 992–1005. https://doi.org/10.1080/13691058.2017.1404643.

Cattapan, Alana, Kathleen Hammond, Jennie Haw, and Lesley A. Tarasoff. 2014. "Breaking the Ice: Young Feminist Scholars of Reproductive Politics Reflect on Egg Freezing." *International Journal of Feminist Approaches to Bioethics* 7 (2): 236–47.

Cavanaugh, Lisa A. 2014. "Because I (Don't) Deserve It: How Relationship Reminders and Deservingness Influence Consumer Indulgence." *Journal of Marketing Research* 51 (2): 218–32.

CBC. 2015. "Zain Rajani Is the 1st Baby Born Using Augment IVF Treatment." CBC News, May 8. https://www.cbc.ca/news/canada/toronto/zain-rajani-is-the-1st-baby-born-using-augment-ivf-treatment-1.3067637.

CBO. 2003. *Modelreglement Embryowet, Kwaliteitsinstituut Voor de Gezondheidszorg.* Alphen aan de Rijn: Van Zuiden. https://www.nvog.nl/wp-content/uploads/2018/02/Embryowet-1.0-18-01-2008.pdf.

CBS. 2017. "Geboorte: Vruchtbaarheid, Herkomstgroepering En Generatie Moeder." Centraal Bureau Voor de Statistiek. July 3. http://statline.cbs.nl/Statweb/publication/?DM=SLNL&PA=83307ned&D1=2&D2=0-2&D3=a&D4=a&VW=T.

CCNE. 2017. "CCNE Opinion on Societal Requests for Medically Assisted Reproduction (MAR)." Opinion 126. Paris: National Consultative Ethics Committee for Health and Life Sciences. https://www.ccne-ethique.fr/sites/default/files/publications/ccne_avis_n126_amp.eng_.pdf.

———. 2018. "Contribution Du Comité Consultatif National d'éthique à La Révision de La Loi de Bioéthique, 2018–2019." Avis 129. Paris: Comité consultatif national d'éthique. https://www.ccne-ethique.fr/sites/default/files/avis_129_vf.pdf.

CDC. 2018. "Assisted Reproductive Technology: Fertility Clinic Success Rates Report 2016." Atlanta: Centers for Disease Control and Prevention. ftp://ftp.cdc.gov/pub/Publications/art/ART-2016-Clinic-Report-Full.pdf.

CHA. 2019a. "Egg Freezing & Banking." *CHA Fertility Center* (blog). https://chaivf.com/treatments-services/egg-freezing/.

———. 2019b. "History." CHA. http://en.chamc.co.kr/vision/history.cha.

Chandra, Anjani, Casey Copen, and Elizabeth Hervey Stephen. 2014. "Infertility Service Use in the United States: Data from the National Survey of Family Growth, 1982–2010." Hyattsville, MD: Centers for Disease Control and Prevention.

Chang, C. C., Liesl Nel-Themaat, and Zsolt Peter Nagy. 2011. "Cryopreservation of Oocytes in Experimental Models." *Reproductive BioMedicine Online* 23 (3): 307–13. https://doi.org/10.1016/j.rbmo.2011.01.007.

Chang, C. C., Li-Ying Sung, Tomokazu Amano, Cindy Tian, Xiangzhong Yang, and Zsolt Peter Nagy. 2009. "Nuclear Transfer and Oocyte Cryopreservation." *Reproduction, Fertility, and Development* 21 (1): 37–44.

Chang, C. C., G. Wright, T. K. Elliott, D. B. Shapiro, A. A. Toledo, and Z. P. Nagy. 2018. "Long Distance/Cross Border Egg Donation: A Model to Have the Best of Both Worlds." *Fertility and Sterility* 110 (4): e192–93. https://doi.org/10.1016/j.fertnstert.2018.07.563.

Chappel, James. 2017. "Modern Family." *Dissent* 64 (3): 147–51. https://doi.org/10.1353/dss.2017.0082.

Chen, Christopher. 1986. "Pregnancy after Human Oocyte Cryopreservation." *Lancet* 327 (8486): 884–86. https://doi.org/10.1016/s0140-6736(86)90989-x.

Chen, Tiantian. 2020. "Spiral Society: An Exploratory Study of the Ban on Single Women's Egg Freezing in China." PhD dissertation. Cambridge: University of Cambridge.

Chian, Ri-Cheng, Lucy Gilbert, Jack Y. J. Huang, Ezgi Demirtas, Hananel Holzer, Alice Benjamin, William M. Buckett, Togas Tulandi, and Seang Lin Tan. 2009. "Live Birth after Vitrification of in Vitro Matured Human Oocytes." *Fertility and Sterility* 91 (2): 372–76. https://doi.org/10.1016/j.fertnstert.2007.11.088.

Christensen, Kaare, Gabriele Doblhammer, Roland Rau, and James Vaupel. 2009. "Ageing Populations: The Challenges Ahead." *Lancet* 374 (9696): 1196–1208. https://doi.org/10.1016/S0140-6736(09)61460-4.

Christopher, Martin, Adrian Payne, and David Ballantyne. 2013. *Relationship Marketing*. Burlington, MA: Taylor & Francis.

Chung, Young Gie, Jin Hee Eum, Jeoung Eun Lee, Sung Han Shim, Vicken Sepilian, Seung Wook Hong, Yumie Lee, et al. 2014. "Human Somatic Cell Nuclear Transfer Using Adult Cells." *Cell Stem Cell* 14 (6): 777–80. https://doi.org/10.1016/j.stem.2014.03.015.

Chung, Young Gie, Shogo Matoba, Yuting Liu, Jin Hee Eum, Falong Lu, Wei Jiang, Jeoung Eun Lee, et al. 2015. "Histone Demethylase Expression Enhances Human Somatic Cell Nuclear Transfer Efficiency and Promotes Derivation of Pluripotent Stem Cells." *Cell Stem Cell* 17 (6): 758–66. https://doi.org/10.1016/j.stem.2015.10.001.

Cibelli, Jose. 2009. "The Human Egg Is Back." *Cell Stem Cell* 5 (4): 345–46. https://doi. org/10.1016/j.stem.2009.09.009.

Clarke, Jacqueline. 2012. "Dying to Be Mommy: Using Intentional Parenthood as a Proxy for Consent in Posthumous Egg Retrieval Cases." *Michigan State Law Review* 2012: 1331.

Coe, Cynthia, and Matthew Altman. 2012. "Mandatory Ultrasound Laws and the Coercive Use of Informed Consent." *Techné: Research in Philosophy and Technology* 16 (1): 16–30.

Cohen, Jacques. 2013a. "Patenting Time: A Response to Professor Reijo Pera's Argument That the Cell Cycle of an Embryo Developing in Vitro Is Not Natural." *Reproductive Biomedicine Online* 27 (2): 115. https://doi.org/10.1016/j.rbmo.2013.05.011.

———. 2013b. "On Patenting Time and Other Natural Phenomena." *Reproductive Bio-Medicine Online* 27 (2): 109–10. https://doi.org/10.1016/j.rbmo.2013.05.001.

Cohen, Philip. 2012. "Births to Mothers in Their Forties Are Less Common Now Than in the Old Days." *Family Inequality* (blog). December 20. https://familyinequality. wordpress.com/2012/12/20/births-to-mothers/.

Cohen, Richard. 1978. "The Clock Is Ticking for the Career Woman: Biological Time Clock Can Create Real Panic." *Washington Post*, March 16.

Cook, Michael. 2018. "In Post-One-Child-Policy China Posthumous Conception Is a Matter of Desperation." BioEdge. April 14. https://www.bioedge.org/bioethics/in-post-one-child-policy-china-posthumous-conception-is-a-matter-of-despera/12654.

Cooper, Melinda. 2006. "Resuscitations: Stem Cells and the Crisis of Old Age." *Body & Society* 12 (1): 1–23. https://doi.org/10.1177/1357034X06061196.

———. 2017. *Family Values: Between Neoliberalism and the New Social Conservatism.* New York: Zone Books.

Cooper, Melinda, and Catherine Waldby. 2014. *Clinical Labor: Tissue Donors and Research Subjects in the Global Bioeconomy.* Durham, NC: Duke University Press Books.

Corrigan, Oonagh. 2003. "Empty Ethics: The Problem with Informed Consent." *Sociology of Health & Illness* 25 (7): 768–92. https://doi. org/10.1046/j.1467-9566.2003.00369.x.

Cromer, Risa. 2019. "Racial Politics of Frozen Embryo Personhood in the US Antiabortion Movement." *Transforming Anthropology* 27 (1): 22–36. https://doi.org/10.1111/ traa.12145.

Crunchbase. 2019. "List of Progyny's 10 Funding Rounds Totaling $99.5M." Crunchbase. https://www.crunchbase.com/search/funding_rounds/field/organizations/ funding_total/progyny.

Cryoport. 2014. "IVF Frozen Shipping FAQ and What to Expect from Shipping." Cryoport. http://www.cryoport.com/in-vitro-fertilization-frozen-shipping/ faq_ivf_frozen_shipping/.

Culley, L., N. Hudson, F. Rapport, E. Blyth, W. Norton, and A. A. Pacey. 2011. "Crossing Borders for Fertility Treatment: Motivations, Destinations, and Outcomes of

UK Fertility Travellers." *Human Reproduction*, June: 1–9. https://doi.org/10.1093/humrep/der191.

Curchoe, Carol Lynn, and Charles Bormann. 2019. "Artificial Intelligence and Machine Learning for Human Reproduction and Embryology Presented at ASRM and ESHRE 2018." *Journal of Assisted Reproduction and Genetics* 36 (4): 591–600. https://doi.org/10.1007/s10815-019-01408-x.

Cyranoski, David. 2004. "Crunch Time for Korea's Cloners." *Nature* 429 (6987): 12–14. https://doi.org/10.1038/429012a.

———. 2013a. "US Scientists Chafe at Restrictions on New Stem-Cell Lines." *Nature News*, June. https://doi.org/doi:10.1038/nature.2013.13114.

———. 2013b. "Stem Cells: Egg Engineers." *Nature News* 500 (7463): 392–94. https://doi.org/10.1038/500392a.

Daar, Judith, Jean Benward, Lee Collins, Joseph Davis, Leslie Francis, Elena Gates, Elizabeth Ginsburg, et al. 2016. "Financial Compensation of Oocyte Donors: An Ethics Committee Opinion." *Fertility and Sterility* 106 (7): e15–19. https://doi.org/10.1016/j.fertnstert.2016.09.040.

Daniels, Cynthia, and Erin Heidt-Forsythe. 2012. "Gendered Eugenics and the Problematic of Free Market Reproductive Technologies: Sperm and Egg Donation in the United States." *Signs: Journal of Women in Culture and Society* 37 (3): 719–47. https://doi.org/10.1086/662964.

Daniluk, Judith C., and Emily Koert. 2013. "The Other Side of the Fertility Coin: A Comparison of Childless Men's and Women's Knowledge of Fertility and Assisted Reproductive Technology." *Fertility and Sterility* 99 (3): 839–46. https://doi.org/10.1016/j.fertnstert.2012.10.033.

Darwin Life. 2019. "Nuclear Transfer." Darwin Life. https://www.darwinlife.com/nuclear-transfer.php.

Davda, Priya. 2019. "The Biomedicalisation, Stratification, and Racialisation of Reproduction through Matching in UK Egg Donation." PhD, London: Royal Holloway, University of London. https://ethos.bl.uk/OrderDetails.do?uin=uk.bl.ethos.792902.

De Arellano, Ramírez. 2007. "Patients without Borders: The Emergence of Medical Tourism." *International Journal of Health Services: Planning, Administration, Evaluation* 37 (1): 193–98.

De Pater, Irene, Timothy Judge, and Brent Scott. 2014. "Age, Gender, and Compensation: A Study of Hollywood Movie Stars." *Journal of Management Inquiry* 23 (4): 407–20. https://doi.org/10.1177/1056492613519861.

De Persgroep Advertising. 2012. "De Volkskrant." http://www.persgroepadvertising.nl/landelijk/de-volkskrant.

De Wert, Guido. 1999. "Met Het Oog Op de Toekomst: Voortplantingstechnologie, Erfelijkheidsonderzoek En Ethiek [Looking Ahead: Reproductive Technologies, Genetics, and Ethics]." PhD, Rotterdam: Erasmus MC: University Medical Center Rotterdam. https://repub.eur.nl/pub/19895/.

DEBU. 2019. "Our Egg Donation Locations." Donor Egg Bank USA. https://donoreggbankusa.com/our-program/locations.

Deomampo, Daisy. 2016. "Race, Nation, and the Production of Intimacy: Transnational Ova Donation in India." *Positions: Asia Critique* 24 (1): 303–32. https://doi.org/10.1215/10679847-3320161.

Depmann, M., S. Broer, M. Eijkemans, I. van Rooij, G. Scheffer, J. Heimensem, B. Mol, and F. Broekmans. 2017. "Anti-Müllerian Hormone Does Not Predict Time to Pregnancy: Results of a Prospective Cohort Study." *Gynecological Endocrinology* 33 (8): 644–48. https://doi.org/10.1080/09513590.2017.1306848.

Devlin, Hannah. 2019. "Baby with DNA from Three People Born in Greece." *Guardian*, April 11, sec. Science. https://www.theguardian.com/science/2019/apr/11/baby-with-dna-from-three-people-born-in-greece-ivf.

Dickenson, Donna, and Itziar Alkorta Idiakez. 2008. "Ova Donation for Stem Cell Research: An International Perspective." *International Journal of Feminist Approaches to Bioethics* 1 (2): 125–44.

Dispatches. 1998. *Granny's Having a Baby*. Videorecording. Channel 4. http://search.wellcomelibrary.org/iii/encore/record/C__Rb1666657__Sgranny%27s%20having%20a%20baby__Orightresult__X7;jsessionid=8381A884CE99E3DDE7EBBF9ED1F51B6F?lang=eng&suite=cobalt.

Ditkowsky, Lisa. 2018. "White Paper: The Fertility Field Mergers & Acquisitions (M&A): Frothy or the Next Frontier?" *Pllush Capital Management* (blog). August 17. http://www.pllush.com/blog/fertility-ivf-donor-eggs-shady-grove-fertility-centers-illinois-private-equ.

DL-Nadiya. 2019. "Nuclear Transfers." *DL-Nadiya*. http://dl-nadiya.com/nuclear-transfers.

Dong-seok, Sah. 2016. "Resumed Stem Cell Study." *Korea Times*, July 13. http://www.koreatimes.co.kr/www/opinion/2019/07/202_209306.html.

Donnez, Jacques, and Marie-Madeleine Dolmans. 2014. "Transplantation of Ovarian Tissue." *Best Practice & Research Clinical Obstetrics & Gynaecology* 28 (8): 1188–97. https://doi.org/10.1016/j.bpobgyn.2014.09.003.

Dresner Partners. 2018. "Staying Ahead of the Curve: Healthcare—Women's Health Sector." Dresner Partners. June. http://www.dresnerpartners.com/ace-files/Fertility_June_2018.pdf.

Dunson, David, Donna Baird, and Bernardo Colombo. 2004. "Increased Infertility with Age in Men and Women." *Obstetrics and Gynecology* 103 (1): 51–56.

Dyer, Owen. 2019. "Dutch Physician Sues FDA for Blocking Her Abortion Services in United States." *BMJ* 366 (September): l5511. https://doi.org/10.1136/bmj.l5511.

Earle, Sarah. 2003. "Is Breast Best? Breastfeeding, Motherhood, and Identity." In *Gender, Identity, and Reproduction: Social Perspectives*, edited by Sarah Earle and Gayle Letherby, 135–50. London: Palgrave. http://www.palgrave.com/products/Catalogue.aspx?is=140390281X.

Economist. 2017. "The Business of Sperm Banks." *Economist*, September 14. https://www.economist.com/business/2017/09/14/the-business-of-sperm-banks.

Edelman, Lee. 2004. *No Future: Queer Theory and the Death Drive*. Durham, NC: Duke University Press.

Effting, Maud. 2011. "Late Abortus Om Sociale Reden Niet van Deze Tijd." *Volkskrant*, February 26. http://www.volkskrant.nl/wetenschap/late-abortus-om-sociale-reden-niet-van-deze-tijd~a1852737/.

Eggbanxx. 2015. "Egg Freezing Informational Events & Egg Freezing Cocktail Parties." EggBanxx: Smart Women Freeze. https://www.eggbanxx.com/events.

Eggfreezer. 2008. "Picture of My Frozen Egg." *My Egg Freezing Process* (blog). April 12. http://eggfreeze.blogspot.co.uk/2008/12/mine.html.

———. 2015. "All the Vitrified Eggs Died on Thaw." *Eggfreezer* (blog). June 27. http://eggfreeze.blogspot.com/2015/06/update-7-years-later-i-went-to-use.html.

European Union. 2004. "Directive 2004/23/EC." *Official Journal of the European Union*, April, L102/48–58.

Extend Fertility. 2003. "Extend Fertility Home." Extend Fertility. October 23. http://www.extendfertility.com:80/. Available on Internet Archive, https://web.archive.org/web/20031023185731/http://www.extendfertility.com:80/.

———. 2016. "FAQs." Extend Fertility. https://extendfertility.com/facts-figures/faq.

———. 2017a. "Egg Freezing Cost." Extend Fertility. https://extendfertility.com/pricing.

———. 2017b. "Extend Fertility: A Premier Egg Freezing Service." Extend Fertility. https://extendfertility.com/.

———. 2017c. "Are There Benefits to Having Children Later in Life?" *Extend Fertility* (blog). June 5. https://extendfertility.com/blog/benefits-of-delayed-motherhood.

———. 2018. "How Frozen Eggs Are Used." Extend Fertility. https://extendfertility.com/your-fertility/how-frozen-eggs-are-used.

———. 2019a. "About Extend Fertility." Extend Fertility. https://extendfertility.com.

———. 2019b. "Extend Fertility Announces $15M Series A Investment by Regal Healthcare Capital Partners and Names Anne Hogarty CEO." PR Newswire. February 4. https://www.prnewswire.com.

Fahmy, Shahira, and Daekyung Kim. 2008. "Picturing the Iraq War: Constructing the Image of War in the British and US Press." *International Communication Gazette* 70 (6): 443–62. https://doi.org/10.1177/1748048508096142.

Faludi, Susan. 1991. *Backlash: The Undeclared War against Women*. London: Random House.

Ferla, Ruth La. 2018. "These Companies Really, Really, Really Want to Freeze Your Eggs." *New York Times*, September 6, sec. Style. https://www.nytimes.com.

FertilityIQ. 2017a. "An Overview of Egg Freezing." FertilityIQ. https://www.fertilityiq.com.

———. 2017b. "IVF Refund and Package Programs." FertilityIQ. https://www.fertilityiq.com/cost/ivf-refund-and-package-programs.

———. 2017c. "The Costs of Egg Freezing." FertilityIQ. https://www.fertilityiq.com/egg-freezing/the-costs-of-egg-freezing.

Fleck, Robert, and F. Andrew Hanssen. 2016. "Persistence and Change in Age-Specific Gender Gaps: Hollywood Actors from the Silent Era Onward." *International Review of Law and Economics* 48 (October): 36–49. https://doi.org/10.1016/j.irle.2016.08.002.

Foucault, Michel. 2003. *Society Must Be Defended: Lectures at the Collège de France, 1975–76.* Edited by Mauro Bertani and Alessandro Fontana. New York: Picador.

Franklin, Sarah. 1997. *Embodied Progress: A Cultural Account of Assisted Conception.* London: Routledge.

———. 2000. "Life Itself: Global Nature and the Genetic Imaginary." In *Global Nature, Global Culture,* edited by Celia Lury, Jackie Stacey, and Sarah Franklin, 188–227. London: Sage.

———. 2001. "Culturing Biology: Cell Lines for the Second Millennium." *Health* 5 (3): 335–54. https://doi.org/10.1177/136345930100500304.

———. 2006a. "The Cyborg Embryo: Our Path to Transbiology." *Theory, Culture & Society* 23 (7–8): 167–87. https://doi.org/10.1177/0263276406069230.

———. 2006b. "Embryonic Economies: The Double Reproductive Value of Stem Cells." *Biosocieties* 1 (1): 71–90.

———. 2007. *Dolly Mixtures: The Remaking of Genealogy.* Durham, NC: Duke University Press.

———. 2011. "Not a Flat World: The Future of Cross-Border Reproductive Care." *Reproductive BioMedicine Online* 23 (7): 814–16. https://doi.org/10.1016/j.rbmo.2011.09.016.

———. 2013a. "Embryo Watching: How IVF Has Remade Biology." *TECNOSCIENZA: Italian Journal of Science & Technology Studies* 4 (1): 23–44.

———. 2013b. *Biological Relatives: IVF, Stem Cells, and the Future of Kinship.* Durham, NC: Duke University Press.

———. 2014a. "Analogic Return: The Reproductive Life of Conceptuality." *Theory, Culture & Society* 31 (2–3): 243–61. https://doi.org/10.1177/0263276413510953.

———. 2014b. "Rethinking Reproductive Politics in Time, and Time in UK Reproductive Politics: 1978–2008." *Journal of the Royal Anthropological Institute* 20 (April): 109–25.

———. 2019. "A Tale of Two Halves? IVF in the UK in the 1970s and 1980s." In *The Reproductive Industry: Intimate Experiences and Global Processes,* edited by Vera Mackie, Nicola Marks, and Sarah Ferber. London: Lexington Books.

Franklin, Sarah, and Celia Roberts. 2006. *Born and Made: An Ethnography of Preimplantation Genetic Diagnosis.* Princeton, NJ: Princeton University Press.

Fraser, Nancy, and Rahel Jaeggi. 2018. *Capitalism: A Conversation in Critical Theory.* Medford, MA: Polity Press.

Freeman, Elizabeth. 2010. *Time Binds: Queer Temporalities, Queer Histories.* Durham, NC: Duke University Press.

Freya. 2017. "Monitor Leeftijdsgrenzen." Freya. https://www.freya.nl/monitor-fertiliteitszorg/monitor-leeftijdsgrenzen/.

Friese, Carrie, Gay Becker, and Robert Nachtigall. 2006. "Rethinking the Biological Clock: Eleventh-Hour Moms, Miracle Moms, and Meanings of Age-Related Infertility." *Social Science & Medicine* 63 (6): 1550–60. https://doi.org/10.1016/j.socscimed.2006.03.034.

———. 2008. "Older Motherhood and the Changing Life Course in the Era of Assisted Reproductive Technologies." *Journal of Aging Studies* 22 (1): 65–73. https://doi.org/10.1016/j.jaging.2007.05.009.

Galkin, Fedor, Bohan Zhang, Sergey Dmitriev, and Vadim Gladyshev. 2019. "Reversibility of Irreversible Aging." *Ageing Research Reviews* 49 (January): 104–14. https://doi.org/10.1016/j.arr.2018.11.008.

Geelen, Jean-Pierre. 2010. "Eitje." *Volkskrant*, November 2. http://www.volkskrant.nl/vk/nl/2844/Archief/archief/article/detail/1044794/2010/11/02/Eitje.dhtml.

GEN. 2015. "Astellas to Acquire Ocata Therapeutics for $379M." GEN. November 10. https://www.genengnews.com/topics/drug-discovery/astellas-to-acquire-ocata-therapeutics-for-379m/.

Gerrits, Trudie. 2016. *Patient-Centred IVF: Bioethics and Care in a Dutch Clinic.* Fertility, Reproduction, and Sexuality. New York: Berghahn Books.

GFA. 2018. "Overview of the GFA." Global Fertility Alliance. http://www.globalfertility-alliance.org/index.php/about-the-gfa/overview.

Gill, Rosalind. 2007. "Postfeminist Media Culture: Elements of a Sensibility." *European Journal of Cultural Studies* 10 (2): 147–66. https://doi.org/10.1177/1367549407075898.

Goisis, Alice, and Wendy Sigle-Rushton. 2014. "Childbearing Postponement and Child Well-Being: A Complex and Varied Relationship?" *Demography* 51 (5): 1821–41. https://doi.org/10.1007/s13524-014-0335-4.

Gold, E., K. Copperman, G. Witkin, C. Jones, and A. B. Copperman. 2006. "A Motivational Assessment of Women Undergoing Elective Egg Freezing for Fertility Preservation." *Fertility and Sterility* 86 (3, Supplement): S201. https://doi.org/10.1016/j.fertnstert.2006.07.537.

Gook, Debra. 2011. "History of Oocyte Cryopreservation." *Reproductive BioMedicine Online* 23 (3): 281–89. https://doi.org/10.1016/j.rbmo.2010.10.018.

Goold, Imogen, and Julian Savulescu. 2008. "Freezing Eggs for Lifestyle Reasons." *American Journal of Bioethics* 8 (6): 32–35. https://doi.org/10.1080/15265160802248492.

———. 2009. "In Favour of Freezing Eggs for Non-Medical Reasons." *Bioethics* 23 (1): 47–58. https://doi.org/10.1111/j.1467-8519.2008.00679.x.

Gootman, Elissa. 2012. "Would-Be Grandparents Nudge Daughters to Egg-Freezing Clinic." *New York Times*, May 13. https://www.nytimes.com/2012/05/14/us/eager-for-grandchildren-and-putting-daughters-eggs-in-freezer.html.

Gorman, Gráinne, Robert McFarland, Jane Stewart, Catherine Feeney, and Doug Turnbull. 2018. "Mitochondrial Donation: From Test Tube to Clinic." *Lancet* 392 (10154): 1191–92. https://doi.org/10.1016/S0140-6736(18)31868-3.

Gosden, Roger. 2011. "Cryopreservation: A Cold Look at Technology for Fertility Preservation." *Fertility and Sterility* 96 (2): 264–68. https://doi.org/10.1016/j.fertnstert.2011.06.029.

Gosden, Roger, and Bora Lee. 2010. "Portrait of an Oocyte: Our Obscure Origin." *Journal of Clinical Investigation* 120 (4): 973–83. https://doi.org/10.1172/JCI41294.

Gottweis, Herbert, and Byoungsoo Kim. 2010. "Explaining Hwang-Gate: South Korean Identity Politics between Bionationalism and Globalization." *Science, Technology & Human Values* 35 (4): 501–24. https://doi.org/10.1177/0162243909345840.

Gow, Rachel, Janet Lydecker, Jennifer Lamanna, and Suzanne Mazzeo. 2012. "Representations of Celebrities' Weight and Shape during Pregnancy and Postpartum: A Content Analysis of Three Entertainment Magazine Websites." *Body Image* 9 (1): 172–75. https://doi.org/10.1016/j.bodyim.2011.07.003.

Grant, Judith. 1992. "Prime Time Crime: Television Portrayals of Law Enforcement." *Journal of American Culture* 15 (1): 57–68. https://doi.org/10.1111/j.1542-734X.1992.00057.x.

Groenier, Rivka. 2010. "Het Verlangen Naar Een Eigen Bolle Buik." *Het Parool*, October 29.

Groskop, Viv. 2006. "Babies on Ice." *Guardian*, March 14. http://www.guardian.co.uk/society/2006/mar/04/health.familyandrelationships1.

———. 2011. "Born in the Nick of Time!" *Guardian*, May 7. http://www.guardian.co.uk/lifeandstyle/2011/may/07/kasey-edwards-biological-clock-fertility.

Guardian.co.uk. 2012. "The Progressive Guardian Audience." *Guardian*, March 23. http://www.guardian.co.uk/advertising/progressives.

Gürtin, Zeynep. 2017. "Why Are Women Freezing Their Eggs? Because of the Lack of Eligible Men." *Guardian*, July 7, sec. Opinion. https://www.theguardian.com/commentisfree/2017/jul/07/egg-freezing-women-30s-40s-lack-of-eligible-men-knights-shining-armour.

Gürtin, Zeynep, Trina Shah, Jinjun Wang, and Kamal Ahuja. 2019. "Reconceiving Egg Freezing: Insights from an Analysis of 5 Years of Data from a UK Clinic." *Reproductive Biomedicine Online* 38 (2): 272–82. https://doi.org/10.1016/j.rbmo.2018.11.003.

Gutteling, Jan, Cees Midden, Carla Smink, and Annelous Meijnders. 2001. "The Netherlands: Controversy or Consensus?" In *Biotechnology, 1996–2000: The Years of Controversy*, edited by George Gaskell and Martin W. Bauer, 229–36. London: Science Museum.

Hafer, Carolyn, Antonia Mantonakis, Regan Fitzgerald, and Anthony Bogaert. 2018. "The Effectiveness of Deservingness-Based Advertising Messages: The Role of Product Knowledge and Belief in a Just World." *Canadian Journal of Administrative Sciences* 35 (1): 34–46. https://doi.org/10.1002/cjas.1406.

Hamel, Liz, Mira Norton, Karen Pollitz, Larry Levitt, Gary Claxton, and Mollyann Brodie. 2016. "The Burden of Medical Debt." Kaiser Family Foundation. https://www.kff.org/wp-content/uploads/2016/01/8806-the-burden-of-medical-debt-results-from-the-kaiser-family-foundation-new-york-times-medical-bills-survey.pdf.

Hanson, Barbara. 2003. "Questioning the Construction of Maternal Age as a Fertility Problem." *Health Care for Women International* 24 (3): 166–76. https://doi.org/10.1080/07399330390178459.

Han-soo, Lee. 2018. "CHA Medical Group Gets Majority Stake in Australian Fertility Center." *Korea Biomedical Review*, January 31. http://www.koreabiomed.com/news/articleView.html?idxno=2479.

Haraway, Donna. 2010. "When Species Meet: Staying with the Trouble." *Environment and Planning D: Society and Space* 28 (1): 53–55.

———. 2016. *Staying with the Trouble: Making Kin in the Chthulucene.* Durham, NC: Duke University Press.

Harper, Joyce, Kylie Baldwin, Lucy van de Wiel, and Jacky Boivin. 2018. "Campaign for UK Parliament to Extend the 10-Year Storage Limit on Egg Freezing: British Fertility Society." British Fertility Society. *Bionews* (blog). April 24. https://www.britishfertilitysociety.org.uk/2018/04/24/campaign-for-uk-parliament-to-extend-the-10-year-storage-limit-on-egg-freezing/.

Harper, Joyce, Emily Jackson, Karen Sermon, Robert John Aitken, Stephen Harbottle, Edgar Mocanu, Thorir Hardarson, et al. 2017. "Adjuncts in the IVF Laboratory: Where Is the Evidence for 'Add-on' Interventions?" *Human Reproduction* 32 (3): 485–91. https://doi.org/10.1093/humrep/dex004.

Harper, Sarah. 2013. *Ageing Societies.* New York: Routledge.

Harris, Lisa. 2006. "Challenging Conception: A Clinical and Cultural History of in Vitro Fertilization in the United States." PhD dissertation, Ann Arbor: University of Michigan. https://deepblue.lib.umich.edu/handle/2027.42/126046.

———. 2013. "Abortion Politics and the Production of Knowledge." *Contraception* 88 (2): 200–203. https://doi.org/10.1016/j.contraception.2013.05.013.

Harter, Lynn, Erika Kirby, Autumn Edwards, and Andrea McClanahan. 2005. "Time, Technology, and Meritocracy: The Disciplining of Women's Bodies in Narrative Constructions of Age-Related Infertility." In *Narratives, Health, and Healing: Communication Theory, Research, and Practice*, edited by Lynn Harter, Phyllis Japp, and Christina Beck, 83–106. New Jersey: Erlbaum.

Harvey, William. 1651. *Exercitationes de Generatione Animalium. Quibus Accedunt Quaedam de Partu; de Membranis Ac Humoribus Uteri; & de Conceptione.* London: Typis Du-Gardianis; Impensis O. Pulleyn. https://archive.org/details/exercitationesdeooharv.

Harwood, Karey. 2009. "Egg Freezing: A Breakthrough for Reproductive Autonomy?" *Bioethics* 23 (1): 39–46. https://doi.org/10.1111/j.1467-8519.2008.00680.x.

Hashiloni-Dolev, Yael. 2015. "Posthumous Reproduction (PHR) in Israel: Policy Rationales versus Lay People's Concerns, a Preliminary Study." *Culture, Medicine, and Psychiatry* 39 (4): 634–50. https://doi.org/10.1007/s11013-015-9447-6.

Hawkins, Jim. 2009. "Doctors as Bankers: Evidence from Fertility Markets." *Tulane Law Review* 84 (July): 841–98.

———. 2010. "Financing Fertility." *Harvard Journal on Legislation* 47: 115–66.

Hayashi, Katsuhiko, and Mitinori Saitou. 2013. "Generation of Eggs from Mouse Embryonic Stem Cells and Induced Pluripotent Stem Cells." *Nature Protocols* 8 (8): 1513–24. https://doi.org/10.1038/nprot.2013.090.

Health Council of the Netherlands. 1997. "IVF Planning Decree." Health Council of the Netherlands.

Heath, Kay. 2009. *Aging by the Book: The Emergence of Midlife in Victorian Britain.* Albany, NY: SUNY Press.

Heng, B. C. 2006. "The Advent of International 'Mail-Order' Egg Donation." *BJOG: An International Journal of Obstetrics & Gynaecology* 113 (11): 1225–27. https://doi.org/10.1111/j.1471-0528.2006.01057.x.

Herbrand, Cathy. 2019. "Mitochondrial Donation: A New Solution for Infertility in the Reproductive Bioeconomy?" Conference presentation presented at the 4S, New Orleans, September 6. https://convention2.allacademic.com/one/ssss/4s19/.

Herderscheê, Gijs. 2009. "CDA Fel Tegen Plan Eicellen." *Volkskrant*, July 14. http://www.volkskrant.nl/vk/nl/2686/Binnenland/article/detail/339393/2009/07/14/CDA-fel-tegen-plan-eicellen.dhtml.

———. 2011a. "IVF-Klinieken Wachten Met Invriezen Eicellen." *Volkskrant*, April 14. http://www.volkskrant.nl/vk/nl/2686/Binnenland/article/detail/1874879/2011/04/14/IVF-klinieken-wachten-met-invriezen-eicellen.dhtml.

———. 2011b. "PVV Is Eruit: Abortus Moet Soms Moeilijker." *Volkskrant*, April 27. http://www.volkskrant.nl/dossier-archief/pvv-is-eruit-abortus-moet-soms-moeilijker~a1881036/.

Herrmann, Janne Rothmar, and Charlotte Kroløkke. 2018. "Eggs on Ice: Imaginaries of Eggs and Cryopreservation in Denmark." *NORA—Nordic Journal of Feminist and Gender Research* 26 (1): 19–35. https://doi.org/10.1080/08038740.2018.1424727.

HFC. 2019. "United States." Human Fertility Collection. https://www.fertilitydata.org/cgi-bin/country.php?code=usa.

HFEA. 2000. "HFEA to Permit Use of Frozen Eggs in Fertility Treatment." Human Fertilisation and Embryology Authority. January 25. http://www.hfea.gov.uk/969.html.

———. 2010a. "HFEA GS Form—Your Consent to the Storage of Your Eggs or Sperm." Human Fertilisation and Embryology Authority. June 4. http://www.hfea.gov.uk/docs/HFEA_GS_form.pdf.

———. 2010b. "HFEA WD Form—Your Consent to the Use and Storage of Your Donated Eggs." Human Fertilisation and Embryology Authority. June 4. http://www.hfea.gov.uk./docs/HFEA_WD_form_new_green_ver2_Sept_09_new_file.pdf.

———. 2011. "HFEA Agrees New Policies to Improve Sperm and Egg Donation Services." Human Fertilisation and Embryology Authority. October 19. http://www.hfea.gov.uk/6700.html.

———. 2012. "Implementation of Withdrawal of Payment to Donors—HFEA Policy Reviews." Human Fertilisation and Embryology Authority. January 13. http://www.hfea.gov.uk/537.html.

———. 2014. "Egg and Sperm Donation in the UK, 2012–2013." Human Fertilisation and Embryology Authority. 2014. http://www.hfea.gov.uk/docs/Egg_and_sperm_donation_in_the_UK_2012-2013.pdf.

———. 2015. "Your Consent to Donating Your Eggs." Human Fertilisation and Embryology Authority. April 1. https://www.hfea.gov.uk/media/2755/wd-your-consent-to-donating-your-eggs.pdf.

———. 2016. *Fertility Treatment 2014: Trends and Figures*. London: Human Fertilisation and Embryology Authority. http://ifqtesting.blob.core.windows.net/umbraco-website/1111/hfea-fertility-treatment-trends-and-figures-2014.pdfnet.

———. 2017. "State of the Fertility Sector: 2016–17." Human Fertilisation and Embryology Authority. https://www.hfea.gov.uk/media/2437/hfea_state_of_the_sector_report_tagged.pdf.

———. 2018a. "Egg Freezing." Human Fertilisation and Embryology Authority. https://www.hfea.gov.uk/treatments/fertility-preservation/egg-freezing/.

———. 2018b. "Egg Freezing in Fertility Treatment Trends and Figures: 2010–2016." Human Fertilisation and Embryology Authority. https://www.hfea.gov.uk/media/2656/egg-freezing-in-fertility-treatment-trends-and-figures-2010-2016-final.pdf.

———. 2018c. "Pilot National Fertility Patient Survey." Human Fertilisation and Embryology Authority. https://www.hfea.gov.uk/media/2702/pilot-national-fertility-patient-survey-2018.pdf.

———. 2018d. "Treatment Add-Ons." Human Fertilisation and Embryology Authority. https://www.hfea.gov.uk/treatments/explore-all-treatments/treatment-add-ons/.

———. 2018e. *Fertility Treatment, 2014–2016: Trends and Figures*. London: Human Fertilisation and Embryology Authority. https://www.hfea.gov.uk/media/2563/hfea-fertility-trends-and-figures-2017-v2.pdf.

———. 2019a. "Information for Trans and Non-Binary People Seeking Fertility Treatment." Human Fertilisation and Embryology Authority. https://www.hfea.gov.uk/treatments/fertility-preservation/information-for-trans-and-non-binary-people-seeking-fertility-treatment/.

———. 2019b. "Women's Consent to the Use and Storage of Eggs or Embryos for Surrogacy." Human Fertilisation and Embryology Authority. January 2. https://www.hfea.gov.uk/media/2752/wsg-form-v6-2-january-2019.pdf.

———. 2019c. "Your Consent to the Storage of Your Eggs or Sperm." Human Fertilisation and Embryology Authority. January 2. https://www.hfea.gov.uk/media/2758/gs-form-v6-2-january-2019.pdf.

HHS. 2019. "Statement from the Department of Health and Human Services." US Department of Health & Human Services. June 5. https://www.hhs.gov/about/news/2019/06/05/statement-from-the-department-of-health-and-human-services.html.

Hildingsson, Ingegerd. 2008. "How Much Influence Do Women in Sweden Have on Caesarean Section? A Follow-up Study of Women's Preferences in Early Pregnancy." *Midwifery* 24 (1): 46–54. https://doi.org/10.1016/j.midw.2006.07.007.

Himmelstein, David U., Deborah Thorne, Elizabeth Warren, and Steffie Woolhandler. 2009. "Medical Bankruptcy in the United States, 2007." *American Journal of Medicine* 122 (8): 741–46. https://doi.org/10.1016/j.amjmed.2009.04.012.

Hochschild, Arlie. 2000. "Global Care Chains and Emotional Surplus Value." In *On the Edge: Living with Global Capitalism*, edited by W. Hutton and A. Giddens. London: Jonathan Cape.

———. 2001. "The Nanny Chain." *American Prospect*, December 19. http://prospect.org/article/nanny-chain.

Hodes-Wertz, Brooke, Sarah Druckenmiller, Meghan Smith, and Nicole Noyes. 2013. "What Do Reproductive-Age Women Who Undergo Oocyte Cryopreservation

Think about the Process as a Means to Preserve Fertility?" *Fertility and Sterility* 100 (5): 1343–1349.e2. https://doi.org/10.1016/j.fertnstert.2013.07.201.

Hogle, Linda F. 2016. "Data-Intensive Resourcing in Healthcare." *BioSocieties* 11 (3): 372–93. https://doi.org/10.1057/s41292-016-0004-5.

Homanen, Riikka. 2018. "Reproducing Whiteness and Enacting Kin in the Nordic Context of Transnational Egg Donation: Matching Donors with Cross-Border Traveller Recipients in Finland." *Social Science & Medicine* 203 (April): 28–34. https://doi.org/10.1016/j.socscimed.2018.03.012.

Hopewell, Victoria. 2014. "Funding for Freezing Your Eggs." ITunes. In Search of Fertility. June 16. https://itunes.apple.com/us/podcast/in-search-of-fertility-victoria-hopewell/id550153152?mt=2#.

Huxley, Aldous. 2007. *Brave New World*. First published 1932 by Chatto & Windus. London: Vintage Classics.

Hwang, Woo Suk, Sung Il Roh, Byeong Chun Lee, Sung Keun Kang, Dae Kee Kwon, Sue Kim, Sun Jong Kim, et al. 2005. "Patient-Specific Embryonic Stem Cells Derived from Human SCNT Blastocysts." *Science* 308 (5729): 1777–83. https://doi.org/10.1126/science.1112286.

Hwang, Woo Suk, Young June Ryu, Jong Hyuk Park, Eul Soon Park, Eu Gene Lee, Ja Min Koo, Hyun Yong Jeon, et al. 2004. "Evidence of a Pluripotent Human Embryonic Stem Cell Line Derived from a Cloned Blastocyst." *Science* 303 (5664): 1669–74. https://doi.org/10.1126/science.1094515.

Ikemoto, Lisa. 2015. "Egg Freezing, Stratified Reproduction, and the Logic of Not." *Journal of Law and the Biosciences* 2 (1): 112–17. https://doi.org/10.1093/jlb/lsu037.

Inhorn, Marcia. 2013. "Women, Consider Freezing Your Eggs." CNN. April 9. http://www.cnn.com/2013/04/09/opinion/inhorn-egg-freezing/index.html.

———. 2015. *Cosmopolitan Conceptions: IVF Sojourns in Global Dubai*. Durham, NC: Duke University Press.

———. 2017. "The Egg Freezing Revolution? Gender, Technology, and Fertility Preservation in the Twenty-First Century." In *Emerging Trends in the Social and Behavioral Sciences*. New York: Wiley. https://doi.org/10.1002/9781118900772.etrds0428.

Inhorn, Marcia, D. Birenbaum-Carmeli, J. Birger, L. Westphal, J. Doyle, N. Gleicher, D. Meirow, et al. 2018. "Elective Egg Freezing and Its Underlying Socio-Demography: A Binational Analysis with Global Implications." *Reproductive Biology and Endocrinology* 16 (1): 70. https://doi.org/10.1186/s12958-018-0389-z.

Inhorn, Marcia, and Pasquale Patrizio. 2012. "Procreative Tourism: Debating the Meaning of Cross-Border Reproductive Care in the 21st Century." *Expert Review of Obstetrics & Gynecology* 7 (6): 509–11. https://doi.org/10.1586/eog.12.56.

Inhorn, Marcia, Pasquale Patrizio, and Gamal Serour. 2010. "Third-Party Reproductive Assistance around the Mediterranean: Comparing Sunni Egypt, Catholic Italy, and Multisectarian Lebanon." *Reproductive BioMedicine Online* 21 (7): 848–53. https://doi.org/10.1016/j.rbmo.2010.09.008.

Institute of Life. 2019. "Through Pioneering Clinical Research, Institute of Life IVF Center in Greece and Embryotools in Spain Achieve Global Innovation in

Assisted Reproduction." BioSpace. April 9. https://www.biospace.com/article/
through-pioneering-clinical-research-institute-of-life-ivf-center-in-greece-and-
embryotools-in-spain-achieve-global-innovation-in-assisted-reproduction/.

Jackson, Emily. 2016. "'Social' Egg Freezing and the UK's Statutory Storage Time Limits."
Journal of Medical Ethics 42 (11): 738–41. https://doi.org/10.1136/medethics-2016-103704.

———. 2018. "The Ambiguities of 'Social' Egg Freezing and the Challenges of Informed
Consent." *BioSocieties* 13 (1): 21–40. https://doi/org/10.1057/s41292-017-0044-5.

Jacoby, Melissa B. 2009. "The Debt Financing of Parenthood." *Law and Contemporary
Problems* 72 (3): 147–75.

Jain, Tarun. 2006. "Socioeconomic and Racial Disparities among Infertility Patients
Seeking Care." *Fertility and Sterility* 85 (4): 876–81. https://doi.org/10.1016/j.
fertnstert.2005.07.1338.

Jardine, Lisa. 2012. "Chair's Letter CH(12)01." Human Fertilisation and Embryology
Authority. August 17. http://www.hfea.gov.uk/6966.html.

Jent, Karen. 2019. "Stem Cell Niches." Fieldsights: Editor's Forum; Theorizing the
Contemporary. Society for Cultural Anthropology. April 25. https://culanth.org/
fieldsights/stem-cell-niches.

Johnson, Joshua, Jacqueline Canning, Tomoko Kaneko, James K. Pru, and Jonathan L.
Tilly. 2004. "Germline Stem Cells and Follicular Renewal in the Postnatal Mammalian Ovary." *Nature* 428 (6979): 145–50. https://doi.org/10.1038/nature02316.

Kakuk, Péter. 2009. "The Legacy of the Hwang Case: Research Misconduct in
Biosciences." *Science and Engineering Ethics* 15 (4): 545. https://doi.org/10.1007/
s11948-009-9121-x.

Kang, Eunju, Xinjian Wang, Rebecca Tippner-Hedges, Hong Ma, Clifford Folmes,
Nuria Marti Gutierrez, Yeonmi Lee, et al. 2016. "Age-Related Accumulation of So-
matic Mitochondrial DNA Mutations in Adult-Derived Human IPSCs." *Cell Stem
Cell* 18 (5): 625–36. https://doi.org/10.1016/j.stem.2016.02.005.

Kasperkevic, Jana. 2016. "'Eggs in the Bank': How One Clinic Is Making Egg Freezing
Less Expensive." *Guardian*, August 20. http://www.theguardian.com/business/2016/
aug/20/egg-freezing-less-expensive-extend-fertility-clinic.

Kaufman, Sharon. 2015. *Ordinary Medicine: Extraordinary Treatments, Longer Lives,
and Where to Draw the Line*. Durham, NC: Duke University Press.

Kbhandal. 2013a. "Baby Eeva Video—Eeva." Early Embryo Viability Assessment Test.
June 14. http://www.eevaivf.com/video-of-eeva-conception/.

———. 2013b. "Baby Eva Named after Pioneering IVF Test—Eeva." Early
Embryo Viability Assessment Test. June 14. http://www.eevaivf.com/
baby-eva-named-after-pioneering-ivf-test/.

Kelhä, Minna. 2009. "Too Old to Become a Mother? Risk Constructions in 35+
Women's Experiences of Pregnancy, Child-Birth, and Postnatal Care." *NORA—
Nordic Journal of Feminist and Gender Research* 17 (2): 89–103. https://doi.
org/10.1080/08038740902885722.

Kerr, Dara. 2017. "Egg Freezing, So Hot Right Now." CNET. May 22. https://www.cnet.
com/news/egg-freezing-so-hot-right-now/.

Kikuchi, Iwaho, Noriko Kagawa, Yuka Shirosaki, Ikumi Shinozaki, Yasuka Miyakuni, Kyoko Oshina, Michio Nojima, and Koyo Yoshida. 2018. "Early Outcomes of a Municipally Funded Oocyte Cryopreservation Programme in Japan." *Human Fertility*, April 1–7. https://doi.org/10.1080/14647273.2018.1464215.

Kim, Leo. 2008. "Explaining the Hwang Scandal: National Scientific Culture and Its Global Relevance." *Science as Culture* 17 (4): 397–415. https://doi.org/10.1080/09505430802515023.

Kindbody. 2018. "Egg Freezing." Kindbody. https://kindbody.com/egg-freezing/.

———. 2019. "Kindbody—The Future of Women's Health, Fertility, and Wellness." Kindbody. https://kindbody.com/.

Kitazato. 2019. "Vitrification Cryotop." Kitazato and Dibimed. https://www.kitazato-dibimed.com/cryotop-vitrification/.

Klitzman, Robert, and Mark Sauer. 2009. "Payment of Egg Donors in Stem Cell Research in the USA." *Reproductive BioMedicine Online* 18 (5): 603–8. https://doi.org/10.1016/S1472-6483(10)60002-8.

Knill, Christoph, Caroline Preidel, and Kerstin Nebel. 2014. "Brake Rather Than Barrier: The Impact of the Catholic Church on Morality Policies in Western Europe." *West European Politics* 37 (5): 845–66. https://doi.org/10.1080/01402382.2014.909170.

Kondapalli, Laxmi A. 2012. "Ovarian Tissue Cryopreservation and Transplantation." In *Oncofertility Medical Practice: Clinical Issues and Implementation*, edited by C. Gracia and T. K. Woodruff, 63–75. New York: Springer Science+Business Media. http://oncofertility.northwestern.edu/sites/oncofertility.northwestern.edu/files/uploadedfilecontent/ovarian_tissue_cryopreservation_and_transplantation_-_laxmi_a._kondapalli.pdf.

Kopaylopa. 2015. "First Post." *Attempting Single Motherhood* (blog). October 18. http://attemptingsinglemotherhood.blogspot.com/2015/10/first-post.html.

Kortman, M., G. De Wert, B. Fauser, and N. Macklon. 2006. "Zwangerschap Op Oudere Leeftijd Door Middel van Eiceldonatie." *Nederlands Tijdschrift Voor Geneeskunde* 150 (47): 2591–95.

Kowal, Emma, and Joanna Radin. 2015. "Indigenous Biospecimen Collections and the Cryopolitics of Frozen Life." *Journal of Sociology* 51 (1): 63–80. https://doi.org/10.1177/1440783314562316.

Kroløkke, Charlotte. 2018. *Global Fluids: The Cultural Politics of Reproductive Waste and Value*. New York: Berghahn Books.

Kuhn, Annette. 2010. "Memory Texts and Memory Work: Performances of Memory in and with Visual Media." *Memory Studies* 3 (4): 298–313. https://doi.org/10.1177/1750698010370034.

Kuleshova, Lilia, Luca Gianaroli, Cristina Magli, Anna Ferraretti, and Alan Trounson. 1999. "Birth Following Vitrification of a Small Number of Human Oocytes: Case Report." *Human Reproduction* 14 (12): 3077–79. https://doi.org/10.1093/humrep/14.12.3077.

Kupka, M., A. Ferraretti, J. de Mouzon, K. Erb, T. D'Hooghe, J. Castilla, C. Calhaz-Jorge, et al. 2014. "Assisted Reproductive Technology in Europe, 2010: Results Generated from European Registers by ESHRE." *Human Reproduction* 29 (10): 2099–2113. https://doi.org/10.1093/humrep/deu175.

Kuwayama, Masashige, Gábor Vajta, Osamu Kato, and Stanley Leibo. 2005. "Highly Efficient Vitrification Method for Cryopreservation of Human Oocytes." *Reproductive BioMedicine Online* 11 (3): 300–308.

Lacey, Sheryl de. 2005. "Parent Identity and 'Virtual' Children: Why Patients Discard Rather Than Donate Unused Embryos." *Human Reproduction* 20 (6): 1661–69. https://doi.org/10.1093/humrep/deh831.

Lafontaine, Céline. 2009. "Regenerative Medicine's Immortal Body: From the Fight against Ageing to the Extension of Longevity." *Body & Society* 15 (4): 53–71. https://doi.org/10.1177/1357034X09347223.

LaFrenz, Carrie. 2018. "Virtus Health Says Artificial Intelligence Has Potential to Make IVF Babies." *Financial Review*, June 27. https://www.afr.com/business/health/virtus-health-says-artificial-intelligence-has-potential-to-make-ivf-babies-20180627-h11xpl.

Lahad, Kinneret. 2012. "Singlehood, Waiting, and the Sociology of Time." *Sociological Forum* 27 (1): 163–86. https://doi.org/10.1111/j.1573-7861.2011.01306.x.

———. 2014. "The Single Woman's Choice as a Zero-Sum Game." *Cultural Studies* 28 (2): 240–66. https://doi.org/10.1080/09502386.2013.798341.

———. 2016. "Stop Waiting! Hegemonic and Alternative Scripts of Single Women's Subjectivity." *Time & Society*, April. https://doi.org/10.1177/0961463X16639324.

Landau, Elizabeth. 2014. "Cloning Used to Make Stem Cells from Adult Humans." CNN. April 28. http://www.cnn.com/2014/04/28/health/stem-cell-breakthrough/index.html.

Landecker, Hannah. 2006. "Microcinematography and the History of Science and Film." *Isis* 97 (1): 121–32. https://doi.org/10.1086/501105.

———. 2007. *Culturing Life: How Cells Became Technologies*. Cambridge, MA: Harvard University Press.

Lee, Ah-Reum, Kwonho Hong, Seo Hye Choi, Chanhyeok Park, Jae-Kyun Park, Jin-Il Lee, Jae Il Bang, Dong-Won Seol, Jeoung-Eun Lee, and Dong-Ryul Lee. 2019. "Anti-Apoptotic Regulation Contributes to the Successful Nuclear Reprogramming Using Cryopreserved Oocytes." *Stem Cell Reports* 12 (3): 545–56. https://doi.org/10.1016/j.stemcr.2019.01.019.

Lee, Bruce. 2016. "Mercer Forms Strategic Alliance with Progyny." Mercer. January 7. https://www.mercer.com/newsroom/mercer-progyny-alliance.html.

Lee, Claire. 2018. "More Korean Women Choose to Freeze Their Eggs." *Korea Herald*. October 23. http://www.koreaherald.com/view.php?ud=20181023000585.

Lee, Katarina. 2018. "An Ethical and Legal Analysis of Ovascience—A Publicly Traded Fertility Company and Its Lead Product, AUGMENT." *American Journal of Law & Medicine* 44 (4): 508–28. https://doi.org/10.1177/0098858818821135.

Leeming, David. 2005. *The Oxford Companion to World Mythology*. New York: Oxford University Press.

Lemke, Thomas. 2011. *Biopolitics: An Advanced Introduction*. New York: NYU Press.

Lesnik-Oberstein, Karín. 2008. *On Having an Own Child: Reproductive Technologies and the Cultural Construction of Childhood*. London: Karnac Books.

Lezaun, Javier. 2013. "The Escalating Politics of 'Big Biology.'" *BioSocieties* 8 (December): 480–85. https://doi.org/10.1057/biosoc.2013.30.

Lichtenstein, Bronwen, and Joe Weber. 2016. "Losing Ground: Racial Disparities in Medical Debt and Home Foreclosure in the Deep South." *Family & Community Health* 39 (3): 178–87.

Lijing, Jiang. 2010. "Advanced Cell Technology, Inc." The Embryo Project Encyclopedia. June 25. https://embryo.asu.edu/pages/advanced-cell-technology-inc.

Linders, Annulla. 1998. "Abortion as a Social Problem: The Construction of 'Opposite' Solutions in Sweden and the United States." *Social Problems* 45 (4): 488–509. https://doi.org/10.2307/3097209.

Lock, Margaret. 1995. *Encounters with Aging: Mythologies of Menopause in Japan and North America*. Berkeley: University of California Press.

———. 2003. "On Making up the Good-as-Dead in a Utilitarian World." In *Remaking Life & Death: Toward an Anthropology of the Biosciences*, edited by Sarah Franklin and Margaret Lock, 165–92. Santa Fe, NM: School of American Research Press.

Loe, Meika. 2006. *The Rise of Viagra: How the Little Blue Pill Changed Sex in America*. New York: NYU Press.

Luciano, Dana. 2007. *Arranging Grief: Sacred Time and the Body in Nineteenth-Century America*. New York: NYU Press.

Luijt, Marleen. 2010. "Ik Heb Mijn Kop Weer Uit Het Zand." *NRC Next*, October 29.

Ma, Hong, Ryan O'Neil, Nuria Marti-Gutierrez, Manoj Hariharan, Zhuzhu Zhang, Yupeng He, Cengiz Cinnioglu, et al. 2017. "Functional Human Oocytes Generated by Transfer of Polar Body Genomes." *Cell Stem Cell* 20 (1): 112–19. https://doi.org/10.1016/j.stem.2016.10.001.

Mack, Heather. 2016. "Progyny Rebrands, Launches New Website for Fertility Health Services." MobiHealthNews. October 19. http://www.mobihealthnews.com/content/progyny-rebrands-launches-new-website-fertility-health-services.

Maguire, Laurie. 2009. *Helen of Troy: From Homer to Hollywood*. Southern Gate, Chichester: Wiley-Blackwell. http://onlinelibrary.wiley.com/doi/10.1002/9781444308624.ch/summary.

Maheshwari, Abha, Maureen Porter, Ashalata Shetty, and Siladitya Bhattacharya. 2008. "Women's Awareness and Perceptions of Delay in Childbearing." *Fertility and Sterility* 90 (4): 1036–42. https://doi.org/10.1016/j.fertnstert.2007.07.1338.

Mann, Alice. 2014. "Eggs or Embryos?" *Egged On* (blog). May 17. https://eggedonblog.com/2014/05/17/eggs-or-embryos/.

———. 2015a. "In a Year's Time . . ." *Egged On* (blog). March 18. https://eggedonblog.com/2015/03/18/in-a-years-time/.

———. 2015b. "What Am I Waiting For?" *Egged On* (blog). July 30. https://eggedonblog.com/2015/07/30/what-am-i-waiting-for/.

———. 2016a. "Permission to Procrastinate . . ." *Egged On* (blog). April 10. https://eggedonblog.com/2016/04/10/permission-to-procrastinate/.

———. 2016b. "A, B, C . . ." *Egged On* (blog). October 21. https://eggedonblog.com/2016/10/21/a-b-c/.

———. 2016c. "Defrosting . . ." *Egged On* (blog). November 20. https://eggedonblog.com/2016/11/20/defrosting/.

———. 2016d. "Emotional Fuckwittery . . ." *Egged On* (blog). December 31. https://eggedonblog.com/2016/12/31/emotional-fuckwittery/.

———. 2017a. "Doing Things Differently . . ." *Egged On* (blog). February 6. https://eggedonblog.com/2017/02/06/doing-things-differently/.

———. 2017b. "Little Victories . . . and Little Disappointments. . . ." *Egged On* (blog). March 5. https://eggedonblog.com/2017/03/05/little-victories-and-little-disappointments/.

Manna, Claudio, Loris Nanni, Alessandra Lumini, and Sebastiana Pappalardo. 2013. "Artificial Intelligence Techniques for Embryo and Oocyte Classification." *Reproductive BioMedicine Online* 26 (1): 42–49. https://doi.org/10.1016/j.rbmo.2012.09.015.

Market Cube. 2015. "Fertility Treatments in the United States: Sentiment, Costs, and Financial Impact." *Prosper* (blog). May 20. https://blog.prosper.com/2015/05/20/fertility-treatments-in-the-united-states-sentiment-costs-and-financial-impact/.

Martin, Emily. 2001. *The Woman in the Body: A Cultural Analysis of Reproduction.* Boston: Beacon.

Martin, Joyce, Brady Hamilton, Michelle Osterman, Anne Driscoll, and T. Mathews. 2017. "Births: Final Data for 2015." *National Vital Statistics Reports* 66 (1): 1–70.

Martin, Lauren Jade. 2010. "Anticipating Infertility: Egg Freezing, Genetic Preservation, and Risk." *Gender & Society* 24 (4): 526–45. https://doi.org/10.1177/0891243210377172.

———. 2017. "Pushing for the Perfect Time: Social and Biological Fertility." *Women's Studies International Forum* 62 (Supplement C): 91–98. https://doi.org/10.1016/j.wsif.2017.04.004.

Martin, Neil. 2018. "UNSW Student's Pioneering Artificial Intelligence Boosts IVF Success." Text. UNSW Newsroom. July 4. https://newsroom.unsw.edu.au.

Matoba, Shogo, and Yi Zhang. 2018. "Somatic Cell Nuclear Transfer Reprogramming: Mechanisms and Applications." *Cell Stem Cell* 23 (4): 471–85. https://doi.org/10.1016/j.stem.2018.06.018.

Mazur, Pavlo, Lada Dyachenko, Viktor Veselovskyy, Yuliya Masliy, Maksym Borysov, Dmytro O. Mykytenko, and Valery Zukin. 2019. "Mitochondrial Replacement Theraphy [sic] Give [sic] No Benefits to Patients of Advanced Maternal Age." *Fertility and Sterility* 112 (3): e193. https://doi.org/10.1016/j.fertnstert.2019.07.623.

McAuliffe, Naomi. 2012. "Egg Freezing—for the Woman Who Can Never Win." *Guardian*, November 27. http://www.guardian.co.uk/commentisfree/2012/nov/27/egg-freezing-women-having-children.

McCormack, Donna, and Suvi Salmenniemi. 2016. "The Biopolitics of Precarity and the Self." *European Journal of Cultural Studies* 19 (1): 3–15. https://doi.org/10.1177/1367549415585559.

McGee, Suzanne. 2014. "Silicon Valley Tries Egg-Freezing Perks: How About Just Hiring More Women?" *Guardian*, October 19, sec. Money.

https://www.theguardian.com/money/us-money-blog/2014/oct/19/silicon-valley-egg-freezing-perks-hiring-women.

McGinley, Ann. 2016. "Subsidized Egg Freezing in Employment: Autonomy, Coercion, or Discrimination." *Employee Rights and Employment Policy Journal* 20: 331–64.

MCK. 2014. "Behandelovereenkomst Cryopreservatie Eicellen." Medisch Centrum Kinderwens. Informed consent contract, in author's possession.

Mediatique. 2018. "Overview of Recent Dynamics in the UK Press Market." London: Mediatique. https://assets.publishing.service.gov.uk/government/uploads/system/uploads/attachment_data/file/720400/180621_Mediatique_-_Overview_of_recent_dynamics_in_the_UK_press_market_-_Report_for_DCMS.pdf.

Menken, J., J. Trussell, and U. Larsen. 1986. "Age and Infertility." *Science* 233 (4771): 1389–94. https://doi.org/10.1126/science.3755843.

Mercer. 2016. "Mercer Survey: Health Benefit Cost Growth Slows to 2.4% in 2016 as Enrollment in High-Deductible Plans Climbs." Mercer. October 26. https://www.mercer.com/newsroom/national-survey-of-employer-sponsored-health-plans-2016.html.

Merck. 2011. "Fertility Research Policy." September. http://www.merckgroup.com/company.merck.de/en/images/FertilityResearchPolicy_EN_tcm1612_105601.pdf?Version=.

———. 2015. "The Eeva™ Test." Merck. November 2015. https://www.professionalsinfertility.com/en_GB/our-fertility-news-technology/the-eeva-test.html.

———. 2016. "Fertility—Merck Biopharma." Merck Biopharma. May 9. http://biopharma.merckgroup.com/en/products/fertility/fertility.html.

———. 2018. "Merck Launches Two New Technologies for Improved Efficiency in Fertility Labs." Merck Fertility. July 8. https://www.merckgroup.com/en/news/improved-efficiency-fertility-02-07-2018.html.

Merleau-Ponty, Noémie. 2019. "A Hierarchy of Deaths: Stem Cells, Animals, and Humans Understood by Developmental Biologists." *Science as Culture*, March, 1–21. https://doi.org/10.1080/09505431.2019.1579787.

Mertes, Heidi, and Guido Pennings. 2011. "Social Egg Freezing: For Better, Not for Worse." *Reproductive BioMedicine Online* 23 (7): 824–29. https://doi.org/10.1016/j.rbmo.2011.09.010.

Miller, Claire Cain. 2018a. "Freezing Eggs as Part of Employee Benefits: Some Women See Darker Message." *New York Times*, March 14, sec. The Upshot. https://www.nytimes.com/2014/10/15/upshot/egg-freezing-as-a-work-benefit-some-women-see-darker-message.html.

———. 2018b. "Americans Are Having Fewer Babies: They Told Us Why." *New York Times*, July 7, sec. The Upshot. https://www.nytimes.com/2018/07/05/upshot/americans-are-having-fewer-babies-they-told-us-why.html.

Mills, Tracey, Rebecca Lavender, and Tina Lavender. 2015. "'Forty Is the New Twenty': An Analysis of British Media Portrayals of Older Mothers." *Sexual & Reproductive Healthcare* 6 (2): 88–94. https://doi.org/10.1016/j.srhc.2014.10.005.

Mills, Tracey A., and Tina Lavender. 2011. "Advanced Maternal Age." *Obstetrics, Gynaecology & Reproductive Medicine* 21 (4): 107–11. https://doi.org/10.1016/j.ogrm.2010.12.003.

Minter, Harriet. 2014. "By Offering to Freeze Their Employees' Eggs, Apple and Facebook Make It Clear They Don't Know What Women Want." *Guardian*, October 15, sec. Women in Leadership. https://www.theguardian.com/women-in-leadership/2014/oct/15/apple-facebook-egg-freezing-employee-perk.

Mladovsky, Philipa, and Corinna Sorenson. 2010. "Public Financing of IVF: A Review of Policy Rationales." *Health Care Analysis* 18 (2): 113–28. https://doi.org/10.1007/s10728-009-0114-3.

Monk, Daniel. 2014. "The Pleasures and Perils of Inheritance." *Studies in Gender and Sexuality* 15 (3): 239–43. https://doi.org/10.1080/15240657.2014.939026.

Montag, Markus. 2015. "How a Decision Support Tool Based on Known Implantation Data Can Enhance Embryo Selection." Vitrolife. August 20. http://blog.vitrolife.com/togetheralltheway/how-a-decision-support-tool-based-on-known-implantation-data-can-enhance-embryo-selection.

Moore, Lisa Jean. 2003. "'Billy, the Sad Sperm with No Tail': Representations of Sperm in Children's Books." *Sexualities* 6 (3–4): 277–300. https://doi.org/10.1177/136346070363002.

Moscucci, Ornella. 1993. *The Science of Woman: Gynaecology and Gender in England, 1800–1929*. Cambridge: Cambridge University Press.

Mr & Mrs M vs HFEA. 2016. [2016] EWCA Civ 611 United Kingdom, Court of Appeal. In the Court of Appeal (civil division). On appeal from The High Court of Justice Queen's Bench Division Administrative court. Mr Justice Ouseley CO30772014.

Mukherjee, Manjeer, and Sarojini Nadimipally. 2006. "Assisted Reproductive Technologies in India." *Development* 49 (4): 128–34. https://doi.org/10.1057/palgrave.development.1100303.

Mulkerrins, Jane. 2017. "Elisabeth Moss on *The Handmaid's Tale*: 'It Is a Feminist Story.'" *Guardian*, June 10, sec. Television & Radio. https://www.theguardian.com/tv-and-radio/2017/jun/10/elisabeth-moss-handmaids-tale-feminist-story.

Mullin, Emily. 2019a. "Pregnancy Reported in the First Trial of 'Three-Person IVF' for Infertility." *STAT* (blog). January 24. https://www.statnews.com/2019/01/24/first-trial-of-three-person-ivf-for-infertility/.

———. 2019b. "Proponents Start Push to Lift U.S. Ban on 'Three-Parent IVF.'" *STAT* (blog). April 16. https://www.statnews.com/2019/04/16/mitochondrial-replacement-three-parent-ivf-ban/.

———. 2019c. "Controversial '3-Parent Baby' Fertility Technique Fails to Deliver for Older Women." Medium. October 15. https://onezero.medium.com/controversial-3-parent-baby-fertility-technique-fails-to-deliver-for-older-women-1d20d2256767.

Murphy, Heather. 2018. "Lots of Successful Women Are Freezing Their Eggs: But It May Not Be about Their Careers." *New York Times*, September 10, sec. Health. https://www.nytimes.com/2018/07/03/health/freezing-eggs-women.html.

Murphy, Michelle. 2011. "Distributed Reproduction." In *Corpus: An Interdisciplinary Reader on Bodies and Knowledge*, edited by Monica J. Casper and Paisley Currah. New York: Palgrave Macmillan.

———. 2017. *The Economization of Life*. Durham, NC: Duke University Press.

Murray, Clare, and Susan Golombok. 2003. "To Tell or Not to Tell: The Decision-Making Process of Egg-Donation Parents." *Human Fertility* 6 (2): 89–95. https://doi.org/10.1080/1464770312331369123.

Myung, Jin-Sook. 2006. "Stem Cell Research and Women." In *Envisioning the Human Rights of Women in the Age of Biotechnology and Science*. Seoul, Korea. http://2006forum.womenlink.or.kr/Myung20060921.pdf.

Nahman, Michal. 2018. "Migrant Extractability: Centring the Voices of Egg Providers in Cross-Border Reproduction." *Reproductive Biomedicine & Society Online*, Symposium: Making Families—Transnational Surrogacy, Queer Kinship, and Reproductive Justice, 7 (November): 82–90. https://doi.org/10.1016/j.rbms.2018.10.020.

National Research Council. 2005. *Guidelines for Human Embryonic Stem Cell Research*. Washington, DC: National Academies Press. http://www.nap.edu/catalog.php?record_id=11278.

———. 2008. *2008 Amendments to the National Academies' Guidelines for Human Embryonic Stem Cell Research*. Washington, DC: National Academies Press. https://doi.org/10.17226/12260.

Neilson, Brett. 2003. "Globalization and the Biopolitics of Aging." *CR: The New Centennial Review* 3 (2): 161–86. https://doi.org/10.1353/ncr.2003.0025.

NHS Choices. 2013. "IVF—NHS Choices." NHS Choices. October 15. http://www.nhs.uk/Conditions/IVF/Pages/Introduction.aspx.

NICE. 2013. "Fertility: Assessment and Treatment for People with Fertility Problems; NICE Clinical Guideline." London: Royal College of Obstetricians and Gynaecologists. http://www.nice.org.uk/nicemedia/live/14078/62770/62770.pdf.

Nightlight Christian Adoptions. 2015. "Snowflakes Embryo Adoption and Donation—Snowflake Babies!" Nightlight Christian Adoptions. https://www.nightlight.org/snowflakes-embryo-donation-adoption/.

NOM. 2019. "NOM Mediamerken 2019-III." NOM Dashboard. https://dundasbi.reports.nl/NOM/Dashboard/Dashboard?guidinput=cc9f473d-5c10-46fa-ba36-fc5abbc587e0.

Nowak, Rachel. 2007. "A Reproductive Revolution." *New Scientist* 193 (2596): 8–9. https://doi.org/10.1016/S0262-4079(07)60707-6.

NVOG. 2010. "Addendum Bij NVOG/KLEM Standpunt 'Vitrificatie van Humane Eicellen En Embryo's.'" Utrecht: Nederlandse Vereniging voor Obstetrie en Gynaecologie. http://www.nvog-documenten.nl/index.php?pagina=/richtlijn/item/pagina.php&richtlijn_id=803.

———. 2016. "Standpunt: Geassisteerde voortplanting met gedoneerde gameten en gedoneerde embryo's en draagmoederschap." Utrecht: Nederlandse Vereniging voor Obstetrie en Gynaecologie. http://www.nvog-documenten.nl/uploaded/docs/standpunt%20geassisteerde%20voortplanting%20met%20gedoneerde%20gameten,%20gedoneerde%20embryos%20en%20draagmoederschap%20ws.pdf.

NVOG & KLEM. 2018. "Modelreglement Embryowet." Nederlandse Vereniging voor Obstetrie en Gynaecologie en Vereniging voor Klinische Embryologie. https://

www.rijksoverheid.nl/binaries/rijksoverheid/documenten/richtlijnen/2018/08/27/
modelreglement-embryowet/modelreglement-embryowet.pdf.

O'Brien, Y., C. Kelleher, and M. Wingfield. 2018. "The Psychological and Emotional Impact of AMH Testing." *Fertility and Sterility* 110 (4): e323. https://doi.org/10.1016/j.fertnstert.2018.07.909.

Ocata. 2015. "RPE Cell Therapy." Ocata Therapeutics. https://www.ocata.com/research-development/regenerative-ophthalmology/rpe-cell-therapy.

OED. 2019. "Precarious, Adj." *Oxford English Dictionary*. https://www.oed.com/viewdictionaryentry/Entry/149548.

Office of the Press Secretary. 2005. "President Discusses Embryo Adoption and Ethical Stem Cell Research." The White House. May 24. https://georgewbush-whitehouse.archives.gov/news/releases/2005/05/20050524-12.html.

OHSU Center for Women's Health. 2015a. "Women's Health Research Unit | About Us." Oregon Health & Science University. 2015. http://www.ohsu.edu.

———. 2015b. "Women's Health Research Unit | Clinical Trials." Oregon Health & Science University. http://www.ohsu.edu/xd/health/services/women/clinical-trials/.

O'Kelly, Lisa. 2005. "This Was Plan B, Actually." *Guardian*. December 6. https://www.theguardian.com/lifeandstyle/2005/dec/04/familyandrelationships.features.

Oktay, K., B. A. Aydin, K. Economos, and J. Rucinski. 2000. "Restoration of Ovarian Function after Autologous Transplantation of Human Ovarian Tissue in the Forearm." *Fertility and Sterility* 74 (3): S90–91. https://doi.org/10.1016/S0015-0282(00)00967-5.

Oliver, Kelly. 2010. "Motherhood, Sexuality, and Pregnant Embodiment: Twenty-Five Years of Gestation." *Hypatia* 25 (4): 760–77.

ONS. 2016. "Births by Parents' Characteristics in England and Wales." Office for National Statistics. November 29. https://www.ons.gov.uk/peoplepopulationandcommunity/birthsdeathsandmarriages/livebirths/bulletins/birthsbyparentscharacteristicsinenglandandwales/2015.

Oudshoorn, Nelly. 1994. *Beyond the Natural Body: An Archaeology of Sex Hormones*. London: Routledge.

Pacheco, Fernanda, and Kutluk Oktay. 2017. "Current Success and Efficiency of Autologous Ovarian Transplantation: A Meta-Analysis." *Reproductive Sciences* 24 (8): 1111–20. https://doi.org/10.1177/1933719117702251.

Paik, Young-Gyung. 2010. "Return of the Sibaji?" *Asian Women* 26 (3): 73–92.

Pande, Amrita. 2011. "Transnational Commercial Surrogacy in India: Gifts for Global Sisters?" *Reproductive BioMedicine Online* 23 (5): 618–25. https://doi.org/10.1016/j.rbmo.2011.07.007.

Parreñas, Rhacel Salazar. 2000. "Migrant Filipina Domestic Workers and the International Division of Reproductive Labor." *Gender & Society* 14 (4): 560–80. https://doi.org/10.1177/089124300014004005.

Pavone, Vincenzo, and Sarah Lafuente Funes. 2017. "Selecting What? Pre-Implantation Genetic Diagnosis and Screening Trajectories in Spain." In *Selective Reproduction in the 21st Century*, edited by Ayo Wahlberg and Tine M. Gammeltoft. Switzerland: Palgrave Macmillan.

Payne, Jenny Gunnarsson. 2013. "Reproduction in Transition: Cross-Border Egg Donation, Biodesirability, and New Reproductive Subjectivities on the European Fertility Market." *Gender, Place & Culture* 22 (1): 1–16. https://doi.org/10.1080/0966 369X.2013.832656.

Peeren, Esther. 2007. *Intersubjectivities and Popular Culture: Bakhtin and Beyond*. Stanford, CA: Stanford University Press.

Pennings, G., G. de Wert, F. Shenfield, J. Cohen, P. Devroey, and B. Tarlatzis. 2006. "ESHRE Task Force on Ethics and Law 11: Posthumous Assisted Reproduction." *Human Reproduction* 21 (12): 3050–53. https://doi.org/10.1093/humrep/del287.

Petchesky, Rosalind Pollack. 1987. "Fetal Images: The Power of Visual Culture in the Politics of Reproduction." *Feminist Studies* 13 (2): 263–92.

Pew Research Center. 2014. "Where *New York Times*'s Audience Fits on the Political Spectrum." *Pew Research Center's Journalism Project* (blog). October 21. http://www.journalism.org/interactives/media-polarization/outlet/new-york-times/.

Pfeffer, Naomi. 2011. "Eggs-Ploiting Women: A Critical Feminist Analysis of the Different Principles in Transplant and Fertility Tourism." *Reproductive BioMedicine Online* 23 (5): 634–41. https://doi.org/10.1016/j.rbmo.2011.08.005.

Pickard, Susan. 2018. *Age, Gender, and Sexuality through the Life Course: The Girl in Time*. London: Routledge

Plunkett, Jack. 2008. *Plunkett's Biotech & Genetics Industry Almanac 2009*. Houston, TX: Plunkett Research.

Pollock, Anne. 2003. "Complicating Power in High-Tech Reproduction: Narratives of Anonymous Paid Egg Donors." *Journal of Medical Humanities* 24 (3–4): 241–63.

Pompei, Marybeth, and Francesco Pompei. 2019. "Overcoming Bioethical, Legal, and Hereditary Barriers to Mitochondrial Replacement Therapy in the USA." *Journal of Assisted Reproduction and Genetics* 36 (3): 383–93. https://doi.org/10.1007/s10815-018-1370-7.

Powell, Jason L. 2010. "The Ageing Body: From Bio-Medical Fatalism to Understanding Gender and Biographical Sensitivity." In *Culture, Bodies, and the Sociology of Health*, edited by Elizabeth Ettorre. Farnham, UK: Ashgate.

Prelude Fertility. 2015. *Martin Varsavsky on Prelude at SIME Miami 2015*. Miami. https://www.youtube.com/watch?v=I_a4Pwwusaw&t=515s.

———. 2016. "Press Pause." Prelude Fertility, Inc. https://www.preludefertility.com/save/.

———. 2017a. "Prelude Fertility." Prelude Fertility, Inc. https://www.preludefertility.com/.

———. 2017b. "Prelude Fertility Expands Network with Pacific Fertility Center in San Francisco." PR Newswire. September 25. https://www.prnewswire.com/news-releases/prelude-fertility-expands-network-with-pacific-fertility-center-in-san-francisco-300524534.html.

———. 2018a. "About—Prelude Fertility." Prelude Fertility, Inc. https://preludefertility.com/about.

———. 2018b. "Options Preserved—Freeze Your Eggs and Have a Baby Now or Later." Prelude Fertility, Inc. https://www.preludefertility.com/freeze-eggs.

Pribenszky, Csaba, Anna-Maria Nilselid, and Markus Montag. 2017. "Time-Lapse Culture with Morphokinetic Embryo Selection Improves Pregnancy and Live Birth Chances and Reduces Early Pregnancy Loss: A Meta-Analysis." *Reproductive Bio-Medicine Online* 35 (5): 511–20. https://doi.org/10.1016/j.rbmo.2017.06.022.

ProFaM. 2019. "ProFaM—Fertility Preservation and Menopause Delay." ProFam. http://www.profam.co.uk/.

Progyny. 2017. "Progyny Raises $10 Million to Support Strong Growth of Fertility Benefits Business." Progyny. May 2. https://progyny.com/wp-content/uploads/2017/09/2017.05.02-Progyny-Raises-10-Million-to-Support-Strong-Growth-of-Fertility-Benefits-Business.pdf.

———. 2019a. "For Providers—Overview." *Progyny* (blog). https://progyny.com/for-providers/.

———. 2019b. "Preliminary Prospectus—Initial Public Offering—Progyny, Inc." Securities and Exchange Commission. October 15. https://www.sec.gov/Archives/edgar/data/1551306/000104746919005727/a2239825zs-1a.htm.

Prothero, Richard. 2013. "Total Household Wealth by Region and Age Group." Office for National Statistics, Regional Economic Analysis. June 4. http://www.ons.gov.uk/ons/rel/regional-trends/regional-economic-analysis/wealth-by-age-group-and-region--june-2013/rep-total-household-wealth-by-region-and-age-group.html.

Qualtrough, Stuart. 1998. "Conceived in the Back of Our Old Maestro: Amazing Story of Mum, 60; Britain's Oldest Mum Tells How Her Baby Was Concieved [sic] in the Back of a Maestro Van." *The People*, January 18.

Radin, Joanna. 2013. "Latent Life: Concepts and Practices of Human Tissue Preservation in the International Biological Program." *Social Studies of Science* 43 (4): 484–508. https://doi.org/10.1177/0306312713476131.

Ramsing, Niels. 2016. "Clinical Relevance of Time-Lapse." Vitrolife. September 20. http://www.vitrolife.com/Global/Corporate/Investors/CMD%202016-09/CEO%20presentation.pdf.

Reijo Pera, Renee A. 2013. "More Than Just a Matter of Time." *Reproductive BioMedicine Online* 27 (2): 113–14. https://doi.org/10.1016/j.rbmo.2013.05.010.

Reno, Jamie. 2017. "Is Human Embryonic Stem Cell Research in Jeopardy?" Healthline. June 14. https://www.healthline.com/health-news/is-human-embryonic-stem-cell-research-in-jeopardy.

Republic of Korea. 2008. "Bioethics and Safety Act." National Law Information Centre. http://law.go.kr/LSW/eng/engLsSc.do?menuId=2&section=lawNm&query=bioethics&x=0&y=0#liBgcolor5.

———. 2009. "Enforcement Decree of Bioethics and Safety Act." National Law Information Centre. http://law.go.kr/LSW/eng/engLsSc.do?menuId=2&section=lawNm&query=bioethics&x=0&y=0#liBgcolor8.

——. 2014. "Enforcement Decree of Bioethics and Safety Act." National Law Information Centre. http://law.go.kr/LSW/eng/engLsSc.do?menuId=2&section=lawNm&query=bioethics&x=0&y=0#liBgcolor11.

Richards, Sarah Elizabeth. 2013. *Motherhood, Rescheduled: The New Frontier of Egg Freezing and the Women Who Tried It*. New York: Simon & Schuster.

——. 2014. "Don't Depend on Those Frozen Eggs." *New York Times*, March 14, sec. Opinion. https://www.nytimes.com/2014/10/17/opinion/dont-depend-on-those-frozen-eggs.html.

Ridley, Jane. 2014. "Career Women Are Having 'Egg-Freezing' Parties." *New York Post*, August 14. http://nypost.com/2014/08/13/nyc-career-women-gather-at-egg-freezing-party/.

Riley, James. 2005. "Estimates of Regional and Global Life Expectancy, 1800–2001." *Population and Development Review* 31 (3): 537–43. https://doi.org/10.1111/j.1728-4457.2005.00083.x.

Robbins. 2017. "Investors See Big Money in Infertility. And They're Transforming the Industry." STAT. December 4. https://www.statnews.com/2017/12/04/infertility-industry-investment/.

Roberts, Celia, and Karen Throsby. 2008. "Paid to Share: IVF Patients, Eggs, and Stem Cell Research." *Social Science & Medicine* 66 (1): 159–69. https://doi.org/10.1016/j.socscimed.2007.08.011.

Roberts, Dorothy. 2017a. *Killing the Black Body: Race, Reproduction, and the Meaning of Liberty*. Second edition. New York: Vintage.

——. 2017b. "Why Baby Markets Aren't Free." Symposium Issue: Baby Markets. *UC Irvine Law Review* 3: 611–22.

Robertson, John, and Theodore Schneyer. 1997. "Professional Self-Regulation and Shared-Risk Programs for in Vitro Fertilization." *Journal of Law, Medicine & Ethics* 25 (4): 283–91. https://doi.org/10.1111/j.1748-720X.1997.tb01410.x.

Rothman, Barbara Katz. 1993. "The Tentative Pregnancy: Then and Now." *Fetal Diagnosis and Therapy* 8 (1): 60–63. https://doi.org/10.1159/000263873.

Rothman, Kenneth, Lauren Wise, Henrik Sørensen, Anders Riis, Ellen Mikkelsen, and Elizabeth Hatch. 2013. "Volitional Determinants and Age-Related Decline in Fecundability: A General Population Prospective Cohort Study in Denmark." *Fertility and Sterility* 99 (7): 1958–64. https://doi.org/10.1016/j.fertnstert.2013.02.040.

Roxland, Beth E. 2012. "New York State's Landmark Policies on Oversight and Compensation for Egg Donation to Stem Cell Research." *Regenerative Medicine* 7 (3): 397–408.

Rudrappa, Sharmila. 2017. "Reproducing Dystopia: The Politics of Transnational Surrogacy in India, 2002–2015." *Critical Sociology*, November, 0896920517740616. https://doi.org/10.1177/0896920517740616.

Sabatello, Maya. 2014. "Posthumously Conceived Children: An International and Human Rights Perspective." Symposium: The Legal and Ethical Implications of Posthumous Reproduction. *Journal of Law and Health* 27: 29–67.

Safier, L. Z., A. Gumer, M. Kline, D. Egli, and M. V. Sauer. 2018. "Compensating Human Subjects Providing Oocytes for Stem Cell Research: 9-Year Experience and Outcomes." *Journal of Assisted Reproduction and Genetics* 35 (7): 1219–25. https://doi.org/10.1007/s10815-018-1171-z.

Sample, Ian. 2006a. "Clinics Prepare for 'Lifestyle' Fertility Treatment." *Guardian*, January 6. http://www.guardian.co.uk/uk/2006/jan/06/health.lifeandhealth.

———. 2006b. "Women Freeze Eggs in Wait for Right Partner, US Study Finds." *Guardian*, October 27. http://www.guardian.co.uk/science/2006/oct/27/medicineandhealth.familyandrelationships.

———. 2007. "Women Urged Not to Use Frozen Eggs as Insurance." *Guardian*, October 18. http://www.guardian.co.uk/science/2007/oct/18/medicalresearch.health.

———. 2009. "Fertility Experts in Moral Warning over Egg Freezing." *Guardian*, February 1. http://www.guardian.co.uk/society/2009/feb/01/egg-freezing-ethics-fertility.

———. 2011. "Have Your Eggs Frozen While You're Still Young, Scientists Advise Women." *Guardian*, October 18. http://www.guardian.co.uk/science/2011/oct/18/eggs-frozen-young-women.

SART. 2018. "National Summary Report 2016." Society for Assisted Reproductive Technology. April 25. https://www.sartcorsonline.com.

Sawicki, Jana. 1999. "Disciplining Mothers." In *Feminist Theory and the Body: A Reader*, edited by Margrit Shildrick and Janet Price. Edinburgh: University of Edinburg Press.

Schellart, Marieke. 2010. *Eggs for Later [Ei voor Later]*. Documentary. Trueworks. http://www.eivoorlater.nl.

———. 2011. "Eggs for Later." Rocky Mountain Women's Film Festival. November 6. http://rmwfilmfest.org/films/eggs-later.

Schippers, E. 2011a. "Kamerbrief vitrificeren van eicellen." Kamerstuk. Rijksoverheid. April 5. http://www.rijksoverheid.nl/documenten-en-publicaties/kamerstukken/2011/04/05/kamerbrief-vitrificeren-van-eicellen.html.

———. 2011b. "Kamerbrief Betreft Vitrificeren van Eicellen." Kamerstuk. Rijksoverheid. May 4. http://www.rijksoverheid.nl/documenten-en-publicaties/kamerstukken/2011/04/05/kamerbrief-vitrificeren-van-eicellen.html.

———. 2012. "Vaststelling Begroting Ministerie van Volksgezondheid: 33000 XVI 188 Brief van de Minister van Volksgezondheid, Welzijn En Sport, Nr. 188." Kamerstuk. Rijksoverheid. June 27, 2012. http://www.rijksbegroting.nl/2012/kamerstukken,2012/7/5/kst172385.html.

Schubert, Charlotte. 2013. "California Bill Poised to Lift Restrictions on Egg Donation." *Nature News*, June. https://doi.org/10.1038/nature.2013.13218.

Schurr, Carolin. 2017. "From Biopolitics to Bioeconomies: The ART of (Re-)Producing White Futures in Mexico's Surrogacy Market." *Environment and Planning D: Society and Space* 35 (2): 241–62. https://doi.org/10.1177/0263775816638851.

Schwartz, D., and M. Mayaux. 1982. "Female Fecundity as a Function of Age: Results of Artificial Insemination in 2193 Nulliparous Women with Azoospermic Husbands."

Obstetrical & Gynecological Survey 37 (8). http://journals.lww.com/obgynsurvey/Fulltext/1982/08000/Female_Fecundity_as_a_Function_of_Age__Results_of.19.aspx.

Segal, Lynne. 2013. *Out of Time: The Pleasures and the Perils of Ageing*. London: Verso.

Shady Grove Fertility. 2016. Egg Freezing Webinar. Webinar. https://www.workcast.com/AuditoriumAuthenticator.aspx?cpak=4227156639769398&pak=6921760491609385.

———. 2017. "The Cost of Freezing Eggs." Shady Grove Fertility. https://www.shady-grovefertility.com/affording-care/egg-freezing-cost/cost-freezing-eggs.

Shaw, Rachel, and David Giles. 2009. "Motherhood on Ice? A Media Framing Analysis of Older Mothers in the UK News." *Psychology & Health* 24 (2): 221–36.

Shenfield, F., J. de Mouzon, G. Pennings, A. Ferraretti, A. Andersen, G. de Wert, and V. Goossens. 2010. "Cross Border Reproductive Care in Six European Countries." *Human Reproduction* 25 (6): 1361–68. https://doi.org/10.1093/humrep/deq057.

Shkedi-Rafid, Shiri, and Yael Hashiloni-Dolev. 2011. "Egg Freezing for Age-Related Fertility Decline: Preventive Medicine or a Further Medicalization of Reproduction? Analyzing the New Israeli Policy." *Fertility and Sterility* 96 (2): 291–94. https://doi.org/10.1016/j.fertnstert.2011.06.024.

Shukman, David. 2014. "China Cloning on 'Industrial Scale.'" *BBC News*. January 14. http://www.bbc.com/news/science-environment-25576718.

Silver, Katie. 2017. "Rita Ora's Egg Freezing in Early 20s 'a Positive Move,' Doctors Say." *BBC News*, November 23, sec. Health. https://www.bbc.com/news/health-42095254.

Smajdor, Anna. 2009. "Between Fecklessness and Selfishness: Is There a Biologically Optimal Time for Motherhood?" *International Library of Ethics, Law, and the New Medicine* 43 (January): 105–17. https://doi.org/10.1007/978-90-481-2475-6_9.

Smietana, Marcin, Charis Thompson, and France Winddance Twine. 2018. "Introduction: Making and Breaking Families—Reading Queer Reproductions, Stratified Reproduction, and Reproductive Justice Together." *Reproductive Biomedicine & Society Online* 7 (November): 112–130. https://doi.org/10.1016/j.rbms.2018.11.001.

Smirnova, Michelle Hannah. 2012. "A Will to Youth: The Woman's Anti-Aging Elixir." *Social Science & Medicine* 75 (7): 1236–43. https://doi.org/10.1016/j.socscimed.2012.02.061.

Smith, Rebecca. 2012. "Fertility Treatment Waiting Times Halve after Increased Payments to Donors." *Telegraph*, November 26. http://www.telegraph.co.uk/health/healthnews/9696083/Fertility-treatment-waiting-times-halve-after-increased-payments-to-donors.html.

Smyth, Lisa. 2008. "Gendered Spaces and Intimate Citizenship: The Case of Breastfeeding." *European Journal of Women's Studies* 15 (2): 83–99. https://doi.org/10.1177/1350506808090305.

Snyder, T., and S. Dillow. 2013. *Digest of Education Statistics 2012*. Washington, DC: National Center for Education Statistics, Institute of Education Sciences, US Department of Education. http://nces.ed.gov/pubs2014/2014015.pdf.

Spar, Debora. 2005. "Reproductive Tourism and the Regulatory Map." *New England Journal of Medicine* 352 (6): 531–33. https://doi.org/10.1056/NEJMp048295.

———. 2006. *The Baby Business: How Money, Science, and Politics Drive the Commerce of Conception.* Boston: Harvard Business Press.

———. 2007. "The Egg Trade: Making Sense of the Market for Human Oocytes." *New England Journal of Medicine* 356 (13): 1289–91. https://doi.org/10.1056/NEJMp078012.

Spivak, Gayatri. 1996. *The Spivak Reader.* Edited by Donna Landry and Gerald Maclean. New York: Routledge.

Squier, Susan M. 1994. *Babies in Bottles.* New Brunswick, NJ: Rutgers University Press.

———. 2004. *Liminal Lives: Imagining the Human at the Frontiers of Biomedicine.* Durham, NC: Duke University Press.

Stephenson, Peter H. 2010. "Age and Time: Contesting the Paradigm of Loss in the Age of Novelty." In *Contesting Aging and Loss,* edited by Janice Elizabeth Graham and Peter H. Stephenson, 87–102. Toronto: University of Toronto Press.

Sterckx, Sigrid, Julian Cockbain, and Guido Pennings. 2017. "Patenting Medical Diagnosis Methods in Europe: Stanford University and Time-Lapse Microscopy." *Reproductive BioMedicine Online* 34 (2): 166–68. https://doi.org/10.1016/j.rbmo.2016.10.014.

Stewart, Catrina. 2011. "Family Drops Efforts to Harvest and Freeze Eggs of Dead Girl." *Independent,* August 9. http://www.independent.co.uk/news/world/middle-east/family-drops-efforts-to-harvest-and-freeze-eggs-of-dead-girl-2334208.html.

Stoop, D., B. Ermini, N. Polyzos, P. Haentjens, M. De Vos, G. Verheyen, and P. Devroey. 2012. "Reproductive Potential of a Metaphase II Oocyte Retrieved after Ovarian Stimulation: An Analysis of 23 354 ICSI Cycles." *Human Reproduction* 27 (7): 2030–35. https://doi.org/10.1093/humrep/des131.

Stoop, D., J. Nekkebroeck, and P. Devroey. 2011. "A Survey on the Intentions and Attitudes towards Oocyte Cryopreservation for Non-Medical Reasons among Women of Reproductive Age." *Human Reproduction* 26 (3): 655–61. https://doi.org/10.1093/humrep/deq367.

Stoop, Dominic, Fulco van der Veen, Michel Deneyer, Julie Nekkebroeck, and Herman Tournaye. 2014. "Oocyte Banking for Anticipated Gamete Exhaustion (AGE) Is a Preventive Intervention, neither Social nor Nonmedical." *Reproductive BioMedicine Online* 28 (5): 548–51. https://doi.org/10.1016/j.rbmo.2014.01.007.

Sunder Rajan, Kaushik. 2006. *Biocapital: The Constitution of Postgenomic Life.* Durham, NC: Duke University Press.

Sung, Li-Ying, Ching-Chien Chang, Tomokazu Amano, Chih-Jen Lin, Misa Amano, Stephen B. Treaster, Jie Xu, et al. 2010. "Efficient Derivation of Embryonic Stem Cells from Nuclear Transfer and Parthenogenetic Embryos Derived from Cryopreserved Oocytes." *Cellular Reprogramming* 12 (2): 203–11. https://doi.org/10.1089/cell.2009.0072.

Sunkara, Sesh. 2018. "Introducing the Concept of Time to Live Birth (TTLB)." Merck—Fertility. February. https://hcp.merckgroup.com/en/fertility/resources/expert-opinion/Introducing-the-concept-of-TTLB.html.

Swanson, Ana. 2015. "Why Men Should Also Worry about Waiting Too Long to Have Kids." *Washington Post*, October 27, sec. Wonkblog. https://www.washingtonpost.com/news/wonk/wp/2015/10/27/men-have-biological-clocks-too-so-why-does-no-one-talk-about-them/.

Tachibana, Masahito, Paula Amato, Michelle Sparman, Nuria Marti Gutierrez, Rebecca Tippner-Hedges, Hong Ma, Eunju Kang, et al. 2013. "Human Embryonic Stem Cells Derived by Somatic Cell Nuclear Transfer." *Cell* 153 (6): 1228–38. https://doi.org/10.1016/j.cell.2013.05.006.

Tachibana, Masahito, Takashi Kuno, and Nobuo Yaegashi. 2018. "Mitochondrial Replacement Therapy and Assisted Reproductive Technology: A Paradigm Shift toward Treatment of Genetic Diseases in Gametes or in Early Embryos." *Reproductive Medicine and Biology* 17 (4): 421–33. https://doi.org/10.1002/rmb2.12230.

Tae-gyu, Kim. 2016. "Stem Cell Research Loses Footing in Korea." *Korea Times*, 17 July. http://www.koreatimes.co.kr/www/tech/2019/07/693_209625.html.

Takahashi, Kazutoshi, Koji Tanabe, Mari Ohnuki, Megumi Narita, Tomoko Ichisaka, Kiichiro Tomoda, and Shinya Yamanaka. 2007. "Induction of Pluripotent Stem Cells from Adult Human Fibroblasts by Defined Factors." *Cell* 131 (5): 861–72. https://doi.org/10.1016/j.cell.2007.11.019.

Tanaka, Atsushi, and Seiji Watanabe. 2019. "Can Cytoplasmic Donation Rescue Aged Oocytes?" *Reproductive Medicine and Biology* 18 (2): 128–39. https://doi.org/10.1002/rmb2.12252.

Taneja, Poonam. 2013. "Asian Egg Donor Shortage in UK 'Forcing Couples Abroad.'" BBC. May 15. http://www.bbc.com/news/uk-22533906.

The London Egg Bank. 2014. "Looking for Donor Eggs?" The London Egg Bank. 2014. http://www.londoneggbank.com/looking-for-donor-eggs/faqs.

The New York Times Company. 2018. "New York Times Company 2017 Annual Report." https://s1.q4cdn.com/156149269/files/doc_financials/annual/2017/Final-2017-Annual-Report.pdf.

The Observer. 2009. "Mother Nature." *Guardian*, September 27. https://www.theguardian.com/lifeandstyle/2009/sep/27/fertility-motherhood.

The World Bank. 2019. "Fertility Rate, Total (Births per Woman)—Korea, Rep." The World Bank. https://data.worldbank.org/indicator/SP.DYN.TFRT.IN?locations=KR&most_recent_value_desc=false.

Thompson, Charis. 2001. "Strategic Naturalizing: Kinship in an Infertility Clinic." In *Relative Values: Reconfiguring Kinship Studies*, edited by Sarah Franklin and Susan Mackinnon, 175–202. Durham, NC: Duke University Press.

———. 2005. *Making Parents: The Ontological Choreography of Reproductive Technologies*. Cambridge, MA: MIT Press.

———. 2011. "Medical Migrations Afterword: Science as a Vacation?" *Body & Society* 17 (2–3): 205–13.

———. 2013. *Good Science: The Ethical Choreography of Stem Cell Research*. Cambridge, MA: MIT Press.

Thurlow, Rebecca. 2015. "A Womb with a View: App to Help Monitor Growing Embryo." *Wall Street Journal*, May 29, sec. Tech. http://www.wsj.com/articles/a-womb-with-a-view-app-to-help-monitor-growing-embryo-1432810802.

Tiffany, Kaitlyn. 2018. "The SoulCycle of Fertility Sells Egg-Freezing and 'Empowerment' to 25-Year-Olds." *Verge*, September 11. https://www.theverge.com/2018/9/11/17823810/kindbody-startup-fertility-clinic-egg-freezing-millennials-location.

Tilly, Jonathan L., and David A. Sinclair. 2013. "Germline Energetics, Aging, and Female Infertility." *Cell Metabolism* 17 (6): 838–50. https://doi.org/10.1016/j.cmet.2013.05.007.

Tober, Diane. 2019. "Are Egg Donors Patients Too? Eggonomics, Bio-Profits, and the Implications for Egg Donor Care." Conference Presentation presented at the 4S, New Orleans, September 6. https://convention2.allacademic.com/one/ssss/4s19/.

Tough, Suzanne, Karen Benzies, Nonie Fraser-Lee, and Christine Newburn-Cook. 2007. "Factors Influencing Childbearing Decisions and Knowledge of Perinatal Risks among Canadian Men and Women." *Maternal and Child Health Journal* 11 (2): 189–98. https://doi.org/10.1007/s10995-006-0156-1.

TWEB. 2009. "The World Egg Bank—About Us." The World Egg Bank. March 24. https://web.archive.org/web/20090324073143/http://www.theworldeggbank.com:80/The%20World%20Egg%20Bank/aboutus/aboutus.aspx.

———. 2014a. *The World Egg Bank: Making Conception Possible!* The World Egg Bank. https://www.youtube.com/watch?v=Dc15PPIgF2Y#t=133.

———. 2014b. "The World Egg Bank." *The World Egg Bank*. http://www.theworldeggbank.com/.

———. 2015a. "The World Egg Bank: Eggs without Borders." The World Egg Bank. http://www.theworldeggbank.com/.

———. 2015b. "Eggs without Borders: US Donor Compensation." *The World Egg Bank* (blog). June 9. http://www.theworldeggbank.com/eggs-without-borders-us-donor-compensation/.

———. 2018. "Options." The World Egg Bank. http://www.theworldeggbank.com/options/.

Twenge, Jean. 2013. "How Long Can You Wait to Have a Baby?" *Atlantic*, July. http://www.theatlantic.com/magazine/archive/2013/07/how-long-can-you-wait-to-have-a-baby/309374/.

Twigg, Julia. 2007. "Clothing, Age, and the Body: A Critical Review." *Ageing & Society* 27 (02): 285–305. https://doi.org/10.1017/S0144686X06005794.

UMCU. 2012. "Overeenkomst Betreffende Het Invriezen En Bewaren van Eicellen." Informed consent form, in author's possession.

United Nations. 2014a. "Ratio of Youth Unemployment Rate to Adult Unemployment Rate, Both Sexes." Millennium Development Goals Indicators. http://unstats.un.org/unsd/mdg/SeriesDetail.aspx?srid=671&crid=840.

———. 2014b. "Youth Unemployment Rate, Aged 15–24, Both Sexes." Millennium Development Goals Indicators. http://unstats.un.org/unsd/mdg/SeriesDetail.aspx?srid=671&crid=840.

———. 2017. "World Population Prospects: Key Findings & Advance Tables. 2017 Revision." New York: United Nations, Department of Economic and Social Affairs Population Division. https://population.un.org/wpp/Publications/Files/WPP2017_KeyFindings.pdf.

Valk, Ülo. 2000. "Ex Ovo Omnia: Where Does the Balto-Finnic Cosmogony Originate?" *Oral Tradition* 15 (1): 145–58.

Van Cuilenburg, J. J., Peter Neijens, and O. Scholten. 1999. *Media in Overvloed*. Amsterdam: Amsterdam University Press.

Van de Pas, Brigitte. 2019. "Netherlands: Average Age of Mother at Birth, 1950–2018." Statista. September 2019. https://www.statista.com/statistics/521023/average-age-mother-at-birth-in-the-netherlands/.

Van de Wiel, Lucy. 2014a. "For Whom the Clock Ticks: Reproductive Ageing and Egg Freezing in Dutch and British News Media." *Studies in the Maternal* 6 (1): 1–28.

———. 2014b. "The Time of the Change: Menopause's Medicalization and the Gender Politics of Aging." *International Journal of Feminist Approaches to Bioethics* 7 (1): 74–98. https://doi.org/10.2979/intjfemappbio.7.1.74.

———. 2015. "Frozen in Anticipation: Eggs for Later." *Women's Studies International Forum* 53 (November–December): 119–28. https://doi.org/10.1016/j.wsif.2014.10.019.

———. 2017. "Cellular Origins: A Visual Analysis of Time-Lapse Embryo Imaging." In *Assisted Reproduction across Borders: Feminist Perspectives on Normalization, Disruptions, and Transmissions*, edited by Nina Lykke and Merete Lie, 288–301. New York: Routledge.

———. 2018. "Prenatal Imaging: Egg Freezing, Embryo Selection, and the Visual Politics of Reproductive Time." *Catalyst: Feminism, Theory, Technoscience* 4 (2): 1–35. https://doi.org/10.28968/cftt.v4i2.29908.

———. 2019. "The Datafication of Reproduction: Time-Lapse Embryo Imaging and the Commercialisation of IVF." *Sociology of Health & Illness* 41 (S1): 193–209. https://doi.org/10.1111/1467-9566.12881.

———. 2020. "The Speculative Turn in IVF: Egg Freezing and the Financialization of Fertility." *New Genetics and Society* 39 (3): 306–26. https://doi.org/10.1080/14636778.2019.1709430.

Van der Valk, J., Karen Bieback, Christiane Buta, Brett Cochrane, Wilhelm Dirks, Jianan Fu, James J. Hickman, et al. 2018. "Fetal Bovine Serum (FBS): Past—Present—Future." *ALTEX* 35 (1): 99–118. https://doi.org/10.14573/altex.1705101.

Van Dijck, José. 2004. "Mediated Memories: Personal Cultural Memory as Object of Cultural Analysis." *Continuum* 18 (2): 261–77.

———. 2005. *The Transparent Body: A Cultural Analysis of Medical Imaging*. Seattle: University of Washington Press.

———. 2007. *Mediated Memories in the Digital Age*. Stanford, CA: Stanford University Press.

———. 2008. "Future Memories: The Construction of Cinematic Hindsight." *Theory, Culture & Society* 25 (3).

Van Erp, Barbara. 2009. "Dilemma's Rond Het Invriezen van Eicellen." Vrij Nederland. July 18. http://www.vn.nl/Standaard-media-pagina/DilemmasRondHetInvriezen-VanEicellen.htm.

Varsavsky, Martin. 2016. "But Daddy, How Are Babies Made?" *Martin Varsavky* (blog). October 7. http://english.martinvarsavsky.net/paternity/but-daddy-how-are-babies-made.html#comments.

Vertommen, Sigrid. 2017. "From the Pergonal Project to Kadimastem: A Genealogy of Israel's Reproductive-Industrial Complex." *BioSocieties* 12 (2): 282–306. https://doi.org/10.1057/biosoc.2015.44.

Vertommen, Sigrid, and Michal Nahman. 2019. "Global Fertility Chains: A New Political Economy Approach to Understanding Transnational Surrogacy and Egg Provision." In *AFEP-IIPPE*, 1. Lille. https://afep-iippe2019.sciencesconf.org/245290/document.

Viloria, Thamara, Nicolas Garrido, Francisco Minaya, José Remohí, Manuel Muñoz, and Marcos Meseguer. 2011. "Report of Results Obtained in 2,934 Women Using Donor Sperm: Donor Insemination versus in Vitro Fertilization according to Indication." *Fertility and Sterility* 96 (5): 1134–37. https://doi.org/10.1016/j.fertnstert.2011.08.016.

Vincent, John. 2006. "Ageing Contested: Anti-Ageing Science and the Cultural Construction of Old Age." *Sociology* 40 (4): 681–98. https://doi.org/10.1177/0038038506065154.

———. 2009. "Ageing, Anti-Ageing, and Anti-Anti-Ageing: Who Are the Progressives in the Debate on the Future of Human Biological Ageing?" *Medicine Studies* 1 (3): 197–208. https://doi.org/10.1007/s12376-009-0016-6.

Virtus Health. 2017. "Annual Report 2017." ABN80129643492. Greenwich, Australia: Virtus Health. http://www.annualreports.com./HostedData/AnnualReports/PDF/ASX_VRT_2017.pdf.

Vitrolife. 2015a. "KIDScore™ D3 & D5 Decision Support Tool." Vitrolife. http://www.vitrolife.com/en/Products/EmbryoScope-Time-Lapse-System/KIDScore-decision-support-tool-/.

———. 2015b. "EmbryoScope™ Counseling App." ITunes App Store. January 10. https://itunes.apple.com/app/fertilitech-counseling-app/id768108306.

———. 2015c. "Summary Annual Report 2014." Gothenburg, Sweden: Vitrolife. http://mb.cision.com/Public/1031/9753413/be2bed7f309b48ed.pdf.

———. 2015d. *KIDScore Decision Support Tool.* Vitrolifetube. https://www.youtube.com/watch?time_continue=74&v=tPtR81sBbzI.

———. 2016. "Vitrolife." http://www.vitrolife.com.

———. 2017. "Interim Report January–June 2017." Interim report. Gothenburg, Sweden: Vitrolife. http://mb.cision.com/Main/1031/9804468/401074.pdf.

———. 2018. "Interim Report January–March 2018." Interim report. Gothenburg, Sweden: Vitrolife. https://mb.cision.com/Main/1031/2503138/827561.pdf.

———. 2019. "Interim Report January–March 2018." Interim report. Gothenburg, Sweden: Vitrolife. https://mb.cision.com/Main/1031/2792295/1028496.pdf.

Von Hagel, Alisa. 2013. "Banking on Infertility: Medical Ethics and the Marketing of Fertility Loans." *Hastings Center Report* 43 (6): 15–17. https://doi.org/10.1002/hast.228.

Vora, Kalindi, and Malathi Michelle Iyengar. 2016. "Citizen, Subject, Property: Indian Surrogacy and the Global Fertility Market." In *Assisted Reproduction across Borders: Feminist Perspectives on Normalization, Disruptions, and Transmissions*, edited by Nina Lykke and Merete Lie, 43–54. New York: Routledge.

Waggoner, Miranda. 2017. *The Zero Trimester: Pre-Pregnancy Care and the Politics of Reproductive Risk*. Oakland: University of California Press.

Wahlberg, Ayo. 2018. *Good Quality: The Routinization of Sperm Banking in China*. Oakland: University of California Press.

Waldby, Catherine. 2002. "Stem Cells, Tissue Cultures, and the Production of Biovalue." *Health* 6 (3): 305–23. https://doi.org/10.1177/136345930200600304.

———. 2008. "Oocyte Markets: Women's Reproductive Work in Embryonic Stem Cell Research." *New Genetics and Society* 27 (1): 19–31. https://doi.org/10.1080/14636770701843576.

———. 2015a. "'Banking Time': Egg Freezing and the Negotiation of Future Fertility." *Culture, Health & Sexuality* 17 (4): 470–82. https://doi.org/10.1080/13691058.2014.951881.

———. 2015b. "The Oocyte Market and Social Egg Freezing: From Scarcity to Singularity." *Journal of Cultural Economy* 8 (3): 275–91. https://doi.org/10.1080/17530350.2015.1039457.

———. 2019. *The Oocyte Economy: The Changing Meaning of Human Eggs*. Durham, NC: Duke University Press.

Waldby, Catherine, and Katherine Carroll. 2012. "Egg Donation for Stem Cell Research: Ideas of Surplus and Deficit in Australian IVF Patients' and Reproductive Donors' Accounts." *Sociology of Health & Illness* 34 (4): 513–28. https://doi.org/10.1111/j.1467-9566.2011.01399.x.

Waldby, Catherine, and Melinda Cooper. 2010. "From Reproductive Work to Regenerative Labour: The Female Body and the Stem Cell Industries." *Feminist Theory* 11 (1): 3–22. https://doi.org/10.1177/1464700109355210.

Walsh, Fergus. 2013. "Time-Lapse Imaging 'Improves IVF.'" BBC, May 17, sec. Health. http://www.bbc.com/news/health-22559247.

Wang, Xiaoqian, Debra A. Gook, Kirsty A. Walters, Antoinette Anazodo, William L. Ledger, and Robert B. Gilchrist. 2016. "Improving Fertility Preservation for Girls and Women by Coupling Oocyte in Vitro Maturation with Existing Strategies." *Women's Health* 12 (3): 275–78. https://doi.org/10.2217/whe-2016-0019.

Wegner, Carole. 2012. "Time Lapse Embryo Imaging: How It May Change IVF." *Fertility Lab Insider* (blog). http://fertilitylabinsider.com/2012/10/time-lapse-embryo-imaging-how-it-may-change-ivf/.

Weigel, Moira. 2016. *Labor of Love: The Invention of Dating*. New York: Farrar, Straus and Giroux.

West, M. 1994. "Ab Ovo." *Classical Quarterly* 44 (2): 289–307. https://doi.org/10.1017/S0009838800043767.

Whittaker, Andrea. 2015. "The Implications of Medical Travel upon Equity in Lower- and Middle-Income Countries." In *Handbook on Medical Tourism and Patient Mobility*, edited by Neil Lunt, Daniel Horsfall, and Johanna Hanefeld, 112–22. Cheltenham, UK: Elgar.

WHO. 2019. "Infertility Definitions and Terminology." WHO. http://www.who.int/ reproductivehealth/topics/infertility/definitions/en/.

Widdows, Heather. 2009. "Border Disputes across Bodies: Exploitation in Trafficking for Prostitution and Egg Sale for Stem Cell Research." *International Journal of Feminist Approaches to Bioethics* 2 (1): 5–24.

Williams, Clare, Jenny Kitzinger, and Lesley Henderson. 2003. "Envisaging the Embryo in Stem Cell Research: Rhetorical Strategies and Media Reporting of the Ethical Debates." *Sociology of Health & Illness* 25 (7): 793–814. https://doi. org/10.1046/j.1467-9566.2003.00370.x.

Williams, Eric, Mark Surowiak, and Matthew Szymanski. 2017. "Fertility Clinics, Q1 2017." Boston: Capstone Partners.

Williams, Zoe. 2010. "How the Inventor of the Pill Changed the World for Women." *Guardian*, October 30. http://www.guardian.co.uk/lifeandstyle/2010/oct/30/ carl-djerassi-inventor-of-contraceptive-pill.

Wiseman, Eva. 2017. "The Real Reason Women Freeze Their Eggs." *Guardian*, July 16, sec. Society. https://www.theguardian.com/society/2017/jul/16/ the-real-reason-women-freeze-their-eggs-fertility-career-family.

Witkin, G., A. Tran, J. Lee, L. Schuman, L. Grunfeld, and J. Knopman. 2013. "What Makes a Woman Freeze: The Impetus behind Patients' Desires to Undergo Elective Oocyte Cryopreservation." *Fertility and Sterility* 100 (3): S24. https://doi. org/10.1016/j.fertnstert.2013.07.1752.

Wolf, Don, Robert Morey, Eunju Kang, Hong Ma, Tomonari Hayama, Louise Laurent, and Shoukhrat Mitalipov. 2017. "Concise Review: Embryonic Stem Cells Derived by Somatic Cell Nuclear Transfer: A Horse in the Race?" *Stem Cells* 35 (1): 26–34. https://doi.org/10.1002/stem.2496.

Wong, Connie C., Kevin E. Loewke, Thomas M. Baer, Renee A. Reijo-Pera, and Barry Behr. 2012. Imaging and Evaluating Embryos, Oocytes, and Stem Cells; Patent US8337387 B2. US8337387 B2, filed November 22, 2011, and issued December 25.

———. 2013. Imaging and Evaluating Embryos, Oocytes, and Stem Cells; Patent EP2430454 B1. EP2430454 B1, filed August 23, 2010, and issued January 23.

Wood, Michelle. 2008. "Celebrity Older Mothers: Does the Media Give Women a False Impression?" *British Journal of Midwifery* 16 (5): 326.

Yamada, Mitsutoshi, James Byrne, and Dieter Egli. 2015. "From Cloned Frogs to Patient Matched Stem Cells: Induced Pluripotency or Somatic Cell Nuclear Transfer?" *Current Opinion in Genetics & Development*, Cell Reprogramming, Regeneration, and Repair, 34 (October): 29–34. https://doi.org/10.1016/j.gde.2015.06.007.

Yamada, Mitsutoshi, Bjarki Johannesson, Ido Sagi, Lisa Cole Burnett, Daniel Kort, Robert Prosser, Daniel Paull, et al. 2014. "Human Oocytes Reprogram Adult

Somatic Nuclei of a Type 1 Diabetic to Diploid Pluripotent Stem Cells." *Nature* 510 (7506): 533–36. https://doi.org/10.1038/nature13287.

Yang, Selena. 2018. "Progyny and Happify Health Give People Dealing with Infertility New Digital Emotional Support Tools." GlobeNewswire News Room. May 16. http://globenewswire.com/news-release/2018/05/16/1507391/0/en/Progyny-and-Happify-Health-Give-People-Dealing-with-Infertility-New-Digital-Emotional-Support-Tools.html.

Ylänne, Virpi. 2016. "Too Old to Parent? Discursive Representations of Late Parenting in the British Press." *Discourse & Communication* 10 (2): 176–97. https://doi.org/10.1177/1750481315611242.

Yoon, Tae K., Hyung M. Chung, Jeong M. Lim, Se Y. Han, Jung J. Ko, and Kwang Y. Cha. 2000. "Pregnancy and Delivery of Healthy Infants Developed from Vitrified Oocytes in a Stimulated in Vitro Fertilization–Embryo Transfer Program." *Fertility and Sterility* 74 (1): 180–81. https://doi.org/10.1016/S0015-0282(00)00572-0.

Yoon, Tae K., Thomas J. Kim, Sung Eun Park, Seung Wook Hong, Jung Jae Ko, Hyung Min Chung, and Kwang Yul Cha. 2003. "Live Births after Vitrification of Oocytes in a Stimulated in Vitro Fertilization–Embryo Transfer Program." *Fertility and Sterility* 79 (6): 1323–26. https://doi.org/10.1016/S0015-0282(03)00258-9.

Zeilmaker, G., A. Alberda, I. van Gent, C. Rijkmans, and A. Drogendijk. 1984. "Two Pregnancies Following Transfer of Intact Frozen-Thawed Embryos." *Fertility and Sterility* 42 (2): 293–96.

Zhang, John, Hui Liu, Shiyu Luo, Zhuo Lu, Alejandro Chávez-Badiola, Zitao Liu, Mingxue Yang, et al. 2017. "Live Birth Derived from Oocyte Spindle Transfer to Prevent Mitochondrial Disease." *Reproductive BioMedicine Online* 34 (4): 361–68. https://doi.org/10.1016/j.rbmo.2017.01.013.

Zorg & Financiering. 2012. "Minister Schippers: Geen Vergoeding Ivf Boven 43." *Zorg & Financiering* 11 (7): 58.

INDEX

abortion: and egg donor profiles, 188; and "embryo adoption," 200–201, 271n92; and fetal imagery, 123–24, 253n1; and IVF, 6, 244n26; legalization, 27; and mandatory ultrasounds, 124; and mitochondrial transfer regulations, 209–10; and regulation of reproductive vs. nonreproductive technologies, 224n26; social vs. medical indications, 39–40, 250n48, 270n81; and stem cell research funding, 6, 200–201; and reproductive timing, 21, 218. *See also* United States

accumulation, 54–57; of capital, 24, 55–56, 95, 110, 142, 186, 225; of data, 140–42; of eggs, 3, 55, 95, 99, 186; of fertility, 24, 99–101, 110, 227–28

Adams, Brigitte, 158, 163, 165–68, 229. See also *Eggsurance*

affect: affective investment in frozen eggs, 168, 178, 228; anticipatory anxiety about future infertility, 24, 43–44, 60–67, 81–86, 103, 111, 231; and egg freezing, 60–66, 84–86, 103, 233; grief and reproductive loss, 164–68; hope, 64–66, 82–85; package plans and reduced anxiety, 101–3; regret, 9, 13–14, 166–68, 178; uncertainty, 13–16. *See also* agency, women's; anticipation

afterlife: and posthumous existence of frozen eggs, 176

age limits: 10-year storage limit, 229, 262n9; 14-day rule in embryo research, 124; for egg freezing, 29, 57–58, 144–46, 153, 221, 262n8; biological clock as limit to liberation, 43, 58, 218; and donor-egg IVF, 151–53, 218; naturalization of reproductive age limits, 22, 28, 36. *See also* age normativities; biological clock; chrononormativities; Netherlands; older motherhood

age normativities: ageism in film and television, 148; egg freezing articulation of, 3–4, 177; egg freezing reconfiguration of, 28, 62; egg freezing transgression of, 4, 28, 56, 58–59, 64, 75–76, 177; gendered, 19–22, 246n68; naturalized, 36, 56; older motherhood as transgression of, 25, 148–55, 177. *See also* age limits; aging; chrononormativities; older motherhood

agency, women's: accessing reproductive healthcare, 39; egg donor selection, 190; and egg freezing, 14, 60, 62, 222; and posthumous use of eggs, 168–76; and reproductive aging, 14, 18, 49, 57, 60–63, 69–72, 77, 117, 208, 219, 222, 229, 254n15; and retrospective regret, 166–68, 178; and singlehood, 161–62; and timing of childbearing, 21, 150–52; and of timing menstruation and maternity, 20–21. *See also* informed consent; older motherhood; reproductive aging; reproductive technologies; willfulness aging: aging societies, 181, 199–200, 204–5; body vs. freezer, 4, 84, 91–99, 116, 165–66, 226–29; and regenerative medicine, 179, 196; and regulation of sexuality, 148–51, 177; "success-ful," 25, 149, 155–57, 177, 181, 216, 234. *See also* age limits; age normativities; biopolitics; body; chrononormativities; distributed reproductive aging; embryonic aging; fertility loss; frozen eggs; gender politics of (reproductive) aging; mortality; older motherhood; reproductive aging

Ahmed, Sara, 66–67, 72–77, 150–51, 174, 177, 265n112. *See also* willfulness

algorithms: for embryo selection, 9, 121, 129–30, 133–37, 140–42, 260n34. *See also* time-lapse embryo imaging

Almeling, Rene, 190, 268n26, 269n40, 272n114

AMC. *See* Amsterdam Medical Centre

American Society for Reproductive Medi-cine (ASRM), 7, 29–30, 97, 136, 169, 185, 203, 219

Amsterdam Medical Centre (AMC), 8, 28–29, 61, 144, 247n3

anticipation, 60–86; as affective state, 60–62; anticipated infertility, 63, 81–86; and bodily futurity, 24, 60–62, 69, 86; and deferral in egg freezing, 109; and hope, 66, 82; and neoliberal-ism, 61, 276n11; and postfertility, 231; "regimes of anticipation," 61, 66–67; of reproductive finitude, 3, 19, 63; and retrospection, 72–77; and uncertain futures, 61, 66, 69, 75. *See also* affect; anticipation work; chrononormativi-ties; informed consent; motherhood; older motherhood; reproductive aging

anticipation work: and imagined future family life, 76; and "memory work," 74–75. *See also* anticipation

anticipatory anxiety. *See* affect

Apple. *See* fertility insurance

artificial gametes. See *in vitro* gameto-genesis

artificial intelligence: used for embryo selection, 136–37, 261n58

ASRM. *See* American Society for Repro-ductive Medicine

assisted reproduction. *See* reproductive technologies

Australia, 136, 185, 193, 200; first children born from frozen embryos and eggs, 5

Baby Eva video, 119–28. *See also* time-lapse embryo imaging

Belgium: egg freezing in, 62, 68, 72, 83

Berlant, Lauren, 15, 62

biocapital, 122, 135–37, 234–35

biodesirability: of egg donors, 189–91, 194, 214; irrelevant in research egg dona-tion, 204, 216, 273n155

biological clock, 21–24, 30–31, 57, 65–68, 247n79; egg freezing to counteract, 12, 80–86, 97, 156–57, 208; as limit to lib-eration, 43, 58, 218; media trope, 41–45, 218. *See also* age limits

biological time, reconfiguration of: with egg freezing, 89–90; with tissue cul-ture, 195–96. *See also* SCNT

biomedicalization: of age-related (in)-fertility, 60, 63; de-/remedicalization, 37–41; of each step in the female repro-ductive life course, 118; of midlife, 18; and neoliberalism, 216; overmedical-ization, 8; and postfertility, 17

bionationalism: and egg donation for SCNT, 198–202; Korea, 198–200; US, 200–202; women and reproduction of the nation, 198

biopolitics, 246n67; of egg freezing, 18; global biopolitics of aging, 26, 181–82, 193, 196, 204–16. *See also* fertility literacy; gender politics of (reproduc-tive) aging; reproductive technologies bioprecarity, 246n61; reproductive, 16, 24, 55–56, 86–87, 225–26; and socioprecarity, 54–55, 225

biopreparation: bioprepared bodies, 180; egg freezing as, 24, 81–85; and fertility, 98, 103, 117, 224, 227, 255n36

biotechnology companies. *See* pharmaceutical and biotechnology companies

biotemporalities: oocyte, 98–99. *See also* temporality

blogs: about egg freezing, 88–95, 158–68

bodily futurity, 24, 60–62, 69–72, 84–86

bodily time: in relation to the egg, 26, 47, 182, 208. *See also* body; temporality

body: age-specific sexualization and desexualization, 148–51; aging, 155–56, 205–6; bioprepared, 81–86, 180; nonreproductive, 59, 150; pathologized, 19, 63; and postfertile condition, 17, 118; pregnant, 84; reproductive, 19–21, 27, 30, 46, 71, 93, 116, 223, 227; site of failure and loss, 47, 72, 91–94, 127. *See also* aging; fertility; ovarian reserve

Briggs, Laura, 32, 224–25; structural infertility, 224, 276n15

Bush, George W., 200–201

Butler, Judith, 14–15, 173–74, 246n68

Buttle, Liz, 147–55, 177, 226. *See also* older motherhood

calculus of fertility, 101–3, 112, 168, 227. *See also* package plans

cancer treatment, and egg freezing, 3, 28–32, 37–40, 170–71, 247n8, 263n31, 265n98

capitalism: chrononormativities and industrialized capitalism, 20; financialized capitalism 54–55, 163, 185. *See also* accumulation; family; fertility industry

Carrel, Alexis, 195–96

child: as "priceless," 102; future child imagined in egg freezing, 74–75, 91, 96, 110, 123, 167–71; future child imagined in time-lapse embryo imaging, 122–26. *See also* frozen eggs

childbearing: and age, 19, 73–75, 144–46, 152–53; delayed, 6, 11–12, 35–36, 77–79, 145, 224; earlier, 57; and family planning, 20–22; fertility without, 13; later, 37, 41, 143–57, 218, 232–34, 262n15, 276n17; timing, 4, 10–11, 17, 41, 153, 157, 263–64n53. *See also* agency; class; race

childlessness: and age-related infertility, 63, 66; finality of, 80, 85; in media, 33–35; risk of "missing out," 57; race- and class-specific trends, 10, 65–66; presented as undesirable, 66–67, 145

China, 169, 190, 232

chrononormativities: and aging, 28, 177; and anticipation, 76; defined, 19–20; gendered, 19–22, 25, 42–43, 56, 219, 246n71; naturalization of, 19–22; and older motherhood, 151; and willfulness, 151, 177. *See also* age normativities; capitalism; contraception

class: and 19th-century gender normativity, 246n71; and childbearing, 10–12, 252n13; and egg donation, 189–92; and egg freezing, 10, 27, 65–66, 105, 112, 157, 160–61, 220, 249n36, 251n73, 252n13, 276–77n23. *See also* selective pronatalism

cloning. *See* SCNT

conception: and age limits 41, 56; and beginning-of-life debates, 38, 128, 201; with future partner, 157–63, 249n31; posthumous, 168–79; video of, 138; willful, 146–53

conflicts of interest: fertility companies, 102–4, 117. *See also* fertility industry; fertility loans; financial inducement; reproductive success

contraception: and chrononormativities, 20–21; controversies, 27, 39; and later reproduction, 42, 218; as nonreproductive technology, 247n1

cryopolitics, 18, 24, 90

datafication: of embryo selection, 25, 129–36, 140–42. *See also* time-lapse embryo imaging

death: changing meanings, 205–6; cryobiology as incomplete, 18; of eggs, 90–92, 176, 227; of egg freezers, 168–77, 230; fertility and life span, 70; hierarchies of, 7. *See also* finitude; mortality; posthumous reproduction

deterritorialization: of egg donation, 182, 186–90, 231

distributed reproductive aging: with egg donation, 191–93; with egg freezing, 16, 24, 88–96, 99, 117, 143, 226–29; with mitochondrial transfer, 210. *See also* aging; reproductive aging

Dolly the Sheep, 151, 194, 275n4. *See also* Franklin, Sarah

donor eggs. *See* egg donation

Dutch Association of Gynecologists (NVOG), 153

Early Embryo Viability Assessment (Eeva), time-lapse system, 119–40. *See also* time-lapse embryo imaging

Edelman, Lee, 74–76. *See also* reproductive futurism

egg(s): age of, 154–55, 164–65; as cellular "fountain of youth," 206–209, 215; chimeric, 209–12, 273n144; "cosmic" egg, 2, 243n1; cytoplasm, 205–15, 273n145; global mobility of, 4, 22–23, 180–216; *in vivo* and *ex vivo* eggs, 84, 92–95, 98–99, 226; invisible, 69; journey in egg freezing, 3, 22–23, 247n84; loss of, 45–47, 51, 92; as measurement of time, 21–22, 98–99; of non-human animals, 2, 6–7; and postfertile condition, 23; as potential progeny, 176; posthumous destruction of, 176; prenatal, 251n68; as "priceless," 103; quality and quantity, 21–22, 51, 68–69, 86, 96–103, 117, 167, 187, 197–200; symbolic meanings of,

2, 168; visualization of, 88–95, 121–23, 254n7. *See also* accumulation; aging; biotemporalities; egg banks; egg donation; egg thawing; fertility; frozen eggs; reproductive time

egg banks, 180–94; and research donation, 212; speeding up reproductive process, 187; and transnational egg flows, 182–94. *See also* egg donation; frozen eggs; World Egg Bank

egg donation, 180–216; "altruistic," 187, 198, 204, 270n81; autologous and heterologous, 230; and bionationalism, 198–202; celebrity, 154–56; and consumer choice, 190, 215; direct and indirect, 212–15; egg donors, 180–94, 197–204, 209–16, 226, 230–31; ethics, 185; fresh eggs, 180, 185–87, 192–215; frozen eggs, 41, 166, 180–216; to future self, 155, 230; health risks, 204; intergenerational, 38; as "kinship compromise," 155; matching donors and recipients, 188–90; networks, 26; political economy of, 191–94; outsourcing, 191–92; and postfertile condition, 17; regulation of, 182–87, 192–94, 196–203, 213–16; for reproduction, 182–94, 216; reproduction vs. research, 203–4, 212; for research, 175–76, 194–215, 230; stratifications in, 191–94, 212; US-UK, 184–91. *See also* abortion; age limits; agency; biodesirability; bionationalism; class; egg banks; deterritorialization; financial inducement; Hwang scandal; race; SCNT

egg freezing: as destabilizing fertility, 17, 22, 153, 226; as ethical instrument, 212–15; extending fertility, 12, 22, 28–29, 33–34, 40–41, 77–81, 96–97, 116–18, 154–68, 226–30; as graduation gift, 19, 68, 220; mainstreaming, 4, 49–52, 68, 96, 106–11, 223–25, 228, 233–34; in media and public discourse, 1–4, 7, 9–13, 17, 23, 27–59, 60–87, 102, 156–58, 208, 217–21, 233; medical risks, 10, 51, 102, 245n36; and neoliberalism, 12, 56, 161–63, 233; as nonreproductive technology, 27, 34; as ongoing fertility management, 25, 50, 90, 97, 102, 108–18, 226–28, 234; peak fertility and last-minute freezing, 4, 63–72, 86, 220–21; political economies of, 88, 95–118, 224; reproductive infrastructures, 95–118, 226–29; as reproductive revolution, 3; as series of incremental steps, 69, 117, 227; "single" vs. "lifestyle," 23, 30–41, 49, 52, 56–57, 249n36, 249n37; "social" vs. "medical," 12, 23, 36–41, 57, 263n31; streamlining, 110–13, 118, 233; success rates, 6–7, 11–12, 51, 64, 78, 97–103, 105, 110, 180, 227, 255n33, 266n1; techno-fix vs. structural change, 11–12, 54, 114; treatment rationales, 24, 72, 88, 90, 96–102, 109–18, 164, 224; women's motivations, 9–10, 30–41, 60, 64, 73, 178, 251n73; women's stories, 30, 49, 60–87, 157–64, 223

Egg Freezing Diary (blog), 158

egg procurement. *See* egg donation

egg thawing, 25, 158–68; frozen-first, fresh-first, and frozen-only approaches, 164–68; motivations for, 158, 164–68. *See also* fertility loss; frozen eggs

Egged On (blog), 159–65

Eggfreezer (blog), 90–97, 116–17, 123, 158, 167–68, 176, 227, 265n97

Eggs for Later (documentary), 24, 60–87, 97. *See also* reproductive time

Eggsurance (blog), 158, 163–68. *See also* Adams, Brigitte

embryo(s): adoption, 200–201, 254n5, 271n92; as collective, 126–29, 139; freezing, 5, 88, 159–60, 244n19, 262n13; as individual, 123, 126–30, 139, 254n3; selection, 119–42. *See also* abortion;

embryonic aging; embryonic stem cell research; prenatal imagery; time-lapse embryo imaging

embryonic aging, 25, 119–42, 259n10; biovalue of, 130–33, 137–40; commercialization, 121–22, 130; knowledge production about, 133–38; patenting, 25, 131–33, 142, 260n46; visualization of, 91, 119–28, 139, 254n3. *See also* embryo(s); patenting; time-lapse embryo imaging

embryonic stem cell research, 194–216; and frozen eggs, 26, 196–204, 212–16; German regulation, 261n73; and IVF, 6; Korean regulation, 197–200, 213, 216; UK regulation, 124; US regulation, 6, 200–202, 273n139. *See also* SCNT

EmbryoScope, time-lapse system, 119, 121, 127, 134–39; KIDScore, 135–36, 141

EmbryoScore, 136, 139

emotions. *See* affect

empowerment, in egg freezing discourses, 11, 50, 56, 69, 103, 233

entrepreneurs. *See* fertility industry

European Society for Human Reproduction and Embryology (ESHRE), 7, 136, 169–71

Facebook. *See* fertility insurance

family: egg freezing pathway to alternative forms of, 178; and financialized capitalism, 54, 163; imagined future family, 72–77, 159–64; hetero-nuclear, 159, 161, 164; intergenerational egg freezing, 38, 171; neoliberal, 162–63, 224; as redistributive unit, 162–63, 178, 224; two-earner, 54, 163; and women's careers, 34–36, 53, 105, 114. *See also* anticipation work; fertility planning; single motherhood

family planning. *See* fertility planning

fatherhood. *See* male partners; older fathers

fertility: assumed, 63–72; becoming
infertile earlier, 220–26; as biologically relative, 245–46n53 (*see also*
Franklin, Sarah); (dis)embodied, 16,
98, 234; dynamic of knowing and not
knowing, 48, 223; extension, 153–54,
166; egg-based model, 15, 68, 82, 225,
246n60; facts, 49, 223; legibility, 12,
15–16, 48, 57, 88, 92, 110, 225–26; and
loss, 15–16, 164–68, 222; medicalization of, 37–41, 60, 63, 118; peak
fertility, 4, 67–72, 86, 220–21; staying
fertile later, 226–31; streamlining,
110–13. *See also* accumulation; aging;
biopreparation; calculus of fertility;
egg freezing; fertility decline; fertility loss; fertility planning; fertility
preservation; finitude; frozen eggs;
IVF; postfertility; precarious fertility; proactive fertility management;
recombinant fertilities; reproductive
aging; will, to fertility; work
fertility apps, 108, 114
fertility companies. *See* fertility industry
fertility decline: not steep, 250n67, 255n22;
in media, 41–48; and naturalization of
gender differences, 33, 42; rhetoric of
failure, 46–48, 51, 72, 84, 168, 234; and
urgency, 43–48. *See also* aging; fertility; fertility loss; fertility marketing;
reproductive aging
fertility industry, 7–8, 95–118, 121–22;
228–31; business models, 186; consolidation, mergers and acquisitions,
8, 96, 118, 137–42, 193, 207, 256n45;
entrepreneurs, 95, 111–13, 225, 255n19;
IVF supply chain, 142; shareholders,
184–85; start-up companies, 96, 106–7,
118, 217; transnational, 192–93. *See also*
conflicts of interest; fertility insurance;
fertility loans; fertility marketing;
financial inducement; financialization
of fertility; private equity

fertility insurance, 7–8, 10–12, 36, 52–53,
113–17, 228–29, 256n49, 257n64; Apple
and Facebook, 28, 52–53, 114, 219;
neoliberal logic, 58, 113, 258n83; as
proactive fertility management, 113–16;
public controversies, 52, 55; speculative
investment, 117. *See also* package plans;
precarious fertility
fertility literacy, 234–35; biopolitical and
biocapitalist projects, 234–35; social
inequalities, 234
fertility loans, 103–6, 117, 227–28, 256n45,
257n67–68, 258n71; conflicts of interest, 104; debt financing of egg freezing,
109–10, 245n38. *See also* fertility industry; financialization
fertility loss: age-related, 41, 164–68;
becoming infertile earlier, 220–26; different points in reproductive life span,
221; and egg thawing, 166; embodied,
89, 229; extended in egg freezing, 164–
68; preemptive, 221; regulatory 229. *See
also* affect; fertility decline
fertility marketing: fertility cocktail
parties, 1, 40, 49–52, 223; fertility
education as, 70, 116, 222–23; fertility
testing, 4, 48, 69, 164–65, 223–25,
333; fertility vans, 49–51, 223, 231;
focus on fertility decline, 50, 107,
154; online platforms, 25, 107, 116,
142; relationship marketing, 109; to
younger women, 4, 49–52, 69–70, 96,
106–8, 221. *See also* fertility industry;
precarious fertility
fertility planning, 69, 72, 85, 218; and
family planning, 20–22, 218. *See also*
childbearing
fertility precarity. *See* precarious fertility
fertility preservation. *See* egg freezing
fetal bovine serum (FBS), 6–7, 244n21
financial inducement: direct and indirect,
in egg donation, 184–87, 191–93, 203,
214–15, 268n25

financialization of fertility, 88–119; and debt, 109–10, 117; financialized capitalism, 54–55, 163, 185; and IVF sector, 96, 107. *See also* capitalism; private equity; reproductive time

finitude: of fertility, 18–22, 44–45, 63–72, 81–85, 90–95, 117, 209–12, 226–31; and posthumous reproduction, 168–76. *See also* anticipation; mortality

Foucault, Michel, 18, 246n67

Franklin, Sarah, 13, 93–94, 127–29, 253n1, 275n4, 260n36, 260n47; analogic return, 98; Dolly the Sheep, 151, 275n4; fertility as biologically relative, 245–46n53

Fraser, Nancy, 54, 185

Freeman, Elizabeth, 19-20. *See also* chrononormativities

frozen eggs: as ageless, 4, 94; and aging, 18–22; "babies on ice," 170–71; "building block" of future child, 90–92, 116, 123, 167, 259n23, 265n98; eggs required per baby, 97–101; and "extended" fertility, 16, 55, 97, 164; frozen in time, 28, 59, 84, 90, 143; individualized, 116, 265n97; as legacy, 174–76; mobility, 7, 9, 26, 182–94, 230–231, 266n4; as "priceless," 103; pricing, 187; residual, 199–200, 213, 216; and SCNT, 199–200, 213; and slowed-down cellular time, 87; and social inequalities, 26, 234; and time, 16–17, 94, 97–98, 117, 176, 231, 235; visual representations, 89–94, 116; as vulnerable, 93. *See also* class; egg(s); egg donation; embryonic stem cell research; individualization; race; temporality

gender politics of (reproductive) aging, 4, 17–19; and biopolitics, 18; and egg freezing, 4, 12, 17, 32, 36, 49, 217, 235; female body as site of, 27; and female fertility, 12, 22, 24, 56, 147; and SCNT,

196, 204–206; and transnational egg donation, 181–82, 193. *See also* age normativities; aging; chrononormativities

genealogical stretch, 155

Geri, time-lapse system, 121, 135–40

global biopolitics of aging. *See* gender politics of (reproductive) aging

global care chain, 215; and transnational egg donation, 193

global cold chains of eggs, 182–83, 191–94, 231, 269n55; and new dependencies, 215; regulation of, 183; and reproductive youth, 215; for research, 199. *See also* Vertommen, Sigrid; Waldby, Catherine

Granny's Having a Baby documentary, 146–51

grief. *See* affect

guarantee packages. *See* package plans

Guardian, The (UK), 27–59, 248n14

Harris, Lisa, 5–6, 66

Human Fertilisation and Embryology Authority (HFEA), UK, 7, 29, 170–72, 184–86, 215, 258n80, 258n5; HFE Act 1990, 7, 29, 172

Hwang scandal, 197–200; frozen egg donation, 213, 216, 270n75, 274n161

in vitro eggs. *See* eggs; frozen eggs

in vitro gametogenesis, 218, 274–75n1

infertility. *See* fertility; fertility decline; fertility loss

informed consent, 2, 23, 26, 146, 168–76, 230–31; and agency, 173; as anticipatory, 169; as authoritative speech acts, 173–75, 179; intended kinship, 175; in the Netherlands, 172–73, 266n115; for posthumous reproduction, 168–76, 265–66n114; in UK, 170–73; as will writing, 169, 174, 265n109. *See also* performativity; posthumous reproduction

Inhorn, Marcia, 157, 244n19; absent partner as motivation for egg freezing, 49, 160, 251n73, 276n15; reproflows, 181

IVF (*in vitro* fertilization): controversies, 2, 30, 41, 60, 143; vs. egg freezing, 13–14, 37, 85, 99–103, 220; egg freezing as two-stage IVF, 3, 79, 217, 255n36; history of, 5–6, 20, 66, 145–46, 218; reactive IVF vs. proactive fertility management, 108, 115–16. See also abortion; class; embryonic stem cell research; fertility industry; financialization; motherhood; pharmaceutical and biotechnological companies; race

kinning extensions: in egg freezing, 157–64, 178

kinship: and aging, 146; egg freezing as kinship technology, 157–59, 163; extending, 157–59; genetic relatedness, 103, 146, 154–64, 168, 175–78, 221, 223, 249n31, 263n47; and informed consent, 26, 174–75, 179, 230; intended kinship bonds, 26, 175, 230; kinship work, 123, 159, 264n61; prenatal, 123; race and "kinship risk," 188; and time-lapse embryo videos, 123; in women's egg freezing narratives, 75–76. See also kinning extensions; older motherhood; posthumous reproduction; race; reproductive aging

Korea, South, 196–201; frozen egg donation, 197–99, 213, 216, 270n75, 274n161; low birth rate, 199–200. See also bionationalism; Hwang scandal; embryonic stem cell research

labor relations, gendered, 21–22, 33, 151, 177. See also work

life expectancy: rising, 70, 205

male partner: absence as motivation for egg freezing, 34–36, 60–87, 152, 160–63,

166, 251n73; imagined future, 159–60, 168–69, 178; patrilineality, 159; subfertile, 245–46n53

medicalization. See biomedicalization

men. See male partner; older fatherhood

menopause: 19th century, 19; early, 38; delaying with ovarian cryopreservation, 274n1; as end of reproductive lifespan, 21. See also older motherhood

menstruation, 18–21, 46, 81; 19th century, 19; timing of, 20. See also agency

Mitalipov, Shoukhrat, 194–97, 200–204, 211, 213, 273n148, 273n154

mitochondrial transfer, 209–11, 218, 273n145, 273n148; and age-related infertility, 209–10; commercialization, 211; and egg donation, 209; legalization in UK, 209; prohibition in US, 209; "three-parent technique," 209. See also abortion; reproductive aging

mortality: bodily, 178; and egg freezing, 26, 230; and fertility, 171; and older motherhood, 149; and reproductive aging, 146; and reproductive finitude, 70, 212. See also finitude; informed consent; posthumous reproduction; reproductive aging

motherhood: anticipation with egg freezing, 24, 74, 152–53; desirability of, 66, 223; through egg freezing, 153–55, 159; "fit and unfit" mothers, 32; future, 64, 67, 73, 76, 79–82, 156, 265n112; idealized, 20, 234; "optimum age," 78; postponement, 11, 24, 32–35, 77–81, 152, 232. See also agency; childbearing; chrononormativities; egg donation; mothering, intensive; older motherhood; posthumous reproduction; single motherhood

mothering, intensive, 157, 263–64n53

National Health Service (NHS), UK, 5, 8–9, 104, 144, 247n8, 249n38

neoliberalism. *See* anticipation; biomedicalization; egg freezing; family; fertility
insurance; reproduction; singlehood
Netherlands, the, 61, 75; age limits for egg
freezing, 28–29, 57–58, 144–46, 153, 221,
252n23, 262n8; egg freezing debates, 23,
28–29, 33–37, 78; health system, 8; legalization of egg freezing, 62, 180; Model
Embryo Act, 2003, 144; regulation of
reproductive technologies, 7–8, 29, 72,
144, 219, 232–33, 249n38, 252n23. *See
also* informed consent
New York Times, 27–59, 158, 248n14

older fatherhood, 145; vs. older motherhood, 12, 150. *See also* male partner
older motherhood, 3, 25–26, 78; anticipation with egg freezing, 152–53; celebrities, 41, 154–56, 177, 218, 250n54; and
children's welfare, 144; controversies, 12,
38, 143–57, 177; and donor-egg IVF, 146,
150–55, 177; and egg freezing, 143–79;
and gendered politics of reproductive
aging, 147; genetically related, 146, 154,
157–64, 168, 178, 263n47; health risks,
144, 152; and IVF, 37, 143, 151; as marker
of technologically interventionist
motherhood, 155; in media, 41–47, 78,
250n54; politicization, 146; postmenopausal, 41, 146; premeditated, 152–53;
and "successful aging," 155–56, 177; as
transgression, 148–55, 177; "unnatural,"
151, 233; and younger women, 25, 152–
53; willful, 26, 145, 150–53, 177. *See also*
age normativities; Buttle, Liz; finitude;
mortality; motherhood; pregnancy;
older fatherhood; reproductive aging;
reproductive technologies; willfulness
oocyte cryopreservation (OC). *See* egg
freezing
ovarian cryopreservation, 71, 218, 274n1
ovarian reserve, 21, 46–47, 51, 69, 97–99,
165, 223, 256n37

package plans, for egg freezing, 24, 96,
106–8, 113, 231, 255n33, 255n36; guarantee plans, 100–104, 117–18; and measures of reproductive success 100–103;
multicycle, 99–104, 117, 227–28, 231;
pricing, 102, 256n40. *See also* affect;
calculus of fertility; fertility insurance;
fertility loans; reproductive success
parental project, 169; intended, 172, 175;
intergenerational, 38, 171; posthumous,
170–75
patenting: embryonic aging, 25, 131–33,
142, 260n46; SCNT, 207; polar body
transfer, 211. *See also* time-lapse embryo imaging
performativity: of gender, 246n68; of informed consent, 173–74; and temporality 173–74
Perry, Emily: first UK frozen egg baby, 8,
29; mother Helen Perry, 68, 249n29
pharmaceutical and biotechnological
companies, 121–22, 135–37; portfolio
expansion to cover each step of IVF,
139–42
postfertile condition, 16–17, 22–23, 118,
231–33, 277n31. *See also* body; egg(s);
egg donation; postfertility
postfertility, 16–17, 110–11, 212, 228, 231;
becoming postfertile, 231–34. *See also*
anticipation; biomedicalization; fertility; postfertile condition; precarious
fertility; retrospection
posthumous reproduction, with frozen
eggs, 25–26, 146, 168–76, 230, 265n98,
265n101; in China, 169; intended kinship, 175, 179; ethics, 169; and familial
continuity after death, 174–75; with
frozen sperm, 175; informed consent,
168–79; as inheritance, 174–75; intergenerational kinship, 174; in Israel,
174–75, 265–66n114. *See also* agency;
death; finitude; informed consent;
parental project

postmenopausal motherhood. *See* older motherhood

precarious fertility, 27–59; defined, 14–16; dynamic of knowing and not knowing, 48, 69; fertility marketing, 69, 223, 233; incremental steps, 69, 117, 227; institutionalization of, 52–53; and insurance, 52–53; intensification with egg freezing, 15, 117; timing of onset, 63–72; and uncertainty, 103, 227; and young women, 47, 49–54, 69. *See also* bioprecarity; fertility; fertility insurance; post-fertility

precarity. *See* bioprecarity

pregnancy: imagined with egg freezing, 82, 165; later with donor eggs, 143–44, 151, 154–55; multiple, 110, 115; temporal hybrid of embryonic and adult aging, 143; ultrasound, 124. *See also* body; childbearing

prenatal imagery, 253n1; and 14-day rule, 124; of eggs, 88–95; of embryos, 119–28, 138, 254n5, 260n31; of fetuses, 123

Primo Vision, time-lapse system, 121, 137, 139

private equity, investments: and consolidation, 8, 118, 193; in egg freezing, 90, 96, 104–18, 221, 225, 233, 257n58, 268n25; in stem cell research, 205–7. *See also* fertility industry; financialization

proactive fertility management: egg freezing as, 50, 56, 69, 102–16, 230. *See also* fertility insurance; fertility marketing; IVF

race: and childbearing, 10–11, 252n13; and egg donation, 184–85, 188–94, 268n36; and egg freezing, 10–12, 65–66, 105, 252n13, 256n54; and financial inequities in US, 256n43; and IVF, 6–8, 65–66. *See also* childlessness; class; kinship; selective pronatalism

readiness, in egg freezing discourses, 110–12, 156–58, 163–65, 263–264n53

recombinant fertilities, and mitochondrial transfer, 209–12

regenerative medicine, 204–9: age-related pathologies, 207–9; capital investments in, 197, 204–7; demand for young women's eggs, 197, 209; biopolitics of aging, 204–6; stem cell research, 206. *See also* aging; embryonic stem cell research; SCNT

relatedness. *See* kinship; older motherhood

reproduction: marketization, 6, 193, 215; neoliberalization, 12, 32, 56, 225; reproductive decision making, 12–14, 23–24, 52, 55, 62, 78, 104, 113, 130–33, 139, 151–52, 162, 165, 185, 189, 229; reproductive health, 40, 57, 69, 113; reproductive infrastructures, 95–118, 192–93, 204, 214, 218, 226–29; reproductive oppression, 247n1; reproductive rights, 11, 244n19; reproductive risk management, 112–13, 122; reproductive timing, 23, 64, 77, 150, 165, 218; respatialization of, 181–82; stratification of, 10, 182, 191–94, 216; transnational, 180–216, 230. *See also* biomedicalization; chrononormativities; egg donation; fertility industry; financial inducement; posthumous reproduction; reproductive technologies

reproductive aging, 27–59: alterable vs. immutable, 28, 56, 58; agentic, 14, 63, 226; anticipating, 3, 224; capitalist reconfiguration of, 110; chrononormativities, 19–22, 28, 42, 56; de-/remedicalization, 37–41; distributed, 94–96; and egg freezing, 14, 16–19, 41, 86–87, 166, 219, 226–29; embodied, 35, 116; in media, 30, 41–48;

norms, 4, 12, 75, 147, 152; reconceptualization with egg freezing, 24, 93, 225; stratification of, 191–94; "successful," 155–57; understood as alterable, 12, 34; understood as immutable, 33–34, 42, 58. *See also* agency; aging; anticipation; biological clock; distributed reproductive aging; gender politics of (reproductive) aging; older motherhood

reproductive bioprecarity. *See* bioprecarity

reproductive body. *See* body

reproductive choice, 1, 39; struggles for, 27; egg freezing as, 11–12, 30, 33–34, 50, 94, 219

reproductive futurism, 74–76. *See also* Edelman, Lee

reproductive-industrial complex, 88–118, 228, 255n19, 276n22. *See also* Vertommen, Sigrid

reproductive orientations, in egg freezing narratives, 72–77

reproductive success: and calculus of fertility, 101–3; conflicts of interest, 102, 117; flexible notion in egg freezing, 99–103, 110, 117, 154, 227, 255n36; "time to live birth," 127

reproductive technologies: and agency, 20–21, 77, 151; and age-related infertility, 5–6, 150–57; biopolitics of, 18; and perceived risk of embodied reproduction, 70; public debates, 27–59; regulation, 7–9, 28–30, 171–72; as visual technologies, 89, 121, 253n1. *See also* egg donation; egg freezing; IVF; Netherlands; reproduction; time-lapse embryo imaging; United Kingdom; United States

reproductive time: in *Eggs for Later*, 81–87; financialization of, 95–99, 117; instrumentalization in egg freezing, 117–18

reproductive value: and capital value, 90, 109–10, 133, 228; of eggs, 101–3; in embryo selection, 133. *See also* accumulation

reproductive will. *See* will

retrospection: and egg freezing, 165–67; and embryo videos, 128–30; and post-fertility, 231; and reproductive orientations, 72–77. *See also* anticipation

Roberts, Dorothy, 10, 192, 245n38; reproductive oppression, 247n1

Schellart, Marieke, 60–87, 97, 103, 226

SCNT (somatic cell nuclear transfer), 194–216; commercialization, 207; compensation of egg donors, 197–203, 271n94; and iPSC, 208–9; regulation, 197–204; rearrangement of biological time, 196; reliance on donor eggs, 196–216. *See also* bionationalism; frozen eggs; patenting

selective pronatalism, 10–11. *See also* Thompson, Charis

sexuality. *See* aging; women

single motherhood, 163–65; as alternative family model, 163–64; and egg freezing, 158–59. *See also* motherhood; older motherhood; singlehood

singlehood: as failure, 161–62; ideology, 168, 178; as motivation for egg freezing, 64, 251n73; and neoliberalism, 162; single egg freezers, 36, 40, 49, 53, 57, 169; as "selfish," 39–40; as "waiting period," 161. *See also* agency; male partner, absent; single motherhood

Smirnova, Michelle, 18, 155

snowflake babies, 254n5, 271n92. *See also* embryo(s)

somatic cell nuclear transfer. *See* SCNT

speculative futures, 66–67; speculative investments and fertility insurance, 117; speculative model of reproductive care, 112. *See also* proactive fertility management

sperm: donation, 157–58, 169–71; failed sperm collection and egg freezing, 38; freezing, 5, 88, 110, 175; intra-cytoplasmic sperm injection (ICSI), 3, 113, 243n7; selection 91, 126; sperm banks, 69, 180, 186, 189, 268n25; "sperm race," 91. *See also* fatherhood; posthumous reproduction
stem cell research. *See* embryonic stem cell research

temporality: of female bodies, 3, 16, 18–22, 232; hormones and cyclical time, 20–21, 247n75; "politics of temporality," 61; of postfertility, 16, 231–32; of precarity, 276n18; and repronormative schemes, 64, 76; temporal plasticity of frozen egg, 93–95, 116–17, 176, 231, 254n15. *See also* anticipation; biotemporalities; egg freezing; reproductive aging; reproductive time; time-lapse embryo imaging
Thompson, Charis, 102–3, 201–4, 263n47, 264n61; selective pronatalism, 10–11
time-lapse embryo imaging, 3, 119–42; biovalue of embryonic aging, 130–33, 137–40; as "camera in the womb," 127, 130; commercialization, 130–33, 138, 142; cost, 121, 134; defined, 25, 120, 258n5; and embryo selection, 119–42; embryo videos, 119–29, 259n19; expansion of IVF cycle, 139; institutional genealogy of, 137–40; instrumentaliza-tion of, 25; intended parents' engage-ment with, 123–41; investments in, 119, 121, 135–39, 141; knowledge production of, 133–38, 261n65; live-streaming em-bryo videos, 138–39; patenting, 131–33, 142; patient-driven technology, 139; popularity, 120–21; *in silico* vision, 130; as technocultural "womb," 127, 259n19; temporality, 125–30, 142. *See also* algorithms; datafication; embryo(s); embryonic aging; kinship

transgender people, and egg freezing, 38, 243n10
transnational egg donation, 182–94. *See also* egg banks; egg donation
Trump, Donald, 201, 244n19

ultrasound, 69: fetal, 121–24, 128, 196, 253n1, 259n19; ovarian, 21. *See also* abortion; pregnancy
United Kingdom: 10-year storage limit, 229, 262n9; 14-day rule, 124; egg do-nation, 183, 186; egg freezing, 7–9, 27–59, 97–105; healthcare system, 8; privatization of IVF, 9; regulation of reproductive technologies, 7–9, 29, 247n8, 249n38, 262n9; time-lapse embryo imaging, 120–21, 138. *See also* egg freezing; embryonic stem cell research; Human Fertilisation and Embryology Authority; informed consent; National Health Service
United States: abortion politics, 6, 51, 123–24, 244n26; egg donation, 125, 181–94, 200–204, 209–10; egg freezing, 6–8, 49–52, 68–69, 95–97, 101–6, 158–64, 172; for-profit fertility sector, 6–8, 51, 117; regulation of reproductive tech-nologies, 8, 29–30, 244n26; regulation of stem cell research, 200–202; social inequities, 6, 8, 66. *See also* bionation-alism; class; race; embryonic stem cell research

Vertommen, Sigrid, 95; global fertil-ity chains, 269n55; reproductive-industrial complex, 95, 255n19
vitrification, 6–7, 9, 244n19, 271n88
Volkskrant (NL), 27–59, 248n14, 250n48

Waldby, Catherine, 68, 102–3, 131, 183, 189, 203
will: to fertility, 155–57, 177; reproductive, 150–52, 177 (*see also* Ahmed, Sara); to

youth, 18, 22, 155–156, 177, 234 (*see also* Smirnova, Michelle).

willfulness: defined, 150; of egg freezing, 34, 145–46, 152–53, 169, 177; of older motherhood, 150–51, 177. *See also* Ahmed, Sara

women: egg donors, 182–94; egg freezers, 31–52, 60–87, 88–95, 158–68; "having it all," 31–34, 56–57, 152, 156, 218; motivations for egg freezing, 9–10, 30–41, 60, 64, 73, 178, 251n73; older, 143–57; public scrutiny of, 23, 30, 57, 146; relationships, 36, 157–64; sexualization of, 148–51; traditional gender roles, 33, 43; willful (non) reproduction, 34, 145–51; younger, 4, 25, 49–52, 69–70, 96, 107–8, 152–153, 221. *See also* agency; motherhood; precarious fertility; proactive fertility management

work: "career women," 12, 31–57, 152; and egg freezing, 11, 114, 218, 224, 233; and fertility, 20–21, 32, 42, 54–57, 229; gendered labor relations, 21, 33, 151, 177. *See also* family; older motherhood

World Egg Bank (TWEB), US, 26, 29, 181–94, 213–15, 266n7, 266–67n8. *See also* egg donation

World Health Organization, 14

ABOUT THE AUTHOR

Lucy van de Wiel is a Research Associate in the Reproductive Sociology Research Group (ReproSoc) at the Department of Sociology, University of Cambridge. She is also a Turing Fellow at the Alan Turing Institute in London.

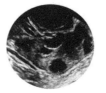